Basic Clinical Neuroscience

SECOND EDITION

PAUL A. YOUNG, Ph.D.

Professor and Chairman Emeritus
Department of Anatomy and Neurobiology
Saint Louis University School of Medicine
St. Louis, Missouri

PAUL H. YOUNG, M.D.

Clinical Professor of Neurosurgery
Department of Surgery
Clinical Professor of Anatomy
Center for Anatomical Science and Education
Department of Surgery
Saint Louis University School of Medicine
St. Louis, Missouri

DANIEL L. TOLBERT, Ph.D.

Professor of Anatomy and Surgery
Director Center for Anatomical Science and Education
Department of Surgery
Saint Louis University School of Medicine
St. Louis, Missouri

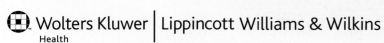

Wolters Kluwer | Lippincott Williams & Wilkins
Health

Philadelphia • Baltimore • New York • London
Buenos Aires • Hong Kong • Sydney • Tokyo

Acquisitions Editor: Crystal Taylor
Managing Editor: Kelly Horvath
Illustration Planner: Jennifer Clements
Production Editor: John Larkin
Compositor: Circle Graphics

Library of Congress Cataloging-in-Publication Data

Young, Paul A., 1926–
   Basic clinical neuroscience / Paul A. Young, Paul H. Young, Daniel L. Tolbert.—2nd ed.
       p. ; cm.
   Rev. ed. of: Basic clinical neuroanatomy. c1997.
   Includes bibliographical references and index.
   ISBN-13: 978-0-7817-5319-7 (pbk.)
   ISBN-10: 0-7817-5319-8 (pbk.)
   1. Neuroanatomy. 2. Neurosciences. I. Young, Paul H. (Paul Henry), 1950– II. Tolbert, Daniel L. (Daniel Lee), 1946– III. Young, Paul A., 1926– . Basic clinical neuroanatomy. IV. Title.
   [DNLM: 1. Nervous System—anatomy & histology. 2. Nervous System—physiopathology. WL 101 Y75b 2008]
   QM451.Y68 2008
   611.8—dc22
                                            2007010589

08 09 10
6 7 8 9 10

To our families and our past, present,
and future students.

PREFACE TO SECOND EDITION

The title of the second edition of this monograph has been changed to *Basic Clinical Neuroscience*. This reflects substantial changes in its organization and content. Building on the fundamental objective of the first edition "to provide the anatomical basis for neurologic abnormalities . . ." so as to be able to answer the question "Where is the lesion located?", the emphasis of this second edition remains to correlate neuroanatomic structures with clinically relevant functions. In addition, fundamental physiologic concepts underlying normal nervous system function and the pathophysiologic basis for abnormal nervous system activity have been included. In this new edition our goal continues to be to describe the subject in a succinct and simple manner so that it will facilitate learning in students of all health science fields.

The chapters in the second edition, as in the first edition, are organized in three main sections. The first includes four chapters that describe the microscopic and macroscopic organization of the brain and spinal cord. Clinically important structures and functional levels are introduced. In the next and largest section of the book (Chapters 5–19), the functional systems are described. The motor and somatosensory paths continue to be described first owing to their paramount importance in localizing injury to the brain or spinal cord. A new vestibular system chapter was taken from disparate information about this system from a number of different chapters in the first edition and brought together to complete the descriptions of the special senses. The final section of the second edition deals with accessory components and more general topics. There are new chapters on the reticular formation, cranial nerves, development, aging, and recovery of function.

The authors are most grateful to Ms. Susan Quinn for her assistance in preparing the manuscript. Mr. Larry Clifford prepared the illustrations used in the first edition, many of which have been modified in the second edition by adding coloring to highlight significant structures and connections. The authors are very grateful and much indebted to the staff of Lippincott Williams & Wilkins for their interest and support, particularly Crystal Taylor and Jennifer Clements, and especially Kelly Horvath for her patience while valiantly attempting to keep us on schedule.

PREFACE TO THE FIRST EDITION

The main objective of this monograph is to provide the anatomical basis for neurologic abnormalities. Knowledge of basic clinical neuroanatomy will enable medical students to answer the first question asked when examining a patient with an injured or diseased nervous system: "Where is the lesion located?" Knowledge of basic clinical neuroanatomy will enable students in health-related fields such as nursing, physical therapy, occupational therapy, physician assistants, to understand the anatomical basis of the neurologic abnormalities in their patients. To accomplish these objectives, the anatomical relationships and functions of the clinically important structures are emphasized. Effort is exerted to simplify as much as possible the anatomical features of the brain and spinal cord.

This monograph is neither a reference book nor a textbook of neuroanatomy. Most neuroanatomy textbooks include much information about anatomical structures that aids in the understanding of a particular system or mechanism, but when these structures are damaged clinical signs or symptoms do not result. Such superfluous information is kept to a minimum in this book.

This basic clinical anatomy book is presented in three main sections: (1) the basic plan, (2) the functional systems, and (3) the associated structures. The basic plan includes the organization of the nervous system, its histologic features and supporting structures, distinguishing anatomical characteristics of the subdivisions of the brain and spinal cord, and an introduction to clinically important brain and spinal cord functional levels. Only those structures needed to identify the subdivisions and their levels are included in this part.

The second section deals with the functional systems and their clinically relevant features. This section is arranged so that the motor and somatosensory systems, of paramount importance because they include structures located in every subdivision of the brain and spinal cord, are described first. The remainder of this section includes the pathways associated with the special senses, higher mental functions, and the behavioral and visceral systems.

In the third section, the vascular supply and the ventricular cerebrospinal fluid system are presented.

The visualization of three-dimensional anatomical relationships plays a key role in localizing lesions and understanding the anatomical basis of neurologic disorders. Every effort has been made to include illustrations that enhance this visualization of three-dimensional images of the clinically important structures. In addition to the three-dimensional illustrations, schematic diagrams of the functional systems and drawings of myelin-stained sections from selected functional levels of the brain and spinal cord are used to provide the anatomical relationships that enhance the understanding of the anatomical basis for neurologic disorders and their syndromes. Clinical relevance is emphasized throughout this book and illustrations of some neurologic abnormalities are included.

Review questions are found at the end of each chapter and an entire chapter is devoted to the principles of locating lesions and clinical illustrations. Answers to the chapter questions are found in the appendixes. Also in the appendixes are a section devoted to cranial nerve components and their clinical correlations, a glossary of terms, a list of suggested readings, and an atlas of the myelin-stained sections used throughout the book.

The authors are most grateful to Mr. Larry Clifford for his artistic skills in creating the illustrations, all of which are an invaluable part of this book. Our deep appreciation is expressed to Ms. Susan Quinn for her superb assistance in preparing the manuscript and to Ms. Susan McClain for her computer expertise in preparing the charts and tables. Finally, the authors are much indebted to the publisher, Williams & Wilkins, and its editorial and marketing staff for their interest, support, and patience throughout the project.

TABLE OF CONTENTS

1

Introduction, Organization, and Cellular Components

Two fundamental properties of animals, irritability and conductivity, reach their greatest development in the human nervous system. Irritability, the capability of responding to a stimulus, and conductivity, the capability of conveying signals, are specialized properties of the basic functional units of the nervous system: the nerve cells or neurons. Neurons respond to stimuli, convey signals, and process information that enable the awareness of self and surroundings; mental functions such as memory, learning, and speech; and the regulation of muscular contraction and glandular secretion.

ORGANIZATION OF THE NERVOUS SYSTEM

The basic functional unit of the nervous system is the neuron. Each neuron has a cell body that receives nerve impulses and an **axon** that conveys the nerve impulse away from the cell body. The nervous system comprises neurons arranged in longitudinal series. The serial arrangement forms two types of circuits: reflex and relay. A reflex circuit conveys the impulses that result in an involuntary response such as muscle contraction or gland secretion (Fig. 1-1A). A relay circuit conveys impulses from one part of the nervous system to another. For example, relay circuits convey

impulses from sensory organs in the skin, eyes, ears, and so forth that become perceived by the brain as sensations (Fig. 1-1B). Relay circuits are categorized according to their functions and are called functional paths, e.g., pain path, visual path, or motor or voluntary movement path. A functional path may consist of a series of only two or three neurons, or as many as hundreds of neurons. Reflex circuits may overlap with parts of relay circuits (Fig. 1-1C).

A functional path may contain thousands or even millions of nerve cell bodies and axons. The nerve cell bodies may form pools or clumps, in which cases they are called nuclei or ganglia, or the nerve cell bodies may be arranged in the form of layers or laminae. The axons in a functional path usually form bundles called tracts, fasciculi, or nerves. Therefore, the entire nervous system is composed of functional paths whose neuronal cell bodies are located in nuclei, ganglia, or laminae and whose axons are located in tracts or nerves.

The human nervous system is divided into central and peripheral parts. The brain and spinal cord form the central nervous system (CNS), and the cranial, spinal, and autonomic nerves and their ganglia form the peripheral nervous system (PNS). The CNS integrates and controls the entire nervous system, receiving information (input) about changes in the internal and external environments,

1

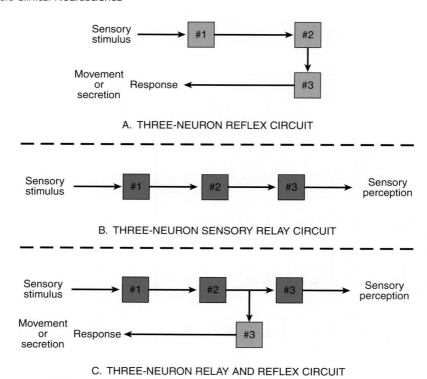

Figure 1-1   Simple reflex and relay circuits. **A.** Three-neuron reflex circuit. **B.** Three-neuron sensory relay circuit. **C.** Combined three-neuron relay and reflex circuits.

interpreting and integrating this information, and providing signals (output) for the execution of activities, such as movement or secretion. The PNS connects the CNS to the tissues and organs of the body. Hence, the PNS is responsible for conveying input and output signals to and from the CNS. Signals passing to the CNS are called **afferent,** whereas those passing away from the CNS are called **efferent.**

NERVOUS SYSTEM SUPPORT AND PROTECTION

Nerve cells are extremely fragile and cannot survive without the protection of supporting cells. The brain and spinal cord, also very fragile, are protected from the surrounding bones of the cranial cavity and vertebral or spinal canal by three coverings or membranes, called the meninges.

THE MENINGES

The CNS is supported and protected by the meninges, three connective tissue membranes located

between the brain and the cranial bones and between the spinal cord and the vertebral column. The meninges are, from external to internal, the **dura mater,** the **arachnoid,** and the **pia mater.** The meninges around the brain and spinal cord are continuous at the foramen magnum, the large opening in the base of the skull where the brain and spinal cord are continuous.

Dura Mater

The dura mater is a strong, fibrous membrane that consists of two layers. In the cranial dura, which surrounds the brain, the two layers are fused and adhere to the inner surfaces of the cranial bones except in those regions where the layers split (Fig. 1-2) to form the venous sinuses that carry blood from the brain to the veins in the neck. The inner layer of the dura forms four folds that extend internally to partially partition various parts of the brain (Fig. 1-3). The sickle-shaped **falx cerebri** lies in the longitudinal groove between the upper parts of the brain, the cerebral hemispheres. The **falx cerebelli,** also oriented longitudinally, separates the upper parts of the hemispheres of the cerebellum, or "little brain." The tentorium cerebelli is a flat

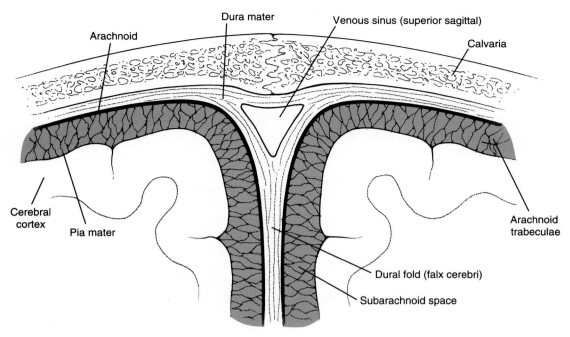

Figure 1-2   Coronal section of cranial meninges showing a venous sinus and dural fold.

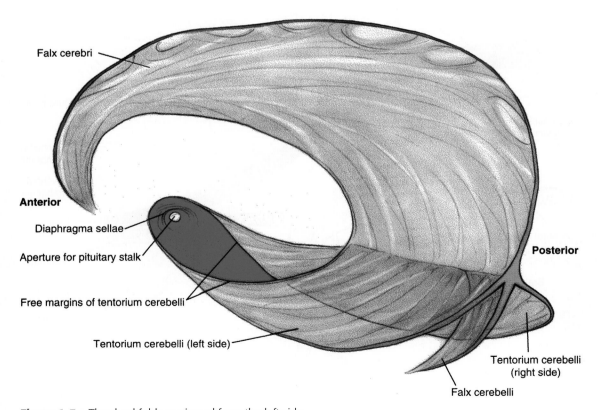

Figure 1-3   The dural folds as viewed from the left side.

dural fold that separates the posterior parts of the cerebral hemispheres above from the cerebellum below. The **diaphragma sellae** is a circular, horizontal fold beneath the brain that covers the sella turcica, in which the pituitary gland is located. The stalk of the pituitary gland pierces the diaphragma sellae and attaches to the undersurface of the brain.

The spinal dura consists of two layers: The outer layer forms the periosteal lining of the vertebral foramina that form the vertebral or spinal canal; the inner layer loosely invests the spinal cord and forms a cuff around the spinal nerves as they emerge from the vertebral canal.

Arachnoid

The arachnoid is a thin, delicate membrane that loosely surrounds the brain and spinal cord. The outer part of the arachnoid adheres to the dura (Fig. 1-4). Extending internally from this outer part are numerous cobweb-like projections or trabeculae that attach to the pia mater.

Pia Mater

The pia mater is the thin membrane that closely invests the brain and spinal cord. The pia is highly vascular and contains the small blood vessels that supply the brain and spinal cord.

Meningeal Spaces

Several clinically important spaces are associated with the meninges (Fig. 1-4). The **epidural space** is located between the bone and the dura mater, and the **subdural space** is located between the dura and arachnoid. Normally, both the epidural and subdural spaces are potential spaces in the cranial cavity. Both may become actual spaces if blood accumulates because of epidural or subdural hemorrhages caused by traumatic tearing of blood vessels that pass through the spaces. In the spinal cord, the subdural space is also potential, but the epidural space is actual and contains semifluid fat and thin-walled veins.

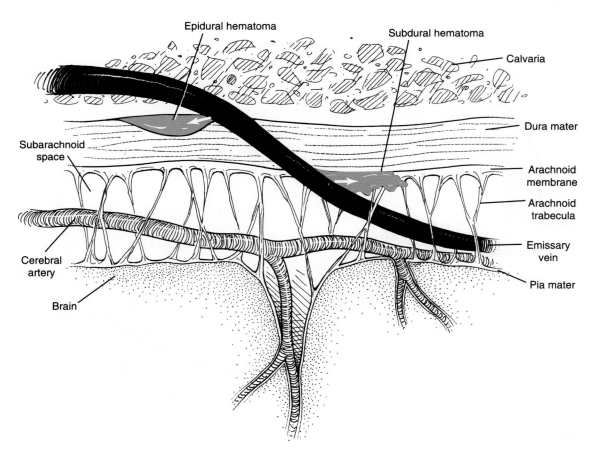

Figure 1-4   Relation of meningeal spaces to blood vessels and hemorrhages.

The **subarachnoid space** is located in the area between the arachnoid and pia mater and contains **cerebrospinal fluid.** The subarachnoid space communicates with the cavities or ventricles of the brain where cerebrospinal fluid is formed. Also located within the subarachnoid space are the initial parts of the cranial and spinal nerves and numerous blood vessels on the surfaces of the brain and spinal cord. Vascular accidents involving the vessels here result in subarachnoid hemorrhage.

SUPPORTING CELLS

Three basic types of supporting or glial cells exist: ependymal, microglial, and macroglial cells. The ependymal cells line the fluid-filled cavities or ventricles of the brain and the central canal of the spinal cord. The microglial cells are phagocytes that arise from macrophages and engulf the debris resulting from injury, infections, or diseases in the CNS. The macroglia consist of four cell types:

astrocytes and **oligodendrocytes** in the CNS and **Schwann cells** and **capsular cells** in the PNS.

Astrocytes

Astrocytes are the most numerous cells in the CNS (Fig. 1-5). Each astrocyte has a star-shaped cell body and numerous irregularly shaped processes, some of which may be extremely long. Processes of some astrocytes have end-feet on the surface of the brain or spinal cord. These end-feet form a protective covering called the external limiting membrane or glial membrane. Many astrocytic processes have vascular end-feet, which surround capillaries. The endothelial cells of CNS capillaries are interconnected by tight junctions and form the **blood-brain barrier,** which selectively governs the passage of materials, including many drugs, from the circulating blood into the CNS.

Astrocytes have other functions as well. They play a major role in the electrolyte balance of the

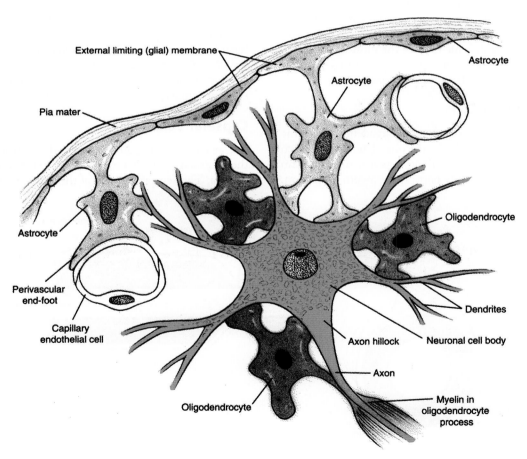

Figure 1-5   Relation of neurons, glia, and capillaries.

CNS, produce neurotrophic factors necessary for neuronal survival, and remove certain neurotransmitters from synaptic clefts. Astrocytes are the first cells to undergo alterations in response to CNS insults such as ischemia, trauma, or radiation. Also, astrocytes form scars resulting from CNS injury. Astrocytes are highly susceptible to the formation of neoplasms.

Oligodendrocytes

The formation and maintenance of CNS myelin are the primary functions of the oligodendrocytes, small glial cells with relatively few processes (Fig. 1-5). The myelin sheath is formed by oligodendrocyte processes, which wrap around the axon to form a tight spiral. The myelin itself is located within the processes. Each oligodendrocyte envelops a variable number of axons depending on the thickness of the myelin sheaths. In the case of thin myelin sheaths, one oligodendrocyte may be related to 40 or 50 axons. Oligodendrocytes may also surround the cell bodies of neurons, but in this location they do not contain myelin. Recent research suggests that oligodendrocytes also produce neurotrophic factors, the most important of which is a nerve growth factor that may promote the growth of damaged CNS axons.

Schwann Cells

The PNS counterpart of the oligodendrocyte is the Schwann cell. Unlike the oligodendrocyte, which envelops many myelinated axons, the Schwann cell envelops only part of one myelinated axon.

During development of the myelin sheath, the Schwann cell first encircles and then spirals around the axon many times, forming multiple layers or lamellae. The myelin is actually located within the Schwann cell lamellae (Fig. 1-6). The outermost layer of the Schwann cell lamellae is called the **neurolemma** or **sheath of Schwann.** Because each Schwann cell myelinates only a small extent of the axon, myelination of the entire axon requires a long string of Schwann cells. Between each Schwann cell, the myelin is interrupted. These areas of myelin sheath interruption are called **nodes of Ranvier** (Figs. 1-6, 1-7). Similar interruptions of myelin sheaths occur in the CNS. In unmyelinated fibers, one Schwann cell envelops many axons.

Schwann cells not only form and maintain the myelin sheath but also are extremely important in the regeneration of damaged axons. When an axon is cut, the part of the axon separated from the cell body degenerates; however, the string of Schwann cells distal to the injury proliferates and forms a tube. Growth sprouts arising from the proximal end of the transected axon enter this tube and travel to the structures supplied by the axon before its injury. Such functional axonal regeneration is common in the PNS. Axonal regeneration has not occurred in the human CNS, and this lack of regeneration may be related, in part, to the absence of Schwann cells.

Capsular Cells

Capsular cells are the glial elements that surround the neuronal cell bodies in sensory and autonomic ganglia. The sensory ganglia of the spinal nerves

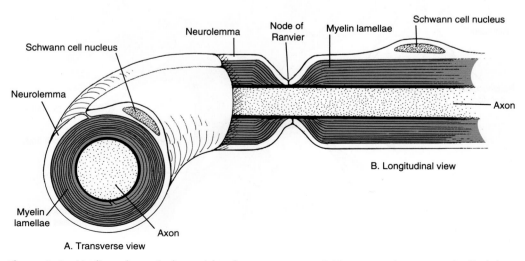

Figure 1-6   Myelinated axon in the peripheral nervous system. **A.** Transverse view. **B.** Longitudinal view.

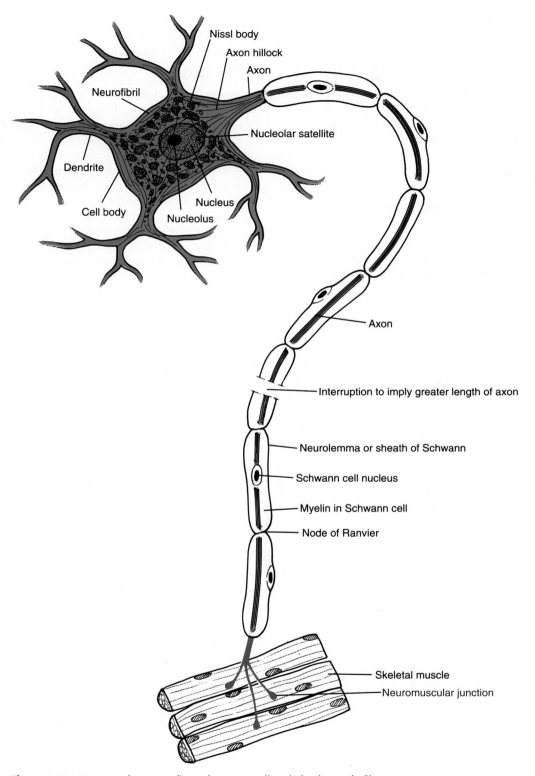

Figure 1-7   Neuron whose myelinated axon supplies skeletal muscle fibers.

and some cranial nerves contain large, round, neurons whose cell bodies are surrounded by a nearly complete layer of flattened capsular or satellite cells, thereby separating the ganglion cell from the nonneural connective tissue and vascular structures. Although capsular cells are present in autonomic ganglia, because of the irregular shapes of these ganglion cells the capsules are less uniform and, hence, incomplete.

NEURONS

MORPHOLOGIC PROPERTIES

A neuron consists of a cell body or soma and of protoplasmic processes called **dendrites** and **axons** (Fig. 1-7). The cell body is the metabolic center of a neuron and contains the nucleus and the cytoplasm. The nucleus contains nucleoplasm, chromatin, a prominent nucleolus and, in the female only, a nucleolar satellite. The cytoplasm contains the usual cellular organelles such as mitochondria, Golgi apparatus, and lysosomes. In addition, various-sized clumps of rough endoplasmic reticulum, called **Nissl bodies,** are prominent in the cytoplasm of neurons. However, the neuronal cytoplasm where the axon emerges is devoid of Nissl bodies; this area is called the axon hillock. Another cytoplasmic characteristic of neurons are neurofibrils, which are arranged longitudinally in the cell body, the axons, and dendrites.

Neurons are classified morphologically as unipolar, bipolar, or multipolar according to their number of protoplasmic processes (Fig. 1-8). The single process of a unipolar neuron is the axon. Unipolar neurons are located almost exclusively in the ganglia of spinal nerves and some cranial nerves. Bipolar neurons have an axon and one

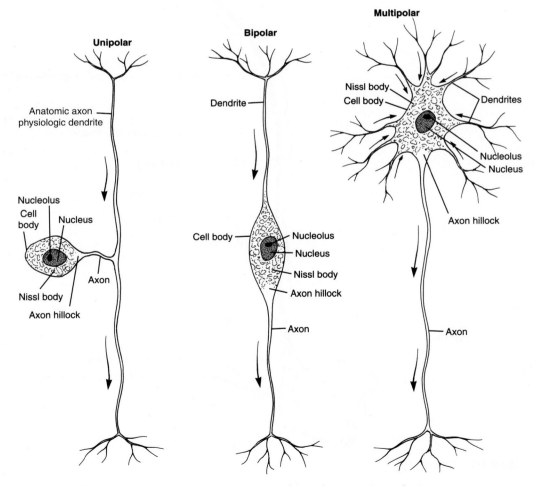

Figure 1-8   Morphologic types of neurons (arrows indicate direction of impulses).

dendrite and are limited to the visual, auditory, and vestibular pathways. All the remaining nerve cells are multipolar neurons and have an axon and between 2 and 12 or more dendrites.

DENDRITES AND AXONS

Dendrites, cytologically similar to the neuronal cell body, are short and convey impulses toward the cell body (Table 1-1). Axons do not contain Nissl bodies, vary in length from microns to meters, and convey impulses away from the cell body.

The integrity of the axon, regardless of its length, is maintained by the cell body via two types of axoplasmic flow or axonal transport. In **anterograde axonal transport,** the cell body nutrients are carried in a forward direction from the cell body to the distal end or termination of the axon. Anterograde axonal transport is vital for axonal growth during development, for maintenance of axonal structure, and for the synthesis and release of **neurotransmitters,** the chemicals that assist in the transfer of nerve impulses from one cell to another.

Besides anterograde transport, **retrograde axonal transport** occurs from the distal end of the axon back to the cell body. The function of retrograde axonal transport is the return of used or worn out materials to the cell body for restoration.

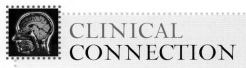

CLINICAL
CONNECTION

Retrograde axonal transport is of clinical importance because it is the route by which toxins such as tetanus and viruses such as herpes simplex, rabies, and polio are transported into the CNS from the periphery.

Axons may be myelinated or unmyelinated. Myelinated axons are insulated by a sheath of myelin that starts near the cell body and stops just before the axon terminates (Fig. 1-7). Myelin is a multilayered phospholipid located within axonal supporting cells. The myelin sheath increases the conduction velocity of the nerve impulse along the axon. The thicker the myelin sheath, the faster the conduction velocity.

SYNAPSES

Axonal endings or terminals occur in relation to other neurons, muscle cells, or gland cells. The junction between the axonal ending and the neuron, muscle cell, or gland cell is called the **synapse.** An important anatomic characteristic of the synapse is that the axonal ending is separated from the surface of the other nerve, muscle, or gland cell by a space, the synaptic cleft. An important physiologic characteristic of a synapse is polarization; that is, the impulse always travels from the axon to the next neuron in the circuit or to the muscle or gland cells supplied by the axon.

When a nerve impulse arrives at the synapse, chemicals called neurotransmitters are released into the synaptic cleft. Neurotransmitters, manufactured and released by the neurons, cross the synaptic cleft to affect the postsynaptic neuron, muscle, or gland cell. The transmitters at neuromuscular and neuroglandular synapses are excitatory; that is, they elicit muscle contraction or glandular secretion. However, the neurotransmitters at synapses between neurons may be excitatory, enhancing the production of an impulse in the postsynaptic neuron, or inhibitory, hindering impulse production in the postsynaptic neuron. All functions of the CNS, that is, awareness of

TABLE 1-1	Comparison of Axons and Dendrites	
	Axons	**Dendrites**
Function	Transport impulses from the cell body	Receive impulses and transport them toward the cell body
Length	Vary from microns to meters	Microns; seldom more than a millimeter
Branching pattern	Limited to collaterals, preterminals, and terminals	Vary from simple to complex arborizations
Surface	Smooth	Vary from smooth to spiny
Coverings	Supporting cells and frequently myelin	Always naked

sensations, control of movements or glandular secretions, and higher mental functions, occur as the result of the activity of excitatory and inhibitory synapses on neurons in various circuits.

PHYSIOLOGIC PROPERTIES

Resting Membrane Potential

Under steady-state conditions neurons are electrically polarized to about–60 mV by the separation of extracellular cationic charges from intracellular anionic charges. This resting membrane potential results from the differential distribution of ions and selective membrane permeability with four major cations and anions contributing to the resting membrane potential. Na^+ and Cl^- ions are concentrated extracellularly, and K^+ and organic anions (proteins and amino acids) are concentrated intracellularly. Transmembranous ion-selective channels or pores allow Na^+, K^+, and Cl^- ions to passively diffuse across the membrane as a result of concentration and electrical gradients. Proteins and amino acids do not move through the membrane as part of the resting membrane potential. The resting membrane potential is determined largely by Na^+ influx and K^+ efflux and their active transport back across the membrane by an ATP-dependent Na^+/K^+ pump, thereby maintaining the membrane potential at about −60 mV.

Electrotonic Conductance in the Soma-Dendritic Membrane

Electrotonic transients in the resting membrane potential can result in the interior of the cell becoming relatively more negative or hyperpolarized or less negative or depolarized. These potential shifts are electrotonically summated, temporally and spatially, as they are conducted passively from the soma and dendrites to the axon hillock-initial segment (Fig. 1-9).

Action Potential Initiation and Conductance

Depolarization of the axon hillock-initial segment region to about −45 mV results in the generation of an action potential. Unlike in the soma and dendrites where membrane transients are graded, membrane conductance at the axon hillock-initial segment becomes self-sustaining with the initia-

tion of an action potential. The initiation or rising phase of an action potential is caused by the rapid influx of Na^+ through voltage-sensitive channels. The subsequent falling phase of the action potential is slightly more prolonged and occurs by the efflux of K^+. Starting at the initial axon segment and continuing through to its terminal branches the propagation of the action potential occurs as a nondecremental voltage change. The velocity of propagation of an action potential is dependent on axonal diameter and myelination.

Saltatory Conduction

In unmyelinated, generally small-diameter (0.2–1.5 μm) axons (type IV motor or type C sensory), Na^+ and K^+ conductances and impulse propagation occur continuously between neighboring axonal membrane segments, resulting in slower impulse transmission (0.5–2 m/s). Conversely, in large-diameter (13–20 μm) myelinated axons (type I or Aα) impulse propagation is much faster (80–120 m/s) because Na^+ and K^+ conductance changes occur discontinuously along the axonal membrane at small gaps (1 μm) between the edges of myelin sheaths, the nodes of Ranvier. In these nodal regions Na^+ channels are many times more numerous than in the internodal axonal membrane whereas K^+ channels are spread along the internodal axolemma. The low internodal capacitance and concentrated Na^+ channels at the nodes allow the action potential to jump (**saltatory conduction**) between nodes, increasing the speed of conduction in myelinated axons (Fig. 1-10).

Action Potential Frequency Encodes Information

Information is transmitted between neurons or between neurons and effector structures by the propagation of action potentials. In many neurons action potential frequency is linearly correlated with stimulus intensity and the resultant degree of depolarization of the soma-dendritic membrane. The more sustained the depolarization, the greater the frequency of action potentials. In other neurons bursts of action potentials are generated by the superimposed action of Ca^{2+} currents that result in the membrane remaining depolarized longer resulting in the repetitive Na^+ influx and K^+ efflux cycles. Yet other neurons associated with neuro-

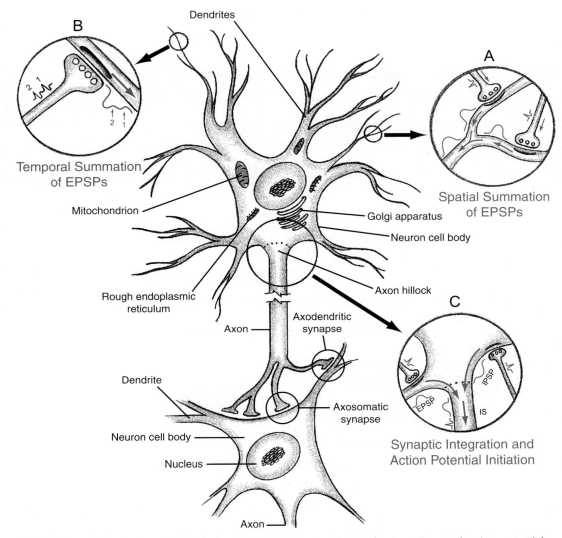

Figure 1-9 Electrotonic conductance in neuron, temporal and spatial summation, and action potential initiation. Synaptic interactions: **A.** Excitatory postsynaptic potentials (EPSPs) can spatially summate when they converge as they are electrotonically conducted from the dendrites to the soma. **B.** EPSPs can summate temporally when the same synaptic input is activated rapidly by multiple presynaptic action potentials. **C.** Excitatory and inhibitory inputs are integrated at the initial segment and sufficient depolarization generates an action potential.

modulatory and autonomic functions fire spontaneously at a relatively slow rate (1–10 Hz).

Synaptic Transmission

The synapse is the point of functional contact between neurons, and the neuromuscular junction is the point of functional contact between axons and skeletal muscle. Most synapses are electrochemical

and mediated by neurotransmitters. Some synapses are characterized as fast when the delay between presynaptic release and postsynaptic action is about 0.5 milliseconds and involve neurotransmitters such as acetylcholine and amino acids stored in vesicles at or attached to the active zone of the presynaptic membrane. Other synapses are characterized as slow (delay is in terms of seconds) and occur when peptidergic and biogenic amines stored

Normal Action Potential Propagation

A.

Saltatory Conduction in Myelinated Axon

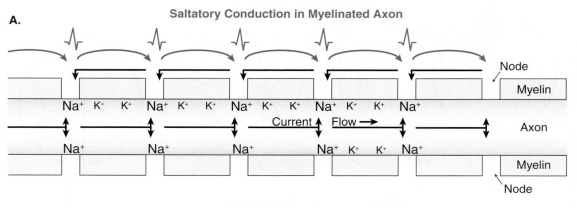

Nonsaltatory Conduction in Unmyelinated Axon

B.

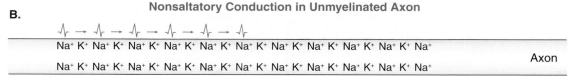

Action Potential Propagation Block

C.

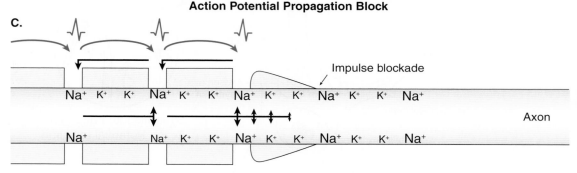

Figure 1-10   Normal and abnormal action potential propagation. **A.** In myelinated axons, action potential propagation is rapid because of saltatory current flow through the nodes of Ranvier where Na^+ channels are concentrated. **B.** In unmyelinated axons, action potential propagation is slower because Na^+ channels are uniformly distributed in the axolemma. **C.** Action potential propagation is blocked in demyelinated axons because current flow dissipates through the denuded membrane before reaching the next cluster of Na^+ channels.

in dense core vesicles away from the terminal membrane are released later and for a longer time. Neurotransmitter release is sequentially triggered by the electrotonic invasion of the action potential into the terminal, the influx of Ca^{2+} ions through voltage-gated channels that trigger the binding of synaptic vesicles at presynaptic active zones, and the subsequent release of neurotransmitter by exocytosis into the synaptic cleft. Each synaptic vesicle contains a quantal amount of neurotransmitter, and the number of quanta released is directly correlated to the amount of Ca^{2+} entering the termi-

nal. Neurotransmitters in the narrow synaptic cleft (~100 nm) effect conformational changes in agent-specific postsynaptic receptors, leading to an opening or closing of ion channels. Transmembrane changes mediated by inotropic receptors that quickly depolarize the postsynaptic neuron generate **excitatory postsynaptic potentials** (EPSPs), whereas ionic changes that hyperpolarize the neuron are classified as **inhibitory postsynaptic potentials** (IPSPs). In the CNS, synaptic contacts can also be formed at en passant axonal swellings along axons.

PATHOPHYSIOLOGY OF DISEASES AFFECTING NEUROTRANSMISSION AND ACTION POTENTIAL PROPAGATION

Relatively common acquired hereditary disorders affect electrochemical transmission at the neuromuscular junction by either reducing the presynaptic release of acetylcholine or the postsynaptic action of acetylcholine.

Acquired autoimmune disorders affect transmission at the neuromuscular junction. **Myasthenia gravis** is an autoimmune disease affecting nicotinic acetylcholine receptors, leading to skeletal muscle weakness and fatigability in orbital, oropharyngeal, and limb musculature. Muscle weakness and fatigability is generally variable in severity and progressive through active hours of the day. Nerve fibers are intact, and acetylcholine release at the nerve terminal is normal. Antibodies attack the acetylcholine receptor in the postjunctional folds, leading to a progressive decrement in amplitude of the evoked end-plate potentials and decreased muscle action potentials with repetitive stimulation. Structural changes of the postjunctional folds and diminished localization of the receptor at the crest of the folds also occur. Increasing the efficacy of the action of acetylcholine in the neuromuscular cleft with acetylcholinesterase inhibitors decreases the severity of the symptoms.

Muscle weakness and fatigability is predominantly in proximal limb and trunk musculature as seen in Lambert-Eaton myasthenic syndrome owing to diminished presynaptic release of acetylcholine from the nerve terminals. Muscle excitability remains normal.

Demyelinating diseases affect PNS Schwann cells or CNS oligodendroglia. **Guillain-Barré syndrome** is prototypical of an acquired, acute-onset inflammatory peripheral demyelinating neuropathy with axonal sparing. Multiple focal areas of demyelination of spinal roots and proximal nerve fibers result in very slow nerve conduction velocities and reduced compound action potential amplitude in electrophysiologic recordings from affected nerves. Symmetric and temporally progressive weakness in movements, first in the legs and then in the arms, gives the impression of an ascending paralysis. Difficulties in walking and rising from a chair are common complaints. Paralysis of respiratory muscles results in a high risk of respiratory failure. After treatment, functional recovery is possible by axonal remyelination. **Charcot-Marie-Tooth disease** (type 1A) is the most common hereditary polyneuropathy resulting in demyelination of sensory and motor axons.

Multiple sclerosis is the most common acquired demyelinating disease in the CNS with an immunologic cause. Symptomatology is dependent on the axonal tracts involved. Adjoining segments of myelin are lost (demyelinating plaques) in the white matter fiber tracts in the cerebrum, cerebellum, brainstem, and spinal cord. Normal impulse conduction occurs proximal and distal to the plaques but is blocked or slowed at the plaques. Biophysical properties of the demyelinated axolemma are altered, thereby affecting impulse propagation. In demyelinated axons, depolarizing currents are no longer focused at the nodes, but rather are dissipated along the demyelinated axolemma owing to the paucity of Na^+ channels in the internodal axolemma and the increased electrical capacitance of the affected segment of the axon. In axons with intact myelin, action potentials jump between nodes of Ranvier because of the high concentration of Na^+ channels at the nodal region. Multiple sclerosis is characterized by chronically protracted cycles of relapse and remission. Remission with improvement of symptoms reflects partial remyelination of the affected axonal segments. Persistent deficits can reflect the failure to remyelinate or, more probably, axonal injury within the plaque and axonal degeneration.

DEGENERATION AND REGENERATION

All cells in the human body are able to reproduce, except nerve cells. As a result, the loss of neurons is irreparable; a neuron once destroyed can never be replaced. Conversely, axons can regenerate and regain their functions even after being completely transected or cut, as long as the cell body remains viable. This capacity to regenerate is limited, however, to axons in the PNS. Functional axonal regeneration has not occurred in the human CNS. Thus, the degeneration of neuronal cell bodies anywhere in the nervous system and the degeneration of CNS axons are irreparable.

Chapter Review Questions

1-1.   What are the two main classes of cells in the CNS?

1-2.   What is a synapse and what are the chief characteristics of synapses in the CNS?

1-3.   What is the significance of axoplasmic transport?

1-4.   What are the chief differences between astrocytes and oligodendrocytes?

1-5.   Between which cranial structures are the following located?
   a. subdural hematoma
   b. cerebrospinal fluid
   c. epidural hematoma

1-6.   Which of the following is most likely involved in a tumor originating from myelin-forming cells in the CNS?
   a. neurons
   b. oligodendrocytes
   c. astrocytes
   d. microglial cells
   e. endothelial cells

1-7.   A common route whereby viruses such as polio or rabies travel to CNS neuronal cell bodies is via:
   a. blood–brain barrier transport
   b. anterograde axonal transport
   c. cerebrospinal fluid transport
   d. retrograde axonal transport
   e. transsynaptic transport

1-8.   The cell most commonly associated with CNS tumors is the:
   a. astrocyte
   b. endothelial cell
   c. microglial cell
   d. neuron
   e. oligodendrocyte

1-9.   Hemorrhage of an artery on the surface of the brain will result in leakage of blood into the:
   a. epidural space
   b. ventricular system
   c. subdural space
   d. cerebral extracellular space
   e. subarachnoid space

CHAPTER 2

Spinal Cord: Topography and Functional Levels

ACCORDING TO THE U.S. Department of Health and Human Services, approximately 10,000 new spinal cord injuries occur in the United States each year, of which at least 50% result in permanent disabilities. Some 200,000 Americans must use wheelchairs because of spinal cord injuries. Most of these injuries result from trauma such as occurs in automobile or sports accidents. An estimated two-thirds of the victims are 30 years of age or younger; the majority are men.

The spinal cord connects with the spinal nerves and is the structure through which the brain communicates with all parts of the body below the head. Impulses for the general sensations such as touch and pain that arise in the limbs, neck, and trunk must pass through the spinal cord to reach the brain, where they are perceived. Likewise, commands for voluntary movements in the limbs, trunk, and neck originate in the brain and must pass through the spinal cord to reach the spinal nerves that innervate the appropriate muscles. Thus, damage to the spinal cord may result in the loss of general sensations and the paralysis of voluntary movements in parts of the body supplied by spinal nerves.

SPINAL CORD GROSS ANATOMY

The spinal cord is located within the vertebral canal, which is formed by the foramina of the 7 cervical (CV), 12 thoracic (TV), 5 lumbar (LV), and 5 sacral (SV) vertebrae that form the vertebral column,

commonly called the spine. The spinal cord extends from the foramen magnum, the large opening in the base of the skull, to the first lumbar vertebra (Fig. 2-1). Superiorly, the spinal cord is continuous with the brain and, inferiorly, it ends by tapering abruptly into the conus medullaris (Fig. 2-1).

CLINICAL CONNECTION

The spinal cord is ordinarily protected by the strong bony ring formed by the vertebral column. However, high-velocity objects (e.g., bullets) or high-velocity impacts against immovable objects (e.g., trees, pavements, or automobile dashboards) can fracture vertebrae or dislocate them at the intervertebral articulations and compress or lacerate the spinal cord. The cervical vertebrae are the smallest and most fragile and, hence, most fractures occur here. Dislocations are most apt to occur at the points of greatest mobility, which are (in descending order of occurrence) the articulations between CV5 and CV6, TV12 and LV1, and CV1 and CV2 (Fig. 2-1).

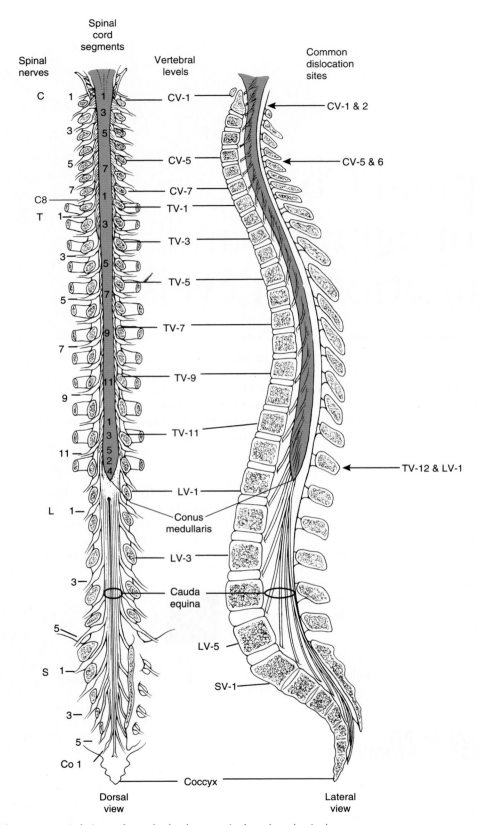

Figure 2-1 Relations of vertebral column, spinal cord, and spinal nerves.

There are 31 spinal cord segments (Fig. 2-1): 8 cervical (C), 12 thoracic (T), 5 lumbar (L), 5 sacral (S), and 1 coccygeal (Co). The segments are named and numbered according to the attachment of the spinal nerves. The spinal nerves are named and numbered according to their emergence from the vertebral canal. Spinal nerves C1 through C7 emerge through the intervertebral foramina above their respective vertebrae. Because there are only seven cervical vertebrae, spinal nerve C8 emerges between CV7 and TV1. The remaining spinal nerves emerge below their respective vertebrae (Fig. 2-1).

Until the third month of fetal development, the position of each segment of the developing spinal cord corresponds to the position of each developing vertebra. After this time, the vertebral column elongates more rapidly than the spinal cord. At birth, the spinal cord ends at the disc between LV2 and LV3. Further growth of the vertebral column results in the inferior or caudal end of the spinal cord being located in adulthood usually at the middle third of LV1. However, variations from the middle third of TV11 to the middle third of LV3 may occur. The approximate relation between spinal levels and vertebral levels is shown in Figure 2-1.

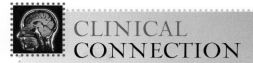

CLINICAL CONNECTION

The relation between spinal cord levels and vertebral levels is clinically important. The level of spinal cord lesions is always localized according to the spinal cord segment. Most spinal cord levels do not, however, correspond to vertebral levels. If neurosurgical procedures are to be performed, the spinal cord level must be correlated with the appropriate vertebral level.

SPINAL MENINGES

The spinal cord is surrounded by three connective tissue membranes called the spinal meninges. From internal to external, the spinal meninges are called the pia mater, arachnoid, and dura mater (Fig. 2-2).

PIA MATER AND ARACHNOID

The pia mater completely surrounds and adheres to the spinal cord. The arachnoid loosely surrounds the spinal cord and is attached to the inner surface of the dura mater. The spinal cord is anchored to the

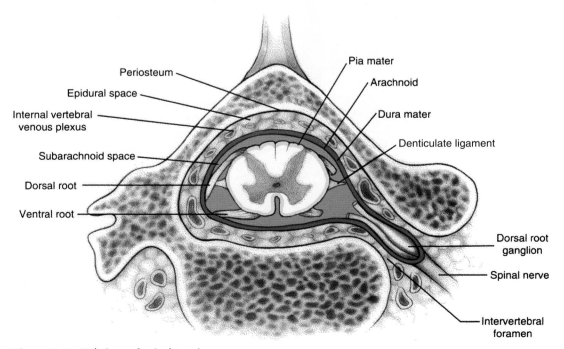

Figure 2-2 Relations of spinal meninges.

dura by the **denticulate ligaments** and by the spinal nerve roots. The denticulate ligaments are 21 pairs of fibrous sheaths located at the sides of the spinal cord. Medially, the ligaments form a continuous longitudinal attachment to the pia mater. Laterally, they form triangular, toothlike processes that attach to the dura. Because of their pial attachments midway between the posterior and anterior surfaces of the spinal cord, the denticulate ligaments can be used as landmarks for surgical procedures. The spinal cord is also anchored by the roots of the spinal nerves, which are ensheathed by a cuff of dura where they perforate it near the intervertebral foramina.

DURA MATER

The spinal dura mater loosely surrounds the spinal cord. The area between the spinal dura and the periosteum lining the vertebral canal is the epidural space. Its contents include loose connective tissue, fat, and the internal vertebral venous plexus.

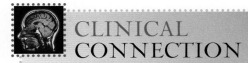

CLINICAL CONNECTION

The internal vertebral venous plexus forms a valveless communication between the cranial **dural sinuses,** which collect blood from the veins of the brain, and the veins of the thoracic, abdominal, and pelvic cavities. It, therefore, provides a direct path for the spread of infections, emboli, or cancer cells from the viscera to the brain.

Inferior or caudal to the spinal cord, the dura mater forms the **dural sac** (Fig. 2-3), which extends inferiorly to the middle third of the second sacral vertebra. Caudal to this point, it surrounds the filum terminale, the threadlike extension of the pia mater, and descends to the back of the coccyx as the coccygeal ligament, which blends with the periosteum. The dural sac is located between the

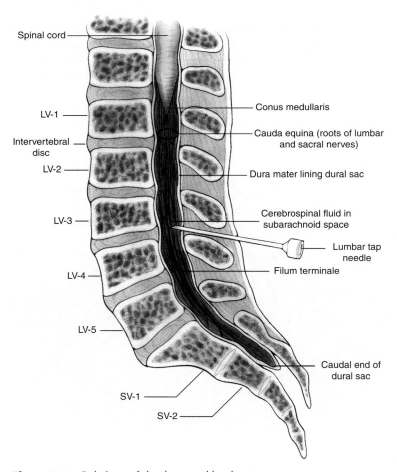

Figure 2-3   Relations of dural sac and lumbar tap.

middle of LV1, where the spinal cord ends as the conus medullaris, and the inferior border of SV2, where the dura ends. Because the arachnoid is attached to the inner surface of the dura lining the dural sac, the contents of the sac are in the subarachnoid space. Therefore, the dural sac contains (a) the filum terminale; (b) the **cauda equina,** consisting of the lumbosacral nerve roots descending from the spinal cord to their points of emergence at the lumbar intervertebral and sacral foramina; and (c) cerebrospinal fluid.

The spinal cord ends just above LV2, whereas the subarachnoid space continues caudally to SV2. A hypodermic needle may be introduced into the subarachnoid space (Fig. 2-3) within the dural sac without danger of accidentally injuring the spinal cord, thereby causing irreparable damage, because

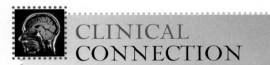

CLINICAL CONNECTION

This procedure, called **lumbar puncture,** may be used to withdraw cerebrospinal fluid for analysis, to measure cerebrospinal fluid pressure, and to introduce therapeutic agents, anesthetics, and contrast media. It is inadvisable to puncture above the LV2–3 interspace in adults and above the LV4–5 interspace in infants or small children.

regeneration or repair to neurons and axons in the spinal cord (or brain) does not occur.

SPINAL NERVES

Each spinal nerve (except the first and last) is attached to a spinal cord segment by posterior (dorsal) and anterior (ventral) roots (Fig. 2-4). Thus, each segment gives rise to four separate roots, one posterior and one anterior on each side. Each of these individual roots is attached to the spinal cord by a series of rootlets. The posterior and anterior roots take a lateral and descending course within the subarachnoid space (Fig. 2-1) and are encased in the dura mater as they approach the intervertebral foramina (Fig. 2-2). The posterior root or spinal ganglia, groups of neurons in the posterior root, are within the thoracic, lumbar, and sacral intervertebral foramina but slightly distal to the cervical foramina. The posterior and anterior roots unite immediately beyond the ganglia to form the spinal nerves, which then exit from the intervertebral foramina and immediately begin to branch.

SPINAL CORD TOPOGRAPHY

On the surface of the spinal cord are several longitudinal grooves (Fig. 2-4). The most prominent

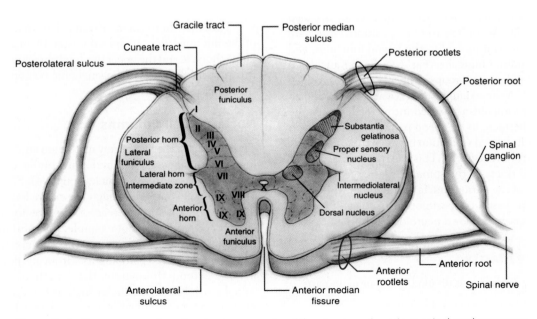

Figure 2-4 Transverse section showing a composite of the structures in various spinal cord segments and the formation of a spinal nerve.

of these is the anterior median fissure, occupied by the anterior spinal artery and the proximal parts of its sulcal branches. On the opposite side is a far less conspicuous groove, the posterior median sulcus. The anterior and posterior rootlets of the spinal nerves arise somewhat lateral to these median grooves, at the anterolateral and posterolateral sulci, respectively. The small posterior spinal arteries are located in the latter sulci.

SPINAL CORD INTERNAL STRUCTURE

The spinal cord has external and internal parts that are similar throughout its extent. The external part is the white matter, which consists of millions of axons transmitting impulses superiorly or inferiorly. A large number of the fibers are myelinated, thus accounting for the white color in the fresh or unstained state.

The internal part is the gray matter, which consists of nerve cell bodies and the neuropil that includes the dendrites, preterminal and terminal axons, capillaries, and glia between the neurons. It contains some entering and exiting myelinated fibers but has a grayish color in the fresh or unstained state because of the virtual absence of myelin.

WHITE MATTER

The white matter is divided into three areas, called funiculi. According to their positions, these are the posterior funiculus, the lateral funiculus, and the anterior funiculus (Fig. 2-4). Each funiculus is subdivided into groups of fibers called fasciculi or tracts. As an example, at cervical levels each posterior funiculus is divided into a medial part, the gracile tract, and a lateral part, the cuneate tract. A well-defined separation between these two tracts is not always evident. This is generally true of most of the tracts in the spinal cord; hence, the locations of the various tracts in the spinal white matter are based on postmortem studies of human subjects with known neurologic abnormalities.

GRAY MATTER

The gray matter is divided into four main parts:

1. The posterior or dorsal horns;
2. The anterior or ventral horns;
3. The intermediate zones;
4. The lateral horns.

For descriptive purposes, an imaginary horizontal line passing from side to side through the deepest part of each posterior funiculus and extending laterally through the gray matter defines the anterior boundary of the posterior horns (Fig. 2-4). The posterior horns contain groups of neurons that are influenced mainly by impulses entering the spinal cord via the posterior roots. Hence, the posterior horns are primarily the "sensory" parts of the spinal gray matter, and many of their neurons give rise to axons that enter the white matter and ascend to the brain.

The anterior horns are located between the anterior and lateral funiculi. Most of their neurons play roles in voluntary movement and many of them give rise to axons that emerge in the anterior roots. Hence, the anterior horns are primarily the "motor" parts of the spinal gray matter.

The intermediate zones are located between the anterior and posterior horns and are continuous medially with the gray matter that crosses the midline at the central canal. The intermediate zones are composed mainly of association or interneurons for segmental and intersegmental integration of spinal cord functions. Hence, the intermediate zones are the "association" parts of the spinal gray matter, and most of the axons arising from their neurons remain in the spinal cord; some, however, do project to the brain.

The lateral horn is a small triangular extension of the intermediate zone into the lateral funiculus of the thoracic and the upper two lumbar segments. It contains cell bodies of preganglionic neurons of the **sympathetic** nervous system.

Nuclei or Cell Columns

The neurons of the spinal gray matter are arranged in longitudinal groups of functionally similar cells referred to as columns or nuclei (Fig. 2-4). Some of these nuclei extend through the entire length of the spinal cord, whereas others are found only at certain levels. For example, the substantia gelatinosa and the proper sensory nucleus, which are related to pain impulses from all spinal nerves, extend throughout the length of the spinal cord, but other nuclei such as the dorsal nucleus and the intermediolateral nucleus, which are related to the cerebellar and autonomic systems, respectively, exist only in certain spinal cord segments.

Laminae

The spinal gray matter can also be divided into laminae or layers based on layerings of morphologically similar neurons (Fig. 2-4). Laminae provide a more precise identification of areas within the spinal gray matter and are very useful in describing the locations of the origins or terminations of the functional paths. Ten laminae make up the spinal gray matter and, in general, they are numbered from posterior to anterior. The posterior horn includes laminae I through VI; the intermediate zone is mainly lamina VII; and the anterior horn contains part of lamina VII and all of laminae VIII and IX. Lamina X is in the commissural area surrounding the central canal.

REGIONAL DIFFERENCES

Myelin-stained transverse sections of the four major regions of the spinal cord can be distinguished from each other most readily by the size and shape of the respective gray matter (Figs. 2-5 to 2-8). Because of the large size of the lower limbs, the lumbar and sacral segments have massive posterior and anterior horns. In lumbar segments, the anterior horn has a distinct medial extension, whereas in sacral segments the anterior horn extends laterally. In addition, the rim of white matter surrounding the sacral gray matter is much thinner than that in the lumbar spinal cord.

The posterior horn in both thoracic and cervical segments is narrow compared with lumbar and sacral segments. However, owing to the muscular volume of the upper limbs, the cervical anterior horn is much larger than the thoracic, which mainly supplies the relatively small intercostal and subcostal muscles. The thoracic segments have the least amount of gray matter, both anteriorly and posteriorly.

Differences in the amount of white matter are subtle throughout the spinal cord. Nevertheless, because the white matter contains axons transmitting information between the spinal cord segments and the brain, the amount of white matter decreases in each segment proceeding from superior to inferior.

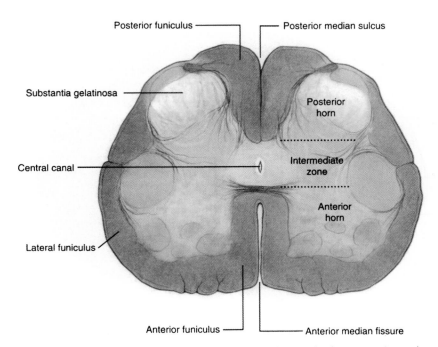

Figure 2-5 Transverse section of sacral spinal cord. Note the huge anterior and posterior horns surrounded by narrow white matter.

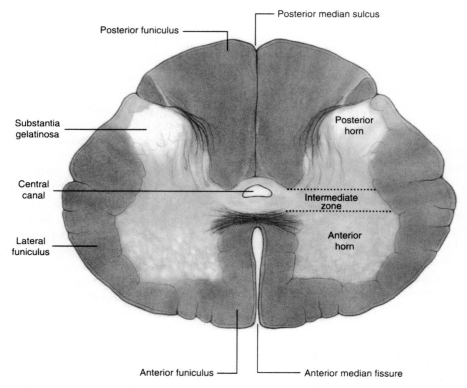

Figure 2-6 Transverse section of lumbar spinal cord. Note the large anterior and posterior horns and the large posterior funiculi.

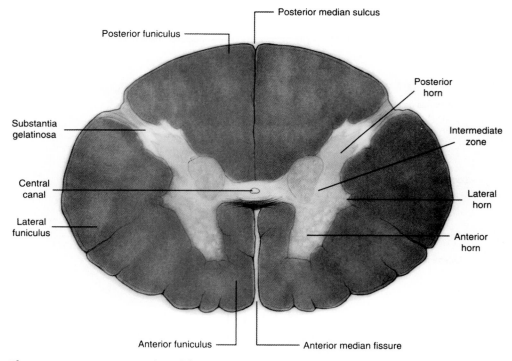

Figure 2-7 Transverse section of thoracic spinal cord. Note the slim anterior and posterior horns and lateral horn indenting the lateral funiculus.

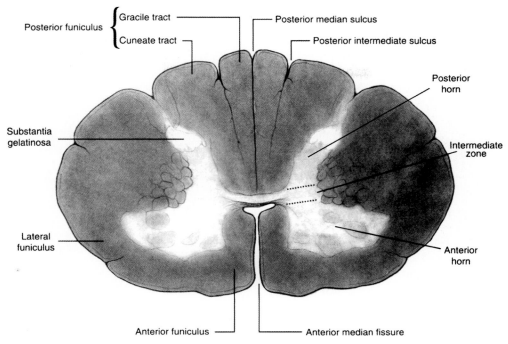

Figure 2-8 Transverse section of cervical enlargement. Note the slim posterior horn, large anterior horn, and the division of the huge posterior funiculus.

Chapter Review Questions

2-1.   What are the contents of the spinal epidural space?

2-2.   What are the contents of the dural sac?

2-3.   At what three intervertebral articulations are dislocations most likely to occur and what spinal cord segments are related to each?

2-4.   Why are lumbar punctures done at the LV3 to LV4 or LV4 to LV5 levels in adults?

2-5.   What are the distinguishing characteristics of transverse spinal cord sections at sacral, lumbar, thoracic, and cervical levels?

2-6.   The C8 nerve emerges between which of the following vertebrae?
   a. CV6 and CV7
   b. CV7 and CV8
   c. CV8 and TV1
   d. CV7 and TV1
   e. TV1 and TV2

2-7.   Each of the following concerning the cauda equina is true except one:
   a. The cauda equina is located within the dural sac.
   b. The cauda equina contains dorsal roots of lumbosacral nerves.
   c. The cauda equina contains ventral roots of lumbosacral nerves.
   d. The cauda equina is located in subarachnoid space.
   e. All are true.

3

Brainstem: Topography and Functional Levels

THE BRAINSTEM CONTAINS FUNCTIONAL centers associated with all but one of the 12 cranial nerves. It also contains the long tracts that transmit somatosensory impulses from all parts of the body to the forebrain, as well as motor impulses for voluntary movements that originate in the forebrain. Damage to the brainstem is manifested by somatosensory or motor dysfunctions or both, accompanied by abnormalities in cranial nerve functions. The level of damage in a brainstem lesion can usually be determined by cranial nerve malfunction. Because of the vital nature of many functional centers located in the brainstem, especially at more caudal levels, brainstem lesions are frequently fatal.

The brainstem is the stalk-like part of the brain that is located in the posterior cranial fossa. It consists of the medulla oblongata, pons, and midbrain (Fig. 3-1). The medulla oblongata is continuous with the spinal cord at the foramen magnum, and the midbrain is continuous with the forebrain at the tentorial notch, the opening at the free margins of the tentorium cerebelli.

The brainstem is covered posteriorly by the cerebellum to which it is connected by huge masses of nerve fibers that form the three pairs of **cerebellar peduncles.** Its anterior surface is closely related to the clivus, the downward sloping basal surface of the posterior cranial fossa between the dorsum sellae and foramen magnum (Fig. 3-2).

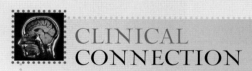

CLINICAL CONNECTION

A life-threatening event involving the brainstem can occur when a lumbar puncture is performed in a patient with increased intracranial pressure. In this circumstance, the brainstem is thrust downward as the overlying mass of the cerebellum herniates through the foramen magnum against the medulla oblongata. Pressure on cardiovascular and respiratory centers in the medulla quickly results in death.

BRAINSTEM ANATOMY

MEDULLA OBLONGATA

The medulla oblongata, more simply called the medulla, extends from the spinal cord to the pons

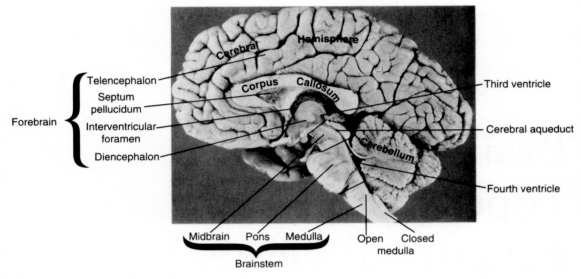

Figure 3-1   Median view of right side of brain showing subdivisions and their parts of the ventricular system.

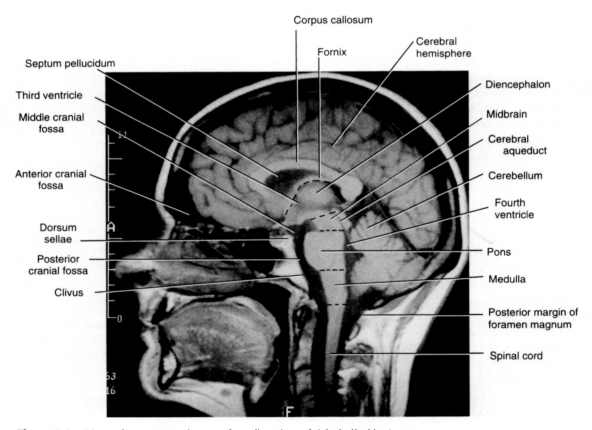

Figure 3-2   Magnetic resonance image of median view of right half of brain.

(Figs. 3-1, 3-2). The posterior surface of its rostral part is anatomically related to the cerebellum to which it is connected by the inferior cerebellar peduncles.

The caudal half of the medulla contains a prolongation of the central canal of the spinal cord and is referred to as the closed part of the medulla. The posterior surface of the rostral half of the medulla forms the caudal or medullary part of the floor of the fourth ventricle, the cerebrospinal fluid-filled cavity between the cerebellum and the pons and open medulla (Fig. 3-2). The rostral half of the medulla is referred to as the open part. The medulla contains nuclei related to the vestibulo-cochlear (VIII), glossopharyngeal (IX), vagus (X), cranial part of the accessory (XI), and hypoglossal (XII) cranial nerves and also contains centers that are associated with equilibrium, audition, degluti-tion, coughing, vomiting, salivation, tongue move-ments, respiration, and circulation.

PONS

The pons extends from the medulla to the mid-brain. Posteriorly, it forms the floor of the rostral part of the fourth ventricle, and it is covered by the cerebellum to which it is attached by the middle cerebellar peduncles or brachii pontis. The pons contains nuclei related to the trigeminal (V), abducens (VI), and facial (VII) cranial nerves and contains centers associated with mastication, eye movements, facial expression, blinking, salivation, equilibrium, and audition.

MIDBRAIN

The midbrain lies between the pons and the fore-brain and is located in the tentorial notch. It is the shortest part of the brainstem and contains the nuclei of the oculomotor (III) and trochlear (IV) cranial nerves as well as centers associated with audi-tory, visual, and pupillary reflexes. It contains the **cerebral aqueduct** (Figs. 3-1, 3-2), the narrow chan-nel that is the only route by which cerebrospinal fluid can exit from the ventricles of the forebrain to the fourth ventricle. An imaginary line passing from side to side through the cerebral aqueduct divides the midbrain into a posterior part or roof, the tec-tum, and an anterior part, the cerebral peduncle.

BRAINSTEM TOPOGRAPHY

As stated in the Preface, before describing the clin-ically important functional paths, it is imperative for the reader to become familiar with the distin-guishing characteristics of the subdivisions of the brain and their functionally important levels. Because only the most conspicuous anatomic land-marks are necessary to distinguish the subdivisions and their functional levels, these alone are described here. Other structures of clinical importance are described with the functional paths.

ANTERIOR SURFACE

Medulla

On the anterior surface of the medulla (Fig. 3-3) are the pyramids, a pair of elongated elevations on either side of the anterior median fissure, which becomes partially obliterated caudally by the pyra-midal decussation. Lateral to the rostral part of each pyramid is a prominent elevation, the olive. The shallow groove between the olive and pyramid is the preolivary sulcus where the hypoglossal (XII) nerve rootlets emerge. The sulcus posterior to the olive is the postolivary sulcus, and this sulcus is where the rootlets of the glossopharyngeal (IX) and vagus (X) nerves attach (from superior to inferior). The cranial rootlets of the accessory (XI) nerve emerge in line with those of the vagus but inferior to the postolivary sulcus. Because these rootlets eventually join and are distributed with the vagus nerve, the so-called cranial part of the accessory nerve is considered by many to be a misnomer.

Pons

The anterior portion of the pons is the basilar part. Its surface consists of transverse bands formed by bundles of fibers that become continuous laterally with the middle cerebellar peduncles. The shallow basilar sulcus near the midline is normally occu-pied by the basilar artery.

The abducens (VI) nerve emerges at the pontomedullary junction, near the lateral border of the pyramid. Attaching more laterally at the pontomedullary junction are the facial (VII) and vestibulocochlear (VIII) nerves. On the antero-lateral surface of the pons about midway between the medulla and midbrain is the attachment of the trigeminal (V) nerve. This nerve consists of a larger inferolateral sensory root (portio major) and a small superomedial motor root (portio minor).

Midbrain

The anterior surface of the midbrain is formed by the cerebral peduncles. These consist of the con-

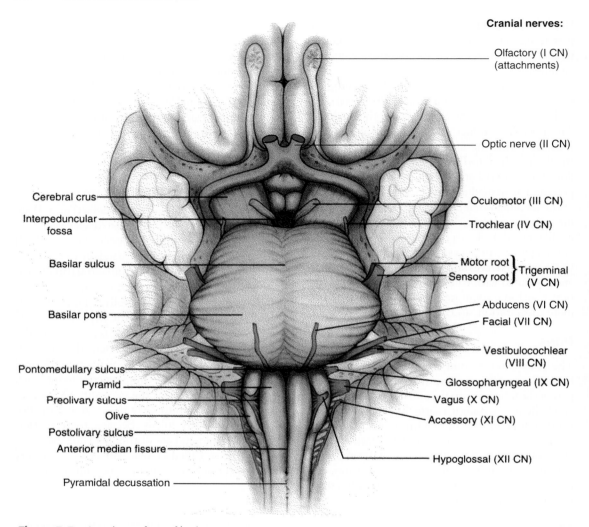

Cranial nerves:

Olfactory (I CN)
(attachments)

Optic nerve (II CN)

Cerebral crus

Interpeduncular
fossa

Basilar sulcus

Basilar pons

Oculomotor (III CN)

Trochlear (IV CN)

Motor root
Sensory root } Trigeminal
(V CN)

Abducens (VI CN)

Facial (VII CN)

Vestibulocochlear
(VIII CN)

Pontomedullary sulcus

Pyramid

Preolivary sulcus

Olive

Postolivary sulcus

Anterior median fissure

Pyramidal decussation

Glossopharyngeal (IX CN)

Vagus (X CN)

Accessory (XI CN)

Hypoglossal (XII CN)

Figure 3-3   Anterior surface of brainstem.

verging cerebral crura (the most anterior parts of the cerebral peduncles), which are separated from each other by the **interpeduncular fossa.** The oculomotor (III) nerves emerge from the walls of the interpeduncular fossa.

POSTERIOR SURFACE

Medulla

The posterior surface of the closed or caudal half of the medulla contains the gracile tubercles on either side of the posterior median sulcus (Fig. 3-4). Lateral to each gracile tubercle and extending slightly more rostral is the cuneate tubercle. The posterior surface of the open half of the medulla

and the posterior surface of the pons form the floor of the fourth ventricle.

Fourth Ventricle

The caudal tip of the fourth ventricle lies between the gracile tubercles and is called the obex. The floor of the fourth ventricle can be divided into medullary and pontine parts by drawing an imaginary horizontal line between the lateral recesses, which are found at the widest point of the fourth ventricle. In most brains, the rostral part of the medullary floor contains a variable number of white strands called the striae medullares, which extend laterally from the median sulcus toward the lateral recess.

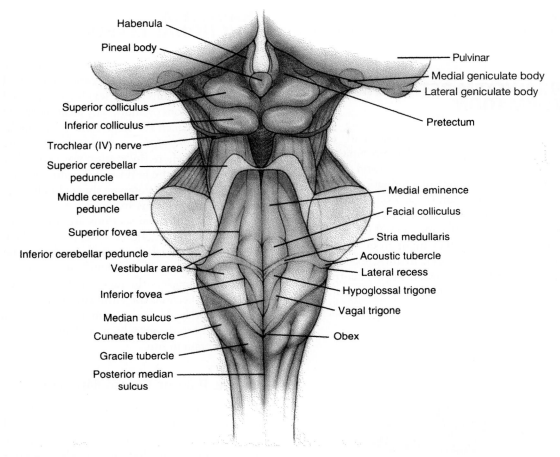

Figure 3-4 Posterior surface of brainstem.

The median sulcus divides the floor of the fourth ventricle into symmetric halves. Each half is further subdivided into medial and lateral parts by the superior and inferior foveae, small depressions at pontine and medullary levels, respectively. These foveae are remnants of the sulcus limitans and indicate the boundary between motor structures, which are medial, and sensory structures, which are lateral. Hence, extending laterally from the two foveae to the lateral recess is the vestibular area, and at the lateral recess is a small eminence, the acoustic tubercle. Both the vestibular area and the acoustic tubercle are sensory structures. Between the inferior fovea and the median sulcus are two small triangular areas, the hypoglossal trigone positioned medially, and the vagal trigone positioned laterally, both of which are motor structures. Between the superior fovea and the median sulcus is the medial eminence. Its caudal part enlarges and is the facial colliculus, which overlies the abducens nucleus.

Cerebellar Peduncles

The cut surfaces of the cerebellar peduncles are at the lateral aspects of the pons and in the roof of the fourth ventricle. The massive **middle cerebellar peduncle** or brachium pontis is continuous with the basilar part of the pons. At its inferomedial part is **the inferior cerebellar peduncle** or restiform body, which connects the medulla to the cerebellum. The **superior cerebellar peduncle** or brachium conjunctivum passes from the roof of the fourth ventricle into the tegmentum of the rostral pons.

Midbrain

The posterior surface of the midbrain is composed of the tectum. The tectum consists of two pairs of mounds, the corpora quadrigemina or inferior and superior colliculi. The trochlear (IV) nerves emerge caudal to the inferior colliculi. The small area rostral to the superior colliculi is the pretectum.

BRAINSTEM RETICULAR FORMATION

Extending through the central part of the medulla, pons, and midbrain is a complex intermingling of loosely defined nuclei and tracts that form the brainstem reticular formation (Fig. 3-5). As its central location (Figs. 3-6 to 3-13) might suggest, it is intimately associated with ascending and descending paths and cranial nerve nuclei. As a result, it receives input from all parts of the nervous system and, in turn, exerts widespread influences on virtually every central nervous system (CNS) function, as described in Chapter 20.

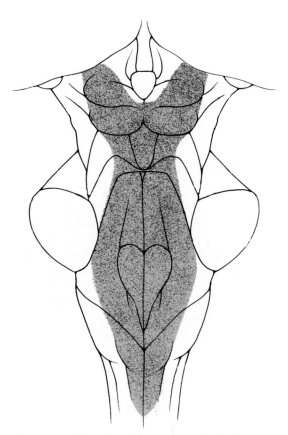

Figure 3-5 Location of brainstem reticular formation (blue shaded area).

BRAINSTEM FUNCTIONAL LEVELS

After the surface features of the brainstem are familiar, these same structures can be identified in transverse sections at the levels that are used in localizing lesions or injuries. By locating on the brainstem specimen the same surface landmarks in a transverse section, one is able to determine precisely from where the section was taken. For example, refer to the brainstem drawings in Figures 3-3 and 3-4 and compare them closely with the transverse sections in Figures 3-6 to 3-13. Because the brainstem sections are referred to repeatedly as the functional systems are studied, knowing precisely where they are located in the brain will enhance the development of a three-dimensional image of the functional paths. This is important because the clinician must project knowledge of the nervous system, no matter what the source, onto the gross brain and ultimately to the living brain in situ.

ROSTRAL PART OF CLOSED MEDULLA

The pyramids are anterior and separated by the anterior median fissure (Fig. 3-6). The gracile and cuneate tubercles are posterior and separated by the posterior intermediate sulcus. The posterior median sulcus is between the gracile tubercles.

CAUDAL PART OF OPEN MEDULLA

Positioned anteriorly are the pyramids and olives with the rootlets of the hypoglossal nerve between them (Fig. 3-7). The preolivary and postolivary sulci are anterior and posterior to the olive, respectively. Posteriorly, the floor of the fourth ventricle contains, from medial to lateral, the hypoglossal and vagal trigones, the inferior fovea, and the vestibular area.

ROSTRAL PART OF OPEN MEDULLA

Anteriorly, the surface of the medulla presents, from medial to lateral, the anterior median fissure, the pyramids, the preolivary sulci, the olives, and the postolivary sulci (Fig. 3-8). Posteriorly, the widest part of the floor of the fourth ventricle is relatively smooth except at the lateral recess where there is an eminence, the acoustic tubercle. Lateral

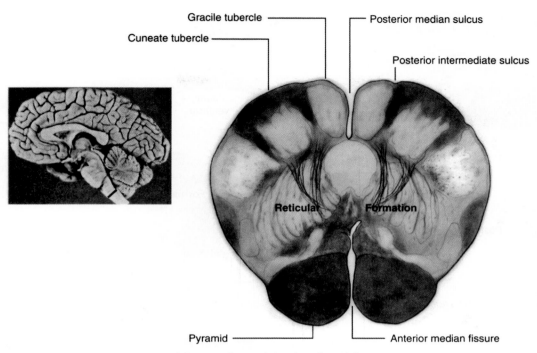

Figure 3-6   Transverse section of the rostral part of the closed medulla.

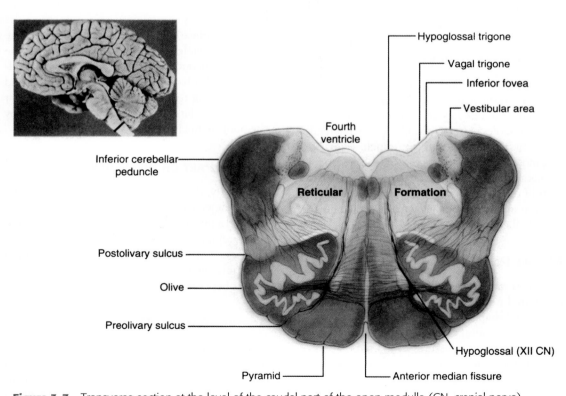

Figure 3-7   Transverse section at the level of the caudal part of the open medulla (CN, cranial nerve).

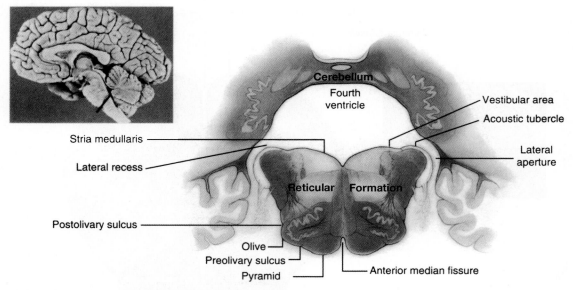

Figure 3-8   Transverse section at the level of the rostral part of the open medulla.

to this tubercle is the lateral aperture, an opening into the subarachnoid space. Most of the ventricular floor consists of the vestibular area. The bundles of myelinated fibers in the floor are the striae medullares of the fourth ventricle.

CAUDAL PART OF PONS

The anterior or basilar part of the pons consists of gray matter, the pontine nuclei, and white matter, large circular bundles of descending fibers and smaller bundles of transverse fibers, which laterally enter the middle cerebellar peduncle (Fig. 3-9). The most conspicuous structures in the posterior or tegmental part of the pons are the intramedullary parts of the abducens (VI) and facial (VII) nerves and the abducens nucleus, which is deep to the facial colliculus.

MIDDLE PART OF PONS

This section is at the midpontine level where the trigeminal nerve attaches (Fig. 3-10). Although its size and shape may vary, the basilar part of the pons appears similar at all pontine levels. The most conspicuous structures in the lateral part of the pontine tegmentum are the large, oval motor trigeminal nucleus and the smaller sensory trigeminal nucleus lateral to it. The superior cerebellar peduncles are in the roof of the fourth ventricle. The **superior medullary velum** is between them.

ROSTRAL PART OF PONS

At the posterior surface of the rostral pons is the decussation and emergence of the trochlear (IV) nerves, the only cranial nerves emerging from the posterior surface of the brainstem (Fig. 3-11). The fourth ventricle has narrowed to become the cerebral aqueduct. The massive superior cerebellar peduncles have entered the tegmentum and are beginning to decussate or cross. The basilar part contains larger bundles of fibers separated by the pontine nuclei.

CAUDAL PART OF THE MIDBRAIN

Posteriorly, the inferior colliculi are separated by the periaqueductal gray matter surrounding the cerebral aqueduct (Fig. 3-12). Anteriorly is located the cerebral peduncle which, from posterior to anterior, consists of the tegmentum, substantia nigra, and cerebral crus. The large interpeduncular fossa is between the **cerebral crura.**

ROSTRAL PART OF MIDBRAIN

Posteriorly, the superior colliculi are partially separated by the periaqueductal gray matter and cerebral aqueduct (Fig. 3-13). The oculomotor nuclei are in the V-shaped anterior part of the periaqueductal gray matter. Anteriorly, the cerebral peduncle is composed of the tegmentum, substantia nigra, and

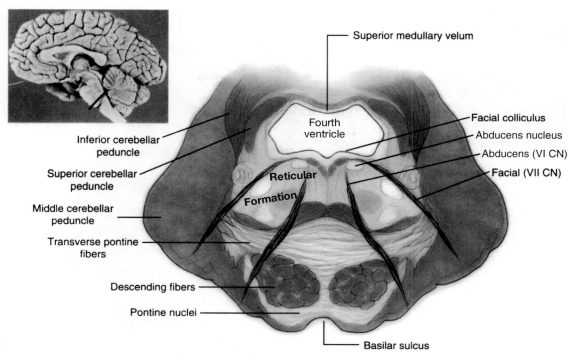

Figure 3-9   Transverse section at the level of the caudal pons (VI and VII cranial nerves [CN]).

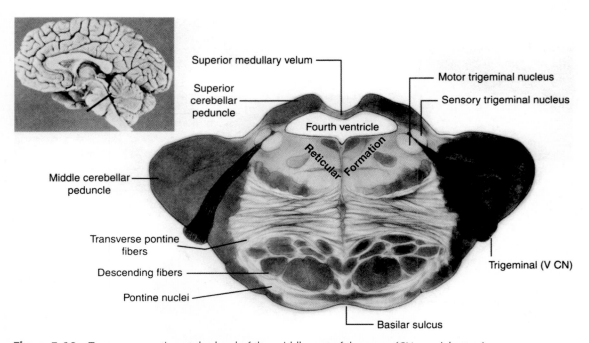

Figure 3-10   Transverse section at the level of the middle part of the pons (CN, cranial nerve).

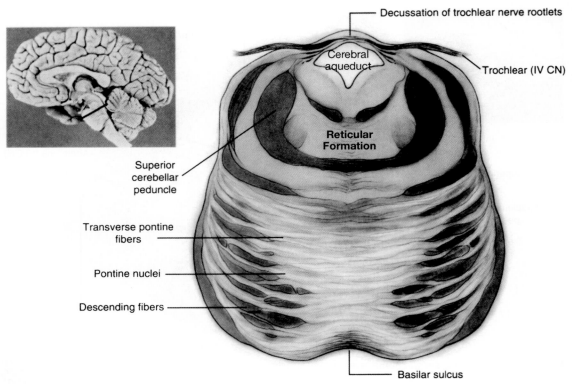

Figure 3-11   Transverse section at the level of the rostral pons (CN, cranial nerve).

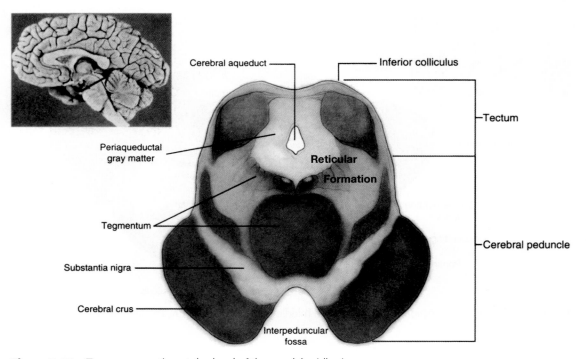

Figure 3-12   Transverse section at the level of the caudal midbrain.

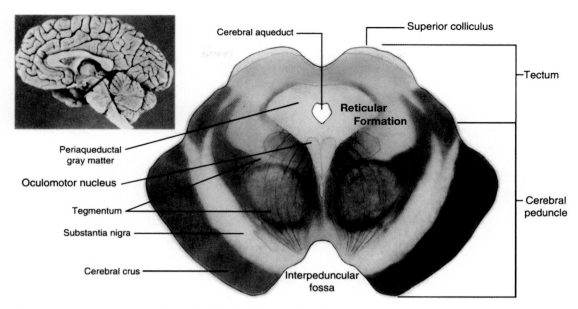

Cerebral aqueduct

Superior colliculus

Reticular Formation

Tectum

Periaqueductal gray matter

Oculomotor nucleus

Tegmentum

Substantia nigra

Cerebral crus

Interpeduncular fossa

Cerebral peduncle

Figure 3-13 Transverse section at the level of the rostral midbrain.

cerebral crus. The oculomotor (III) cranial nerves emerge from the walls of the interpeduncular fossa.

Chapter Review Questions

3-1. What are the distinguishing characteristics of the ventral surface of the (a) medulla, (b) pons, and (c) midbrain?

3-2. What are the distinguishing characteristics of the dorsal surface of the (a) closed medulla, (b) open medulla, (c) pons, and (d) midbrain?

3-3. What and where is the brainstem reticular formation?

3-4. At which specific brainstem level is each of the following?

a. hypoglossal trigone
b. motor trigeminal nucleus
c. superior colliculus
d. decussation of trochlear nerve
e. acoustic tubercle
f. gracile tubercle

g. facial colliculus
h. inferior colliculus

3-5. The brainstem is located in the:

a. anterior cranial fossa
b. middle cranial fossa
c. posterior cranial fossa
d. supratentorial compartment of cranial cavity
e. none of the above

3-6. Motor and sensory structures in the floor of the fourth ventricle are separated by the:

a. anterior median fissure
b. superior and inferior foveae
c. median sulcus
d. preolivary sulcus
e. basilar sulcus

3-7. The cerebral crus, substantia nigra, and adjacent tegmentum are located in the:

a. tectum
b. medulla
c. cerebellar peduncles
d. pons
e. cerebral peduncle

4

Forebrain: Topography and Functional Levels

DAMAGE TO THE FOREBRAIN may result in disturbances involving hormonal imbalance, temperature regulation, emotions, or behavior. Forebrain lesions may also affect sensory perception and voluntary movements as well as memory, judgment, and speech. The most common vascular lesions in the entire nervous system are "capsular strokes" that occur deep within the forebrain.

The forebrain or prosencephalon consists of the telencephalon, the paired cerebral hemispheres, and the diencephalon. The diencephalon contains functional centers for the integration of all information passing from the brainstem and spinal cord to the cerebral hemispheres as well as the integration of motor and visceral activities. The two cerebral hemispheres integrate the highest mental functions such as the awareness of sensations and emotions, learning and memory, intelligence and creativity, and language.

The diencephalon (interbrain) receives the optic (II) nerves and is subdivided into four parts: thalamus, hypothalamus, subthalamus, and epithalamus. The cerebral hemispheres receive the olfactory (I) nerves. The diencephalon contains the third ventricle, and the cerebral hemispheres contain the lateral ventricles, which are separated from each other in part by the septum pellucidum (Figs. 3-1, 3-2, 4-2).

DIRECTIONAL TERMINOLOGY

The forebrain is located in the anterior and middle cranial fossae and is supratentorial in position, that is, superior to or above the tentorium cerebelli. It is oriented almost perpendicularly to the brain and spinal cord (Figs. 3-1, 3-2, 4-1). The change in direction occurs at the junction between the midbrain and forebrain, and at this junction there is a change in directional terms. In descriptions of the spinal cord and brainstem, the terms anterior or ventral indicate toward the front of the body, and the terms posterior or dorsal mean toward the back. Moreover, superior or rostral indicate higher or toward the top or above, and inferior or caudal mean lower or toward the bottom or below.

With the change in direction at the midbrain-forebrain junction, the directional terms used in anatomic descriptions of the forebrain are as follows:

Anterior—toward the front of the skull
Posterior—toward the back of the skull
Ventral or inferior—toward the base of the skull
Dorsal or superior—toward the top of the skull

37

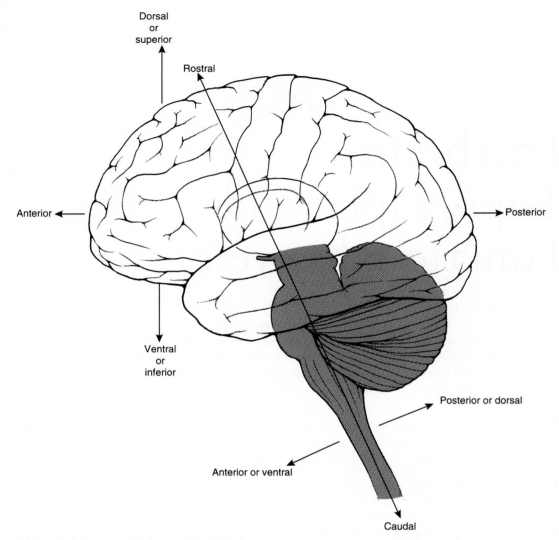

Figure 4-1 Central nervous system directional terminology. The midbrain, hindbrain, and spinal cord (stipples) are oriented almost vertically, whereas the forebrain is oriented horizontally. Because of this change in orientation at the midbrain-forebrain junction, the terms dorsal and ventral have different connotations rostral and caudal to this junction.

DIENCEPHALON

The cerebrospinal fluid–filled cavity found in the middle of the diencephalon is the third ventricle (Figs. 3-1, 3-2, 4-2). Posteriorly, the third ventricle is continuous with the cerebral aqueduct. Anteriorly, it is continuous with the two lateral ventricles at the interventricular **foramina (of Monro).** The hypothalamic sulcus traverses the lateral wall of the third ventricle from the interventricular foramen to the cerebral aqueduct and

separates the thalamus, above, from the hypothalamus, below.

The diencephalon includes the thalamus, a large nuclear mass forming the dorsal part of the wall of the third ventricle; the hypothalamus, which lines the ventral part of the wall of the third ventricle and extends ventrally from the medial part of the thalamus to the base of the brain; the subthalamus, ventral to the lateral part of the thalamus and lateral to the hypothalamus, but not reaching the surface of the brain; and the epithalamus, a small

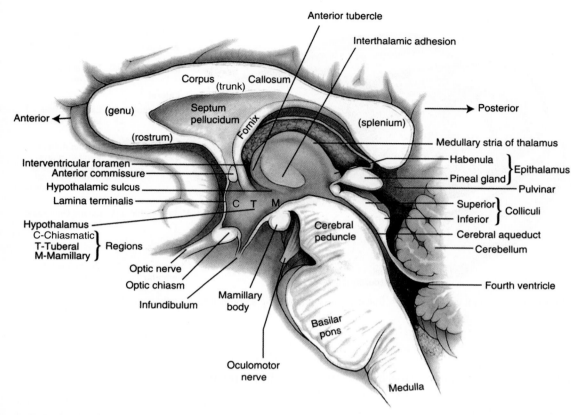

Figure 4-2   Median view of right diencephalon and adjacent parts of the brainstem and cerebral hemisphere.

area dorsal to the most posterior part of the third ventricle.

HYPOTHALAMUS

The only subdivision of the diencephalon on the ventral surface of the brain is the hypothalamus (Fig. 4-2). It is located in the median part of the middle cranial fossa (Fig. 4-2) above the diaphragma sellae. The hypothalamus is subdivided into three main areas in the anterior-posterior plane. Positioned posteriorly is the mamillary region, which is related to the mamillary bodies, paired spherical masses about the size of small peas located in the rostral part of the interpeduncular fossa. Found anteriorly is the chiasmatic region located dorsal to the optic chiasm. Between the mamillary and the chiasmatic regions is the tuber cinereum after which the tuberal region is named. The anterior part of the tuberal region contains the **infundibulum** or stalk of the pituitary gland

and is sometimes referred to as the infundibular region.

THALAMUS

The thalami are two egg-shaped masses bordering the third ventricle, dorsal to the hypothalamic sulcus (Fig. 4-2). In most brains, the right and left thalami are partially fused across the third ventricle by the interthalamic adhesion or massa intermedia. At the interventricular foramen is a swelling, the anterior tubercle, and on the dorsomedial surface of the thalamus is a bundle of fibers, the medullary stria. Posteriorly, the pulvinar overhangs the midbrain like a pillow.

Thalamic Nuclei

The thalamus consists of a large number of nuclei that form eight nuclear masses named according to their anatomic locations (Fig. 4-3). The internal medullary lamina, a thin sheet of bundles of

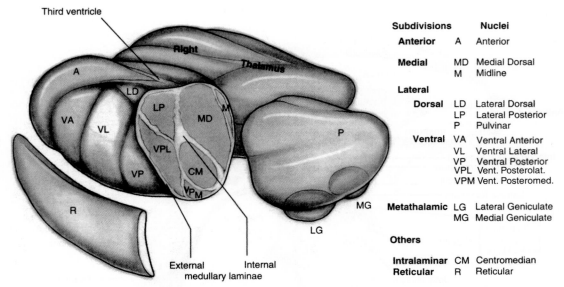

Figure 4-3   Lateral view of the left thalamic nuclei, including a coronal section through the posterior part of the thalamus.

myelinated fibers, separates the thalamus into three major subdivisions: anterior, medial, and lateral. The anterior subdivision is located at the anterior tubercle of the thalamus and consists of the anterior nuclei (A). The medial subdivision chiefly includes a large medial dorsal nucleus (MD) and a thin midline nucleus (M) along the wall of the third ventricle. The interthalamic adhesion is a bridge of midline nuclei.

The lateral subdivision is composed of two nuclear masses. The more ventral nuclear mass is subdivided into ventral anterior (VA), ventral lateral (VL), and ventral posterior (VP) nuclei. The ventral posterior nucleus is further divided into ventral posterolateral (VPL) and ventral posteromedial (VPM) nuclei. The more dorsal mass consists of lateral nuclei, the lateral dorsal (LD) and lateral posterior (LP) anteriorly and the pulvinar (P) posteriorly. On the undersurface of the pulvinar are the metathalamic nuclei, the lateral geniculate (LG) and medial geniculate (MG) nuclei.

Two other nuclear masses are anatomically related to the medullary laminae. Within the internal medullary lamina are several intralaminar nuclei, the most prominent of which is the centromedian (CM). Lateral to the external medullary lamina is the reticular (R) nucleus, a thin nucleus forming the most lateral part of the thalamus.

SUBTHALAMUS

The **subthalamus** consists of a wedge-shaped area ventral to the thalamus and lateral to the hypothalamus. It contains several nuclei, the most prominent of which is the subthalamic nucleus.

EPITHALAMUS

Posteriorly, the dorsal surface of the diencephalon is formed by the epithalamus. The epithalamus consists of the pineal gland and the **habenula** (Figs. 3-4, 4-2).

CEREBRAL HEMISPHERE

The right and left cerebral hemispheres consist of cortical, medullary, and nuclear parts. The cortical portion of each hemisphere is located externally and consists of gray matter that is folded or convoluted to form gyri, which are separated by sulci. Underlying the cortex are masses of nerve fibers that form the white matter or medullary region of the hemisphere, commonly called the centrum semiovale. Embedded deeply in the white matter are the telencephalic nuclei, the most prominent of which are the caudate and lentiform.

LATERAL SURFACE

The lateral surface (Fig. 4-4) is convex and conforms to the concavity of the cranial vault. The most uniform and prominent cleft on the lateral surface of the hemisphere is the lateral sulcus or **fissure of Sylvius,** which begins at the base of the brain, extends to the lateral surface of the hemisphere, and proceeds posteriorly and slightly superiorly. It separates the frontal and parietal lobes (superiorly) from the temporal lobe (inferiorly). The next most uniform and prominent cleft is the central sulcus or fissure of Rolando, which is between the frontal and parietal lobes. This sulcus is oriented in the dorsoventral direction behind the most anterior gyrus that extends uninterruptedly from the lateral sulcus to the superior margin of the hemisphere. The anterior and posterior walls of the central sulcus are formed by the precentral and postcentral gyri, respectively.

The frontal lobe extends anteriorly from the central sulcus to the anterior tip of the hemisphere, called the frontal pole. The parietal lobe is superior to the lateral sulcus and behind the central sulcus. The temporal lobe is inferior to the lateral

sulcus. It is shaped like the thumb of a boxing glove and its most anterior part is called the temporal pole. Posteriorly, the parietal and temporal lobes become continuous with the occipital lobe. The occipital lobe is demarcated from the parietal and temporal lobes by an imaginary line between the parieto-occipital sulcus and the preoccipital notch. The occipital pole is the most posterior part of the cerebral hemisphere.

MEDIAL SURFACE

The medial surfaces of the hemispheres (Fig. 4-5) are flat and vertical and form the walls of the longitudinal fissure between the two hemispheres. The most conspicuous clefts on the medial surface are two horizontally oriented sulci, the callosal and cingulate, and the vertically oriented parieto-occipital sulcus. The callosal sulcus is dorsal to the corpus callosum, the huge mass of nerve fibers connecting the two hemispheres. The cingulate sulcus encircles the cingulate gyrus, which is dorsal to the callosal sulcus. The parieto-occipital sulcus, located a short distance posterior to the corpus callosum, separates the parietal and occipital

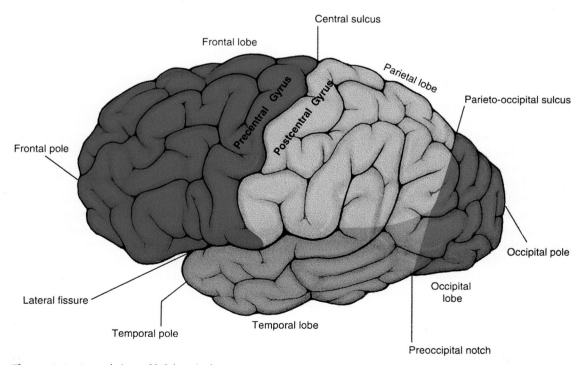

Figure 4-4 Lateral view of left hemisphere.

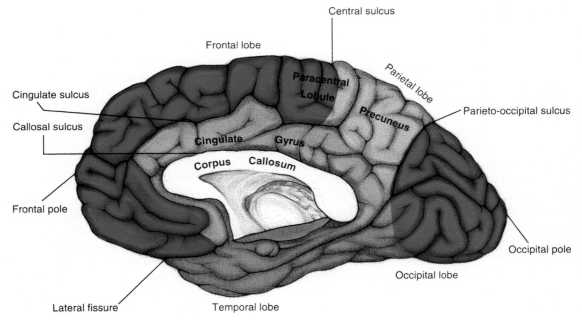

Figure 4-5   Medial view of right hemisphere.

lobes. The central sulcus reaches the medial surface of the hemisphere in the posterior part of the paracentral lobule. Between the paracentral lobule and the parieto-occipital sulcus is the precuneus.

FOREBRAIN FUNCTIONAL LEVELS

POSTERIOR THALAMIC

This level is at the posterior part of the thalamus and the underlying rostral part of the cerebral peduncle (Fig. 4-6). The level also includes parts of the cerebral hemisphere: the corpus callosum, lateral ventricles, and the caudate and lentiform nuclei. The caudate and lentiform nuclei are telencephalic nuclei.

As found in the midbrain sections, the midbrain here also comprises, from anterior to posterior, the cerebral crus, substantia nigra, and tegmentum. Dorsal to the midbrain is the thalamus. The most prominent thalamic nuclei are the round, centrally located centromedian nucleus in the internal medullary lamina and the ventral posteromedial nucleus located ventrolateral to it. The ventral posterolateral nucleus lies lateral and somewhat dorsal to the ventral posteromedial nucleus. Other thalamic nuclei at this level are

the medial dorsal, lateral posterior, and reticular nucleus, which is lateral to the external medullary lamina. In the walls of the third ventricle, medial to the dorsal parts of the thalamus, are the habenulae of the epithalamus and the medullary striae.

MAMILLARY

This level includes the diencephalon at the mamillary bodies and surrounding parts of the cerebral hemispheres (Fig. 4-7). In the midline, from ventral to dorsal, are the hypothalamic area between the mamillary bodies, the third ventricle, the interthalamic adhesion, and the corpus callosum. The walls of the third ventricle are formed by the hypothalamus ventrally and the thalamus dorsally. The thalamus extends laterally to the **internal capsule,** a huge mass of hemispheric white matter or nerve fibers. Many of these fibers are continuous with the cerebral crus. The area bounded by the hypothalamus medially, the thalamus dorsally, the internal capsule laterally, and the cerebral crus ventrally is the subthalamus. The biconvex structure dorsal to the cerebral crus is the subthalamic nucleus.

The lateral ventricle is beneath the lateral part of the corpus callosum. The caudate nucleus is found in the lateral wall of the lateral ventricle. More ventrally, lateral to the internal capsule, is

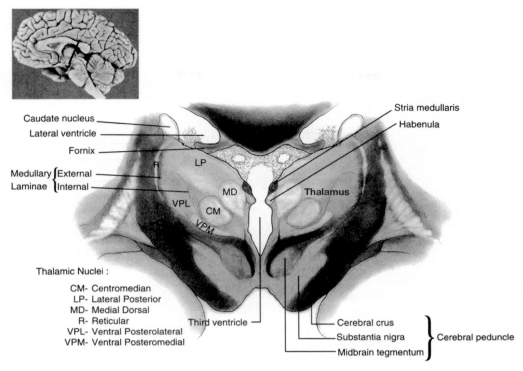

Thalamic Nuclei :

CM- Centromedian
LP- Lateral Posterior
MD- Medial Dorsal
R- Reticular
VPL- Ventral Posterolateral
VPM- Ventral Posteromedial

Figure 4-6   Coronal section at posterior thalamus. Note the overlap with the rostral cerebral peduncle.

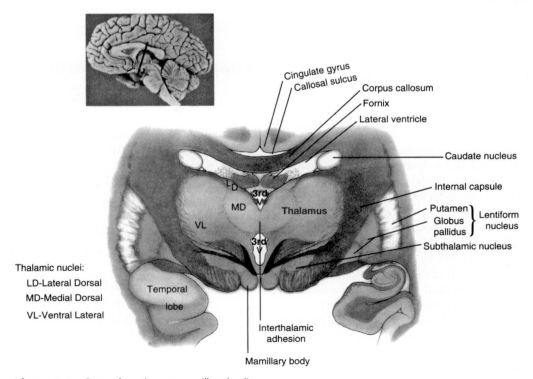

Thalamic nuclei:

LD-Lateral Dorsal
MD-Medial Dorsal
VL-Ventral Lateral

Figure 4-7   Coronal section at mamillary bodies.

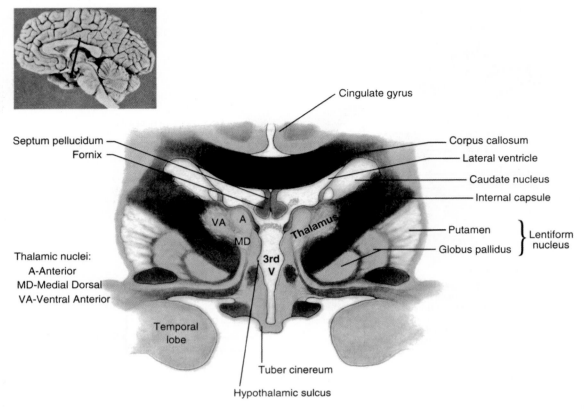

Figure 4-8   Coronal section at tuber cinereum.

the lentiform nucleus, which comprises two more medial segments, the globus pallidus, and a lateral segment—the putamen.

TUBERAL

The tuberal level is at the anterior part of the thalamus and the surrounding cerebral hemisphere (Fig. 4-8). In the midline, from ventral to dorsal, are the tuber cinereum of the hypothalamus, the third ventricle, and the corpus callosum. The fornix, a group of nerve fibers arching beneath the corpus callosum, is suspended from the corpus callosum by the septum pellucidum. The walls of the third ventricle are formed by the hypothalamus ventrally and the thalamus dorsally. Lateral to the thalamus is the internal capsule. In the angle between the internal capsule and corpus callosum is the caudate nucleus and lateral ventricle. Lateral to the internal capsule are the putamen and globus pallidus, the two nuclei that form the lentiform nucleus.

Chapter Review Questions

4-1.   How do cranial nerves differ from spinal nerves?

4-2.   Which cranial nerves attach to the forebrain, which to the midbrain, and which to the hindbrain?

4-3.   In which divisions of the brain are the various parts of the ventricular system located?

4-4.   When are the terms "anterior or ventral" and "posterior or dorsal" synonymous in regard to the CNS?

4-5.   The internal medullary lamina separates which of the following thalamic nuclei?

   a. anterior, medial, and reticular
   b. anterior, lateral, and medial
   c. anterior, medial, and ventral
   d. anterior, lateral, and midline
   e. anterior, medial, and metathalamic

4-6.   Which of the following is the correct anatomic relationship of the regions or levels of the hypothalamus?

a. chiasmatic is posterior to mamillary
b. tuberal is anterior to chiasmatic
c. infundibular is posterior to mamillary
d. mamillary is anterior to tuberal
e. none of the above

4-7.   The most uniform and prominent landmark on the lateral surface of the cerebral hemisphere is the:

a. central sulcus
b. postcentral gyrus
c. parieto-occipital sulcus
d. precentral gyrus
e. lateral fissure

4-8.   The paracentral lobule includes parts of the:

a. temporal and occipital lobes
b. frontal and parietal lobes
c. occipital and parietal lobes
d. parietal and temporal lobes
e. temporal and frontal lobes

CHAPTER 5

Lower Motor Neurons: Flaccid Paralysis

A 22-YEAR-OLD MEDICAL STUDENT awakened one morning and found the left side of his face paralyzed. The left nasolabial groove was smoothed out and his lips were drawn toward the right side. He was unable to retract the left corner of his mouth or to pucker his lips as in whistling. Frowning and raising his eyebrow on the left were impossible, and he was unable to close the left eye tightly. No other motor abnormalities and no sensory abnormalities were present.

The motor system consists of neurons and pathways whose integrated activity allows normal movements to occur. For convenience of description, this complex system is traditionally divided into five groups of neurons: lower motor, pyramidal system, basal ganglia, cerebellar, and brainstem motor centers (Fig. 5-1). All of these participate in the sequence of events that occurs when a voluntary movement is desired. The idea or desire to perform the movement occurs in association areas of the cerebral cortex. Impulses from these areas pass to the basal ganglia and cerebellum. The basal ganglia allow the desired voluntary movements and necessary postural adjustments to occur, whereas the cerebellum controls the programming for coordination of the movements. Both the basal ganglia and cerebellum exert their influences on the premotor and motor areas of the cerebral cortex. The pyramidal system, which arises from the premotor and motor areas, then carries the cortical commands to the lower motor neurons located in the brainstem and spinal cord. In turn, the lower motor neurons carry the commands to the con-

tractile units of the voluntary muscles, and the movement occurs. During the execution of the movement, muscle receptors that record stretch send information back to the lower motor neurons and to the cerebellum to fine-tune the coordination of the movement as it continues. The fine-tuning occurs via connections of the cerebellum with the motor cortex and the brainstem motor centers, both of which influence the lower motor neurons. It should be remembered that even though the five subdivisions are described separately, all participate in commanded movements and all must be intact for normal voluntary movements to occur.

THE MOTOR UNIT

Lower motor neurons are also called **alpha motor neurons.** Whether in the spinal cord or brainstem, alpha motor neurons and their axons are the only connections between the central nervous system (CNS) and skeletal muscle contraction units,

47

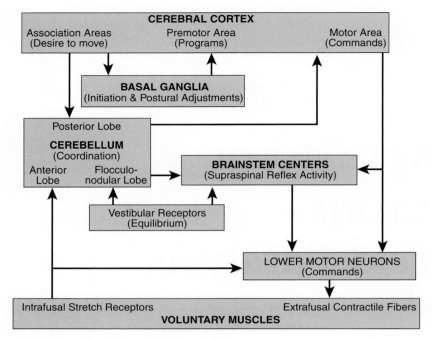

Figure 5-1 Motor system interconnections.

the **extrafusal muscle fibers.** These huge multipolar neurons are influenced by impulses from many sources. Because all CNS influences on the contraction of skeletal muscles must be mediated through these units, they are designated as the **"final common path."** Their large myelinated axons, which may be greater than 1 m in length in tall individuals, synapse as **motor endplates** (myoneural junctions) on muscle fibers. Acetylcholine is the neurotransmitter at these junctions.

The alpha motor neuron, its axon, and the extrafusal muscle fibers it innervates form the **motor unit** (Fig. 5-2). The number of muscle fibers within a motor unit varies considerably and depends on the delicacy or coarseness of the movement produced by the muscle. Thus, motor units in muscles involved in delicate movements such as the extraocular, lumbrical, or interosseus muscles include less than a dozen muscle fibers; motor units in muscles involved in coarse movements such as the biceps, gluteus maximus, or soleus muscles may contain a thousand or so muscle fibers.

In addition to alpha motor neurons, skeletal muscles are also supplied by **gamma motor neurons.** The axons of the gamma motor neurons innervate the intrafusal fibers of the **muscle spindles,** which are sensory organs that are stimulated by

lengthening or stretching the muscle. The intrafusal fibers are located at the poles of the muscle spindles. When activated by the gamma motor neurons, the intrafusal fibers increase the tension on the muscle spindle receptors, thereby decreasing the thresholds of these receptors. The gamma motor neurons play an important role in muscle tone.

BRAINSTEM LOWER MOTOR NEURONS

All cranial nerves, except the olfactory, optic, and vestibulocochlear nerves, contain axons of lower motor neurons. The cell bodies of these lower motor neurons are clumped in paired nuclei located from the level of the superior colliculus to the caudal part of the medulla (Fig. 5-3).

OCULOMOTOR NUCLEUS AND CRANIAL NERVE III

The oculomotor nucleus is located in the V-shaped ventral part of the periaqueductal gray of the midbrain at the level of the superior colliculus

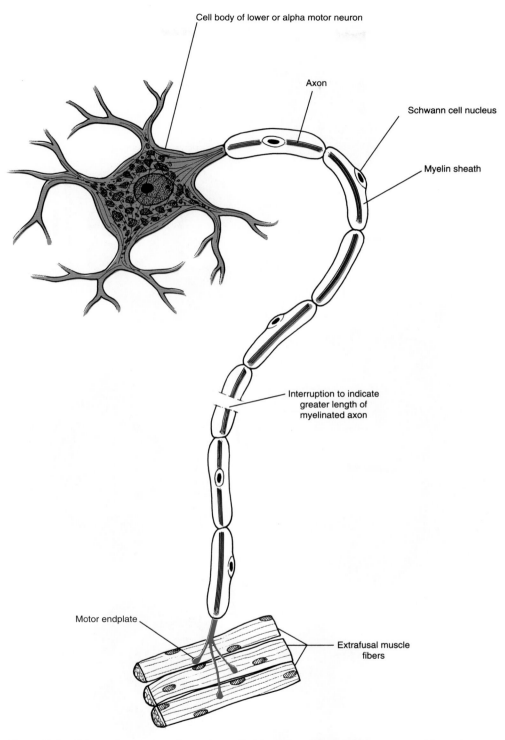

Figure 5-2   Schematic drawing of a motor unit. A lower or alpha motor neuron and the extrafusal muscle fibers it innervates. The cell body is located in the spinal cord or brainstem and its myelinated axon courses in a spinal or cranial nerve to synapse on a variable number of extrafusal muscle fibers. Figure 1-7 contains cellular details.

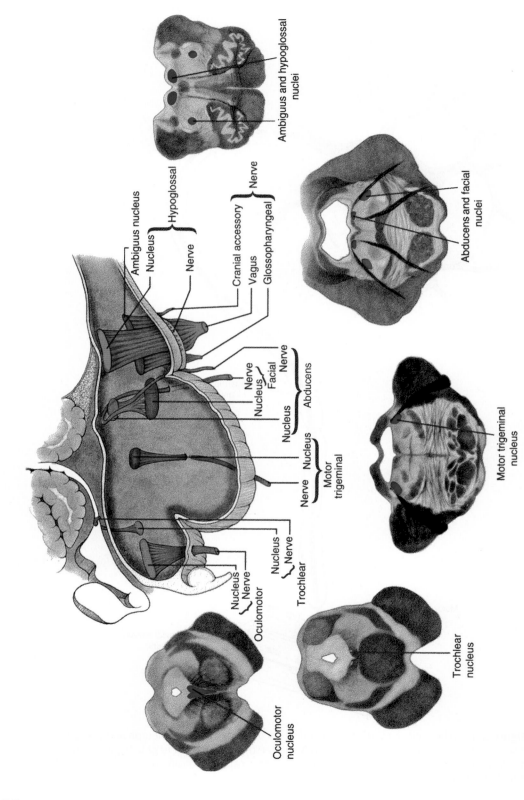

Figure 5-3 Distribution and relationships of brainstem motor nuclei.

Ambiguus nucleus

Nucleus
} Hypoglossal

Nerve

Cranial accessory

Vagus } Nerve

Glossopharyngeal

Ambiguus and hypoglossal nuclei

Abducens and facial nuclei

Nerve
Nucleus } Facial

Nucleus } Abducens

Nucleus

Nerve
Nucleus } Motor trigeminal

Motor trigeminal nucleus

Nucleus
Nerve } Oculomotor

Nucleus
Nerve } Trochlear

Oculomotor nucleus

Trochlear nucleus

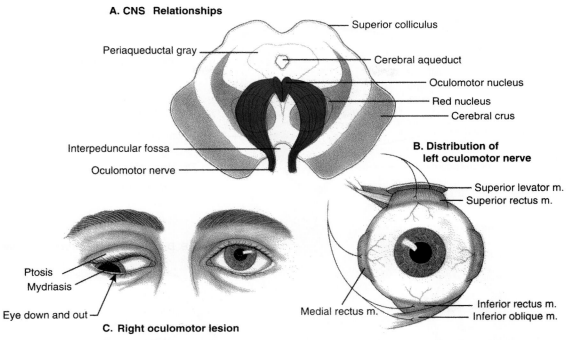

Figure 5-4   Oculomotor nucleus and nerve (cranial nerve III). **A.** Central nervous system (CNS) relationships; **B.** Distribution (m, muscle); **C.** Lesion results.

(Fig. 5-4). The oculomotor (III cranial nerve [CN]) rootlets pass ventrally and emerge in the wall of the interpeduncular fossa, just medial to the cerebral crus. The oculomotor nerve innervates five muscles: four external ocular muscles (superior, medial, and inferior rectus, and inferior oblique) and the levator of the superior eyelid.

CLINICAL CONNECTION

A lesion of the oculomotor nucleus or nerve results in ipsilateral ophthalmoplegia, in which the eye turns downward and outward, and **ptosis,** or sagging of the upper eyelid. In addition, because of the presence of the visceromotor components, an ipsilateral **mydriasis,** a dilated pupil, usually occurs, often as the initial sign of oculomotor **palsy.** Also, accommodation of the lens for near vision is lost. The affected eye is turned downward and outward because of the unopposed actions of the lateral rectus and superior oblique muscles, which are not supplied by the oculomotor nerve. The ptosis occurs because of paralysis of the levator muscle of the superior eyelid.

TROCHLEAR NUCLEUS AND CRANIAL NERVE IV

The trochlear nucleus is located at the ventral border of the periaqueductal gray of the midbrain at the level of the inferior colliculus (Fig. 5-5). The trochlear (IV CN) rootlets arch dorsally and caudally in the outer part of the periaqueductal gray to reach the most rostral part of the pons. Here, they decussate in the superior medullary velum before emerging from the dorsal surface of the brainstem immediately caudal to the inferior colliculus. The trochlear nerve innervates the superior oblique muscle of the eye. The trochlear nerve differs from all other cranial nerves in two ways: It emerges at the dorsal surface of the brainstem, and all of its fibers arise from the trochlear nucleus in the opposite side.

MOTOR TRIGEMINAL NUCLEUS AND MOTOR ROOT OF CRANIAL NERVE V

The motor trigeminal nucleus lies in the dorsolateral part of the tegmentum at the midpontine level (Fig. 5-6). Its axons emerge in the motor

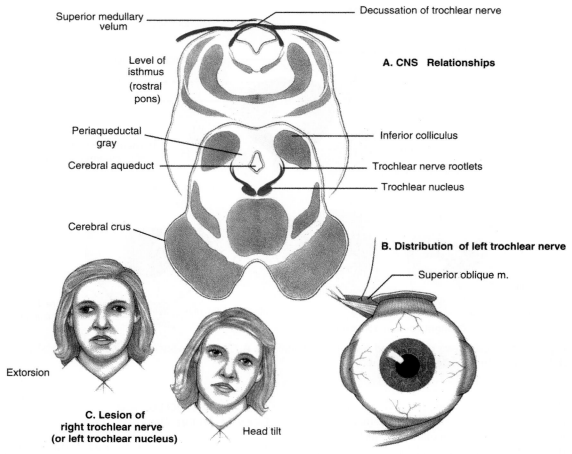

Superior medullary velum

Decussation of trochlear nerve

Level of isthmus (rostral pons)

A. CNS Relationships

Periaqueductal gray

Inferior colliculus

Cerebral aqueduct

Trochlear nerve rootlets

Trochlear nucleus

Cerebral crus

B. Distribution of left trochlear nerve

Superior oblique m.

Extorsion

C. Lesion of right trochlear nerve (or left trochlear nucleus)

Head tilt

Figure 5-5   Trochlear nucleus and nerve (cranial nerve IV). **A.** Central nervous system (CNS) relationships; **B.** Distribution (m, muscle); **C.** Lesion results.

root of the trigeminal nerve, and after entering the mandibular division they innervate mainly the muscles of mastication—the masseter, temporalis, and medial and lateral pterygoid muscles.

ABDUCENS NUCLEUS AND CRANIAL NERVE VI

The abducens nucleus is located beneath the facial colliculus in the floor of the fourth ventricle in the caudal pons (Fig. 5-7). The abducens (VI CN) rootlets pass ventrally near or through the lateral parts of the medial **lemniscus** and pyramidal tract

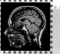

CLINICAL CONNECTION

Lesions of the trochlear nucleus are rare, but when they do happen, two abnormalities occur in the contralateral eye: a slight extorsion or outward rotation of the superior part of the globe, which is compensated for by a tilting of the head slightly downward and toward the contralateral shoulder, and a slight impairment of depression after the eye is adducted. The diplopia resulting from a trochlear palsy is most noticeable to the patient when walking down a stairway. When the trochlear nerve is damaged, these abnormalities are in the ipsilateral eye.

CLINICAL CONNECTION

A lesion of the trigeminal motor nucleus, the motor root, or the mandibular nerve results in paralysis and wasting of the ipsilateral muscles of mastication. The opened jaw may also deviate to the ipsilateral side as a result of the unopposed action of the intact contralateral lateral pterygoid muscle.

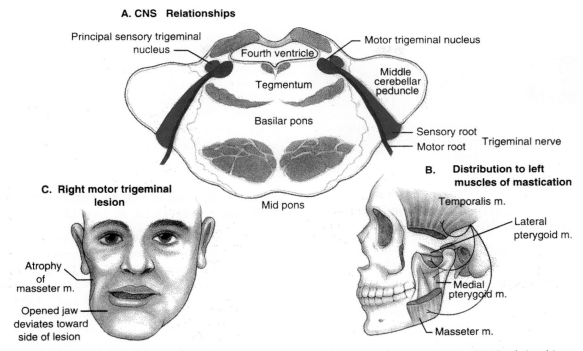

A. CNS Relationships

Principal sensory trigeminal nucleus

Fourth ventricle

Motor trigeminal nucleus

Tegmentum

Middle cerebellar peduncle

Basilar pons

Sensory root

Motor root

Trigeminal nerve

Mid pons

B.   Distribution to left muscles of mastication

Temporalis m.

Lateral pterygoid m.

Medial pterygoid m.

Masseter m.

C. Right motor trigeminal lesion

Atrophy of masseter m.

Opened jaw deviates toward side of lesion

Figure 5-6   Motor trigeminal nucleus and nerve (cranial nerve V). **A.** Central nervous system (CNS) relationships; **B.** Distribution (m, muscle); **C.** Lesion results.

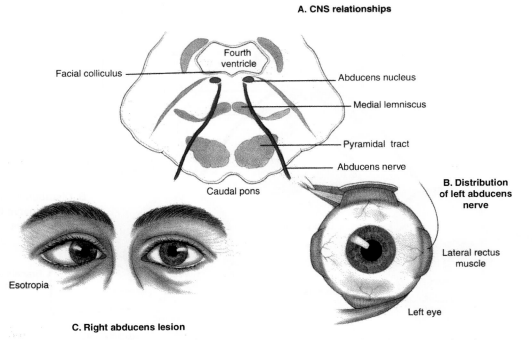

A. CNS relationships

Facial colliculus

Fourth ventricle

Abducens nucleus

Medial lemniscus

Pyramidal tract

Abducens nerve

Caudal pons

B. Distribution of left abducens nerve

Lateral rectus muscle

Left eye

Esotropia

C. Right abducens lesion

Figure 5-7   Abducens nucleus and nerve (cranial nerve VI). **A.** Central nervous system (CNS) relationships; **B.** Distribution; **C.** Lesion results.

and emerge in the ponto-medullary junction, near the pyramid. The abducens nerve innervates the lateral rectus muscle of the eye.

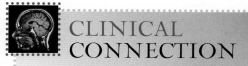

CLINICAL CONNECTION

Lesions of the abducens nucleus or nerve result in medial deviation or **esotropia** and paralysis of abduction of the ipsilateral eye.

FACIAL NUCLEUS AND MOTOR ROOT OF CRANIAL NERVE VII

The facial nucleus lies in the lateral part of the tegmentum of the caudal pons (Fig. 5-8). This motor nucleus is divided into two parts: a small part that innervates the upper facial muscles and a larger part that supplies the lower facial muscles.

The facial root fibers, on emerging from the nucleus, stream dorsomedially as individual fibers or in small groups (unobservable in myelin-stained sections) to the floor of the fourth ventricle where they form the ascending root of the facial nerve, a compact bundle directed rostrally for about 2 mm. The ascending root is located medial to the abducent nucleus, and at the rostral border of this nucleus the fibers of the ascending root arch over it as the genu of the facial nerve. The fibers then course ventrolaterally, passing lateral to the facial nucleus before emerging in the lateral part of the pontomedullary junction in the **cerebellar angle.** The facial nucleus innervates the muscles of facial expression and several other muscles, including the stapedius.

NUCLEUS AMBIGUUS AND MOTOR ROOTS OF CRANIAL NERVES IX, X, AND XI

The nucleus ambiguus is an elongated column of alpha motor neurons in the ventrolateral part of the reticular formation of the medulla (Fig. 5-9). Its axons emerge with the glossopharyngeal and vagus nerves and with the "cranial part" of the accessory nerve. The latter joins the vagus at the jugular foramen. The nucleus ambiguus supplies the skeletal muscles of the palate, pharynx, larynx, and upper esophagus; hence, it is involved in deglutition and phonation.

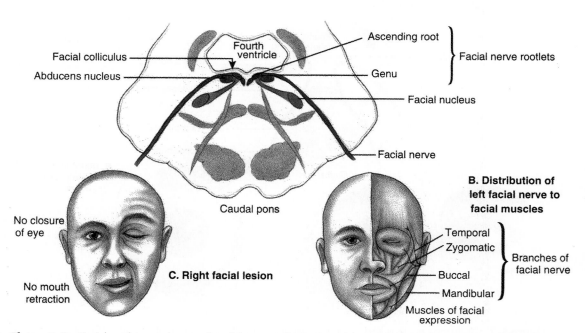

Figure 5-8   Facial nucleus and nerve (cranial nerve VII). **A.** Central nervous system (CNS) relationships; **B.** Distribution; **C.** Lesion results.

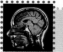

CLINICAL CONNECTION

As given in the case at the beginning of this chapter, lesions of the facial nucleus or nerve result in paralysis of the ipsilateral facial muscles, both upper and lower. The most common lesion of the facial nerve occurs in **Bell palsy,** which produces weakness of both upper and lower facial muscles and inability to close the eye tightly. In addition, lacrimation, salivation, and taste may be impaired (owing to involvement of secretory and gustatory fibers), accompanied by **hyperacusis** (abnormal loudness of hearing because of paralysis of the stapedius muscle). An inflammatory reaction of the nerve as it courses in the facial canal is the presumed cause of Bell palsy. The accompanying abnormalities depend on the location of the inflammation in the facial canal. Fortunately, most Bell palsy patients recover completely within a month or two.

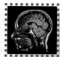

CLINICAL CONNECTION

A lesion of the rostral part of the nucleus, which gives axons to the glossopharyngeal nerve, results in **dysphagia** owing to paralysis of the stylopharyngeus muscle. A lesion of the remainder of the nucleus, which supplies axons to the vagus nerve, results in paralysis of the vocal muscles (causing hoarseness and vocal weakness). Paralysis of the palatal muscles results in sagging of the ipsilateral palatal arch and deviation of the uvula to the contralateral side. Bilateral lesions involving the vagal nerves or vagal components of the nucleus ambiguus may result in a closing of the airway severe enough to require tracheostomy.

HYPOGLOSSAL NUCLEUS AND CRANIAL NERVE XII

This elongated motor nucleus is located in the floor of the medullary part of the fourth ventricle near the midline (Fig. 5-10). The rootlets pass ventrally through the medulla and emerge at the preolivary sulcus. Along their route they lie next to or in the lateral parts of the medial lemniscus and pyramidal tract. The hypoglossal nerve supplies the ipsilateral muscles of the tongue.

SPINAL CORD LOWER MOTOR NEURONS

In the spinal cord, the lower motor neurons make up two main cell columns forming lamina IX in the

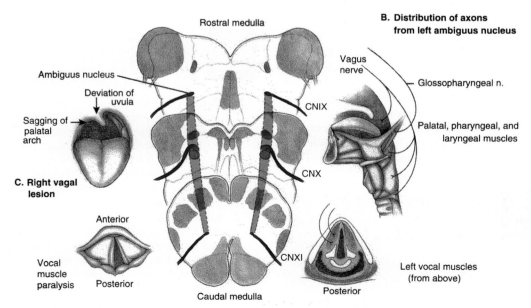

Figure 5-9 Ambiguus nucleus and glossopharyngeal (cranial nerve IX); vagus (cranial nerve X); and cranial accessory (cranial nerve XI) nerves. **A.** Central nervous system (CNS) relationships; **B.** Distribution (n, nerve); **C.** Lesion results (CN, cranial nerve).

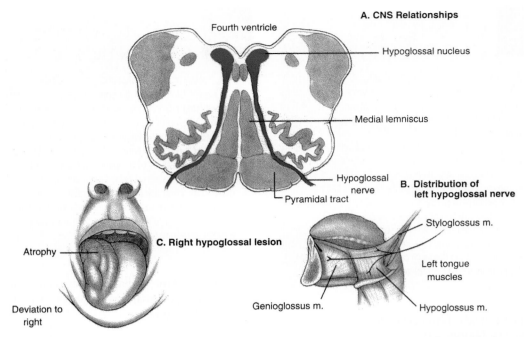

Figure 5-10   Hypoglossal nucleus and nerve (cranial nerve XII). **A.** Central nervous system (CNS) relationships; **B.** Distribution (m, muscle); **C.** Lesion results.

anterior horn. The medial column is uniform in size and, for the most part, extends through the length of the cord; it supplies the paravertebral or paraxial musculature. The lateral column varies segmentally; it is relatively small in the thoracic segments because its neurons here innervate only the intercostal and abdominal muscles. In contrast, the lateral column is extremely large in the cervical and lumbar enlargements, where it is subdivided into a number of nuclei. The more lateral nuclei of the lateral column supply the more distal muscles of the limbs, whereas the more medial nuclei supply muscles located more proximally (Fig. 5-11).

The spinal alpha motor neurons innervating any muscle (other than an intercostal muscle) are found in more than one spinal cord segment. Thus,

in addition to a medial-lateral representation of muscles in the spinal cord, a segmental representation is present as well. The muscles innervated by a single spinal cord segment form a **myotome.** The segmental innervation of some important groups of muscles is given in Table 5-1.

CLINICAL CONNECTION

Three groups of motor neurons, the spinal accessory nucleus and phrenic nucleus in the cervical region and Onuf nucleus in the sacral region, are of special interest. The spinal accessory nucleus is located in upper cervical segments 5 or 6. It gives rise to the accessory nerve, which innervates the sternomastoid and trapezius muscles. Lesions of the accessory nerve result in weakness in turning of the head to the opposite side and in shrugging the ipsilateral shoulder. The phrenic nucleus, whose axons innervate the diaphragm, is located in cervical segments 3, 4, and 5. Lesions of this nucleus, or of the descending fibers to it, result in paralysis of the ipsilateral hemidiaphragm or, if bilateral, in respiratory failure. Onuf nucleus makes up a distinct group of alpha motor neurons in sacral segments 2, 3, and 4. These neurons innervate the external urethral and anal sphincters and, hence, play a major role in continence mechanisms.

CLINICAL CONNECTION

Lesions of the hypoglossal nucleus or nerve result in a paralysis and atrophy of the ipsilateral muscles of the tongue. Moreover, when protruded, the tongue deviates toward the side of the lesion as a result of the unopposed actions of the normal genioglossus and transverse muscles on the other side.

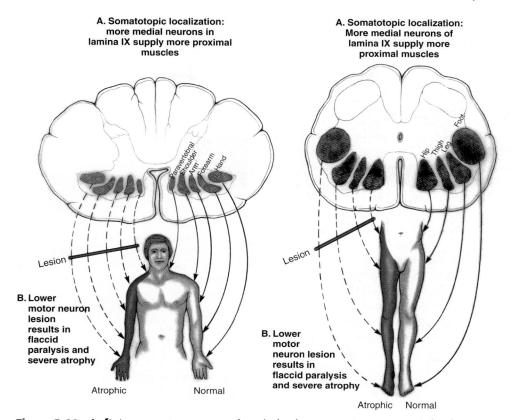

Figure 5-11   Left: Lower motor neurons of cervical enlargement. **A.** Somatotopic localization; **B.** Results of lesions. **Right:** Lower motor neurons of lumbosacral enlargement. **A.** Somatotopic localization; **B.** Results of lesions.

TABLE 5-1 Segmental Innervation of Selected Muscles	
Muscles	**Nerves**
Trapezius	C3, C4 and spinal part of XI CN
Deltoid	**C5,**[a] C6
Biceps	C5, **C6**[a]
Triceps	C6, **C7,**[a] C8
Flexor digitorum profundus	C7, **C8,**[a] T1
Thenar, hypothenar, interossei	C8, **T1**[a]
Abdominal	T6–L1
Quadriceps	L2, L3, **L4**[a]
Extensor hallucis	L4, **L5,**[a] S1
Gastrocnemius	L5, **S1,**[a] S2
Rectal sphincter	S3, S4

[a]**Provides major innervation.**

LOWER MOTOR NEURON SYNDROME

Injury to lower motor neurons interrupts the flow of impulses along the final common path and results in **flaccid paralysis,** or paralysis accompanied by hypotonia (because lower motor neurons maintain normal tone). In addition, decreased or absent superficial and deep reflexes occur (because lower motor neurons form the efferent limbs of all skeletal muscle reflexes). Spontaneous twitches or fasciculation may also take place. Finally, pronounced decrease in bulk (atrophy) occurs in the denervated muscles after weeks to months (Fig. 5-11).

The **lower motor neuron syndrome** may occur from either CNS or peripheral nervous system lesions. In the former, cell bodies or intramedullary rootlets are involved, whereas in the latter the axons within peripheral nerves are involved. Another feature of the lower motor neuron syndrome is that the paralysis and atrophy are segmental, i.e., these abnormalities are limited to the individual muscles denervated by the lesion; no other muscles are involved.

SKELETAL MUSCLE

Skeletal muscle fibers can be classified based on (1) histochemical criteria (type I, type II), (2) physiologic properties such as speed of contraction (slow twitch, fast twitch), and (3) fatigability determined by the aerobic or anaerobic metabolic pathways providing the energy needed for contraction. Type I or slow-twitch muscles respond slowly to neural activation, producing relatively small amounts of tension for a protracted period. Type I muscles use predominately oxidative or aerobic metabolic enzymatic pathways to support sustained contractions. Type I muscles are composed of relatively smaller muscle cells, each containing fewer contractile elements, therefore producing less contractile force. Type II or fast-twitch motor units can be either fatigue-resistant (type IIA) or fatigable (type IIB) depending on their metabolic ability to support sustained muscle contractions. In type II muscles metabolic enzymes are predominantly glycolytic or anaerobic. Type II muscles are relatively larger because they contain more contractile units and produce more-rapid and greater force of contraction. Muscles generally contain groups of different muscle fiber types, but one type may predominate. Histochemical analysis on muscle biopsies is used diagnostically to identify muscle diseases.

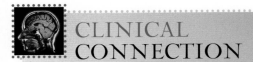

PHYSIOLOGY OF THE MOTOR UNIT

As stated previously, the lower or alpha motor neuron, its axon, and the extrafusal muscle fibers it innervates form the motor unit.

Extrafusal muscle fibers are innervated solely by alpha motor neurons, the final common path. Each motor neuron will innervate only one type of muscle fiber. The three different types of motor units are innervated by different size lower motor neurons. Smaller type I muscles are innervated by the smallest lower motor neurons, type IIB muscle fibers are innervated by intermediate-size lower motor neurons, and type IIA muscle fibers are innervated by the largest motor neurons. Background levels of firing in motor neurons are responsible for normal muscle tone. Muscle contractions above these levels are caused by activation of the motor neurons by peripheral afferents, interneurons, and descending pathways. There is a fixed order in the recruitment of lower motor neurons depending on the force and speed of the commanded muscle action. The sequence of recruitment is correlated with the electrical properties of the lower motor neurons (LMN). Neuronal activation to an excitatory synaptic input is dependent on its electrical resistance, which is inversely related to its size or surface area. Small-diameter LMN somata have greater internal electrical resistance than larger-diameter LMN cell bodies. Correspondingly, small LMNs will reach threshold levels for firing with less excitatory synaptic input than neighboring larger motor neurons. Thus, firing of the smallest LMNs first and the largest LMNs last allows sustained contraction of fatigue-resistant type I muscles fibers throughout a movement. The type II muscles will be held in reserve for superimposed, more rapid, and less sustainable contractions. Initial motor neuron recruitment is characterized by a firing frequency of about 5 to 10 Hz. As the demand for muscle contraction increases, there is an increased firing frequency in the motor neurons and a progressive increase in recruitment of larger motor neurons. Correspondingly, as the need for muscle contraction decreases, firing frequency decreases in the reverse order, and the largest motor neurons are the first to stop firing.

The complexity of neural control of movement is determined by the number of muscles required for the movement, the number and type of joints involved in the movement, and the type of movement. Muscles can only pull when contracting, and so a simple bidirectional movement at a hinge type joint (elbow, finger, and knee) requires the pairing of agonist and antagonist muscles with opposing actions, e.g., the biceps and triceps muscles to respectively flex and extend the forearm at the elbow. Conversely, ball joints (shoulder and hip), because they allow for a much greater range of motion, require the interactions between greater numbers of muscles. Complex movements involving synchronous or sequential movements over multiple joints require the greatest amount of neural control. Furthermore, rapid voluntary movements do not occur by activity in agonist muscles alone. Rather, most rapid movements involve first the overactivation of motor neurons innervating the agonist muscles followed shortly by neural activation of antagonist muscles to counteract the resultant overshoot of the movement as a result of the action of the agonist muscle(s). The lack of coordination of neural firing in agonist and antagonist muscles can be seen in disorders involving the cerebellum (Chapter 9).

PATHOPHYSIOLOGY OF THE MOTOR UNIT

Disorders of the motor unit can be caused by skeletal muscle disorders (myopathic) or motor neuron or axon dysfunction (neuropathic). Both neuropathic and myopathic diseases result in muscle weakness. Generally, distal limb weakness is suggestive of a neuropathic disorder, whereas proximal limb weakness is suggestive of a myopathic disorder. Weakness, muscle wasting (atrophy), and synchronous involuntary contractions of all muscle fibers in a motor unit (fasciculations) are indicative of motor neuron disease. Demyelinating neuropathies affecting action potential propagation and altered neurotransmission at the neuromuscular junction are described in Chapter 1. Weakness and muscle atrophy without paresthesia is indicative of a selective motor axon neuropathy.

CLINICAL CONNECTION

The best known diseases of motor neurons are amyotrophic lateral sclerosis (ALS) or Lou Gehrig disease and poliomyelitis. In ALS spontaneous and involuntary muscle twitching or fasciculation reflects abnormal compound action potential activity in the distal motor nerve, in its terminal arborization, or at the neuromuscular junction. Muscle atrophy (loss of trophic support) follows axonal degeneration. Myopathies are more commonly observed in the inherited muscular dystrophies and less commonly in acquired dermatomyositis or polymyositis.

REFLEX ACTIVITY OF SPINAL MOTONEURONS

The lower motor neurons in the spinal cord are involved in numerous reflex mechanisms, three of which are of clinical importance—the **myotatic,** the **inverse myotatic,** and the **gamma loop reflexes.**

MYOTATIC REFLEX

The myotatic reflex is the contraction of a muscle when it is stretched. The myotatic reflex, which

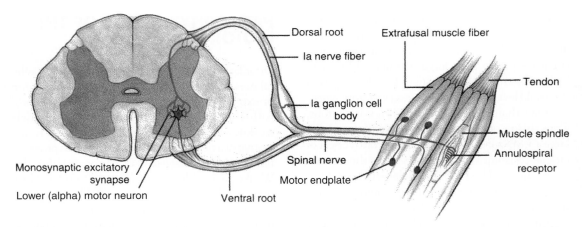

Figure 5-12   The myotatic reflex. Muscle stretch → annulospiral receptor activation → Ia impulse directly excites lower motor neuron → contraction of muscle stretched.

is also called the tendon or stretch reflex, is monosynaptic (Fig. 5-12). To initiate the reflex, the muscle is stretched by tapping either the muscle itself or its tendon with a reflex hammer. The afferent limb of the reflex consists of **Ia afferent fibers** and their **annulospiral stretch receptors** located at the center of muscle spindles. An Ia afferent fiber is the peripheral branch of the axon of a unipolar neuron in a dorsal root or spinal ganglion. The central branch of the unipolar neuron's axon has excitatory synapses on lower motor or alpha motor neurons in lamina IX of the anterior horn. The axons of the lower motor neurons enter the appropriate spinal nerves via their ventral roots and synapse in the muscle that has been stretched, thereby causing it to contract. The Ia fibers from the stretch muscle will also excite interneurons that will synaptically inhibit lower motor neurons innervating antagonist muscles. This stretch reflex–mediated excitation of some motor neurons and inhibition of others is the basis for reciprocal innervation. Rec-

iprocal innervation is important for voluntary movements in which the antagonists to the muscles contracting for the desired movement are relaxed, allowing for greater speed and efficacy of the movement. The more commonly tested myotatic reflexes and their central and peripheral components are given in Table 5-2.

INVERSE MYOTATIC REFLEX

The contraction of voluntary muscle is influenced by tendon receptors that respond to increases in tension. Such receptors are the **Golgi tendon organs,** which are the endings of nerve fibers belonging to the Ib afferent system. The **Ib afferent fibers** decrease the contraction of their own muscles by inactivation or inhibition of the alpha motor neurons that supply these muscles. This alpha motor neuron inactivation occurs through inhibitory interneurons on which the Ib afferent fibers synapse (Fig. 5-13). The inverse myotatic reflex, also called the lengthening or autogenic inhibition reflex,

TABLE 5-2 More Commonly Tested Myotatic Reflexes		
Muscle or Tendon	**Nerve**	**Crucial Spinal Segment**
Biceps	Musculocutaneous	C6
Triceps	Radial	C7
Patellar	Femoral	L4
Achilles	Tibial and sciatic	S1

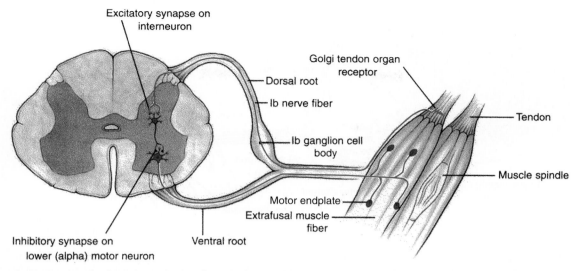

Figure 5-13   The inverse myotatic reflex: tendon tension → Golgi tendon organ activation → Ib impulse excites interneuron which, in turn, inhibits lower motor neuron → relaxation of muscle whose tendon has increased tension. Prevents tendon tear.

protects the tendon from an injury that would result from too much tension. It also plays an important role in mechanisms related to fatigue and hyperextension or hyperflexion of a joint.

THE GAMMA LOOP

In addition to the populations of large lower or alpha motor neurons in the anterior horn of the spinal cord, numerous small gamma motor neurons exist here. The axons of the gamma motor neurons, which are about one-third of the total ventral root fibers, supply the **intrafusal muscle fibers** at the poles of muscle spindles. On contracting, the intrafusal muscle fibers stretch the central parts of the muscle spindles, where the annulospiral stretch receptors are located. By regulating the stretch or tautness in the central receptor part of the muscle spindle, the gamma motor neuron can maintain the sensitivity of the muscle spindles when an entire muscle is contracting or shortening during voluntary or reflex contractions.

The gamma system of motor neurons can participate in the activation and control of movements by producing enough muscle spindle tautness to stimulate the annulospiral stretch receptors, thereby eliciting myotatic reflexes. This mechanism, referred to as the gamma loop (Fig. 5-14), can be influenced by various centers in the brain.

REFLEXES SERVE PROTECTIVE AND POSTURAL FUNCTIONS

The number of neurons interposed between the afferent sensory input and the efferent motor neuron determines the simplicity or complexity of reflexes and their modifiability. Simple reflexes like the myotatic reflex are least modifiable under normal conditions because the reflex requires only the sensory afferent and the motor efferent neuron. When interneurons are located between the afferent sensory signal and the efferent motor output, reflexes become more complex and allow for greater modulation. Reflexes can be protective, such as when the leg is withdrawn after stepping on a painful stimulus. This response is caused by reflex activation of flexor muscles on the side of the stimulus (flexion withdrawal reflex) followed by reflex contraction of extensors on the contralateral side (crossed extension reflex) to provide postural support. The speed, amplitude, and duration of these reflexes are directly correlated with the intensity of the stimulus. Breathing and the baroreceptor reflex are examples of a complex reflex. Breathing needs to be under voluntary control for activities such as speech and singing. One can consciously inhibit breathing for only a relatively short period of time before voluntary control of breathing is overridden by inspiratory and expiratory movements reflexly triggered by a sensory

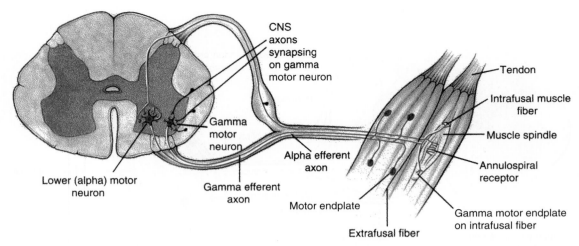

Figure 5-14 The gamma loop. Excitation of gamma motor neuron → contraction of intrafusal muscle fibers at poles of muscle spindle → stretch of annulospiral receptor. Regulates muscle spindle excitability (CNS, central nervous system).

signal of elevated peripheral arterial carbon dioxide levels. Descending motor pathways integrate the myriad of spinal reflexes that coordinate lower motor neuron activity, leading to complex coordinated movements.

Lower motor neuron excitability is affected by inhibitory Renshaw cells. Renshaw cells are excited by collaterals of lower motor neuron axons and then make inhibitory synaptic contacts with the surrounding motor neurons and Ia inhibitory interneurons. This negative feedback helps regulate the firing of lower motor neurons and reciprocal contraction of antagonist muscles.

Chapter Review Questions

5-1. Define the term "motor unit" and compare those involved in delicate and coarse movements.

5-2. Explain the chief abnormalities associated with a spinal lower motor neuron lesion.

5-3. Which skeletal muscle fiber type (I or II) would be ideal for a sustained muscle contraction?

5-4. Rapid movements with relatively greater contractile forces are accomplished generally by which skeletal muscle fiber type (I or II)?

5-5. There are three types of muscle fibers: I, IIA, and IIB. How many of these types are found in an individual motor unit?

5-6. What size lower motor neurons are most excitable?

5-7. Weakness, muscle atrophy, and fasciculations are collectively strongly suggestive of what lower motor neuron disorder?

5-8. Collaterals of lower motor neuron axons excite what interneurons that subsequently inhibit surrounding lower motor neurons?

5-9. What phenomenon results in the inhibition of motor neurons innervating antagonists on the activation of motor neurons innervating agonists?

5-10. What abnormalities result from the lesion, appearing as a cross-hatched area, in each section on page 63?

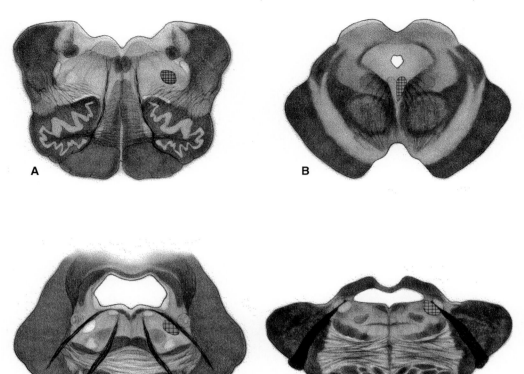

A

B

C

D

The Pyramidal System: Spastic Paralysis

A 60-YEAR-OLD HYPERTENSIVE MAN has sudden headache accompanied by spastic hemiplegia on the right side of the body. An extensor plantar response is present on the right side, tendon reflexes of the right limbs are exaggerated, and resistance to passive movements is increased. Also, the lower facial muscles on the right are weak.

The pyramidal system is composed of the upper motor neurons in the cerebral cortex. Their axons pass without interruption to lower motor neurons or their interneuronal pools for the purpose of initiating and regulating voluntary movements (especially the more skilled movements). Most pyramidal system neuronal cell bodies are located in the precentral gyrus and anterior part of the paracentral lobule.

Axons of the pyramidal system destined for the spinal motor nuclei form the pyramidal or corticospinal tract; those destined for brainstem motor nuclei form the corticobulbar (or corticonuclear) tract.

THE PYRAMIDAL OR CORTICOSPINAL TRACT

The pyramidal tract arises from upper motor neurons mostly in the primary motor cortex (MI) located in the precentral gyrus and anterior part of the paracentral lobule (Figs. 6-1, 6-2). A large number of neurons in the premotor cortex, immediately

anterior to MI, and the primary somatosensory cortex in the postcentral gyrus and posterior part of the paracentral lobule also contribute fibers. Whether the neurons in the primary somatosensory cortex should be considered "upper motor neurons" is questionable because their function is to modulate secondary sensory neurons in the spinal cord.

Those corticospinal neurons influencing the upper limb are located in the more dorsal parts of the precentral gyrus, where contralateral upper limb movements are represented. The corticospinal neurons influencing the lower limb are located in the anterior part of the paracentral lobule, where contralateral lower limb movements are represented.

After leaving the cortex, the pyramidal tract axons descend through the **corona radiata** to reach the posterior limb of the internal capsule (Figs. 6-1, 6-2). After passing through the internal capsule, the pyramidal tract enters the cerebral crus, where it is located in the middle third (Fig. 6-3). The cerebral crus is said to contain about 20 million fibers; only a minority of these, 1 to 2 million, are corticospinal fibers. Most of

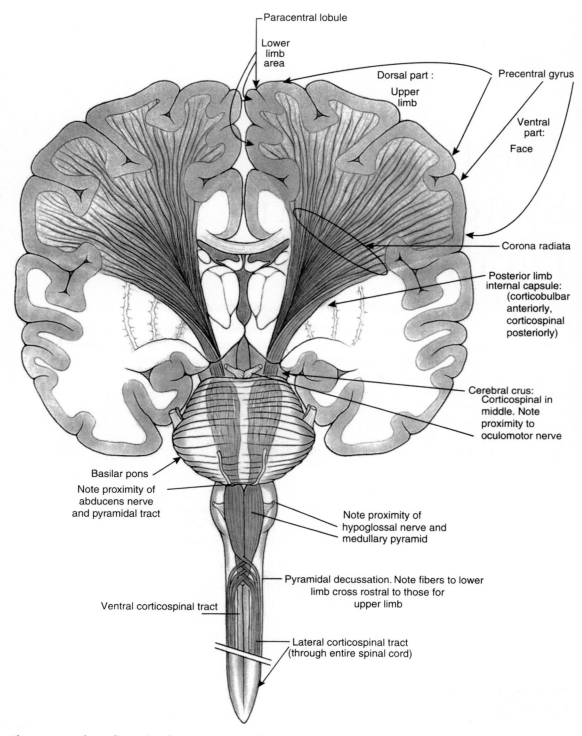

Figure 6-1 Three-dimensional anterior view of the pyramidal system, showing its origin, course, and relations.

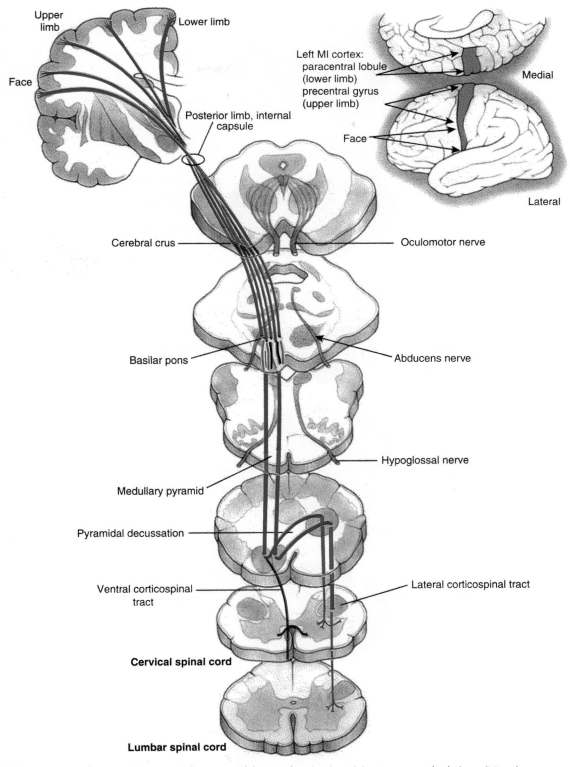

Figure 6-2   Schematic diagram of the pyramidal tract, showing its origin, course, and relations (MI, primary motor cortex).

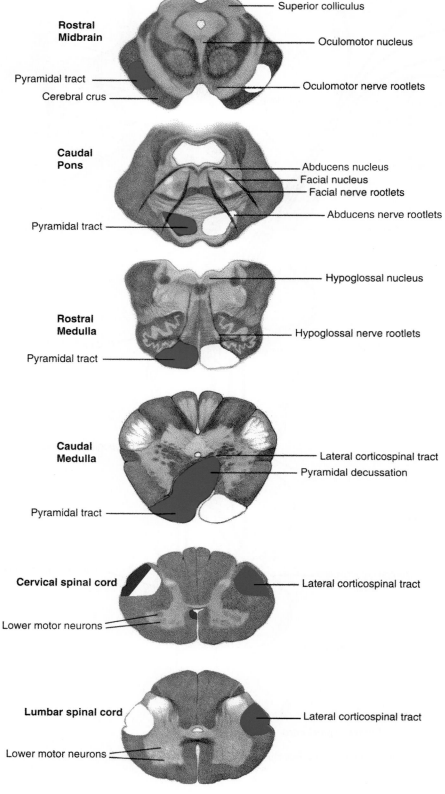

Figure 6-3   Location and relations of pyramidal tract in brainstem and spinal cord sections.

the others are corticopontine fibers that are associated with the cerebellar system.

At the caudal end of the midbrain, the pyramidal tract separates into bundles, which enter the basilar part of the pons. These bundles are separated from one another by the pontine nuclei and the transversely directed pontine fibers. As the pyramidal bundles descend through the pons, they gradually move closer together, so that on entering the medulla, they again form one bundle, the medullary pyramid (after which the pyramidal tract was named).

The pyramid extends through the rostral two thirds of the medulla. In the caudal third of the medulla, its fibers cross in the pyramidal decussation. Here, the decussating fibers (ordinarily composing about 90% of the pyramidal tract) pass dorsolaterally and form the lateral corticospinal tract, which descends through all spinal cord levels in the dorsal half of the lateral funiculus. The uncrossed pyramidal fibers continue directly into the anterior funiculus of the spinal cord as the ventral corticospinal tract (usually limited to the cervical segments). Most fibers of the ventral corticospinal tract decussate in the ventral white commissure at the level at which they terminate. They bilaterally innervate the most medial motor nuclei, which supply paraxial muscles that act in unison with each other. As far as the limbs are concerned, the corticospinal tracts are usually considered to be completely crossed.

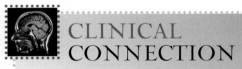

CLINICAL CONNECTION

The percentage of fibers crossing in the pyramidal decussation can vary from totally crossed to totally uncrossed, although these extremes seem to be very rare. Nevertheless, variations in the pyramidal decussation and the crossed and uncrossed components in both the lateral and the ventral corticospinal tracts may account for unusual motor abnormalities after lesions of the corticospinal tracts in the brain or spinal cord.

THE CORTICOBULBAR OR CORTICONUCLEAR TRACT

The corticobulbar tract is formed from the upper motor neurons located primarily in the ventral part of the precentral gyrus, the face region of the motor cortex. The corticobulbar tract accompanies the pyramidal tract through the corona radiata and the internal capsule (Figs. 6-1, 6-2).

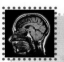

CLINICAL CONNECTION

For many years it was thought that within the internal capsule, the corticobulbar fibers are located at the **genu** whereas the corticospinal fibers are located in the adjacent part of the posterior limb. Recent evidence, based on electrical stimulation in humans and studies of autopsy specimens, suggests that both groups of fibers are located in the posterior half of the posterior limb. Actually, depending on the capsular level, both views are true. Careful dissections show that the tracts gradually shift from anterior to posterior as they descend through the capsule en route from the corona radiata to the cerebral crus. As a result, a lesion in the posterior half of the posterior limb in the dorsal part of the internal capsule does not damage the corticobulbar tract, whereas a similarly located lesion in the ventral part does damage this tract.

Below the internal capsule the corticobulbar fibers are difficult to identify. Some descend in relation to the corticospinal fibers; others descend within the tegmentum of the pons and medulla. As the corticobulbar tract passes caudally through the brainstem, it continuously gives off fibers to the various motor nuclei of the cranial nerves.

Limb movements are controlled by the contralateral cerebral cortex. However, muscles on both sides of the trunk or head that ordinarily act in unison are influenced by the motor cortex of both sides. Thus, the motor nuclei associated with mastication, deglutition, phonation, and lingual movements are influenced by corticobulbar fibers arising from both the contralateral and ipsilateral hemispheres (Fig. 6-4). As a result, unilateral lesions of the corticobulbar tract above the level of the facial nucleus are manifested by abnormalities that are most pronounced in the lower part of the face contralaterally. Because the cerebral cortex exerts a more powerful influence even on contralateral muscles that work in unison with their homologs on the opposite side, transient contralateral abnormalities may occur after acute unilateral cortical or capsular lesions. Such transient abnormalities occur especially in the case of the soft palate and tongue.

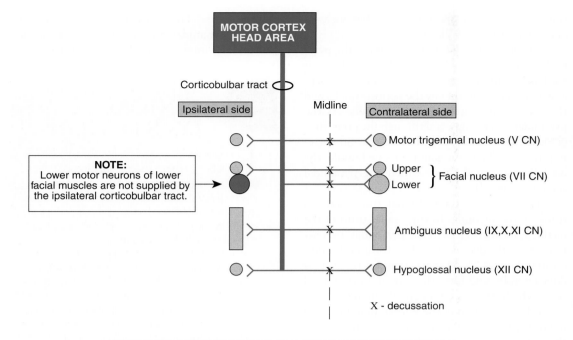

Figure 6-4   Connections of corticobulbar tract with lower motor neurons of cranial nerves (CN) V, VII, IX, X, XI, and XII.

The nuclei innervating the external ocular muscles are not under the direct influence of the cerebral cortex. Voluntary eye movements are so intricate that they are controlled by cortical centers, which influence specialized gaze centers in the brainstem (as is described later with the ocular motor system).

FUNCTION OF THE PYRAMIDAL SYSTEM

Stimulation of the primary motor cortex (MI) activates the pyramidal system, resulting in the excitation of contralateral lower motor neurons and the contraction of *individual* muscles on that side. Individuated and highly skilled movements, particularly of the distal limbs and facial musculature, are commanded solely by MI upper motor neurons by monosynaptic cortical motoneuronal connections. Other types of movements, such as walking and reaching, that involve more proximal muscles acting on multiple joints are frequently mediated by polysynaptic cortical-interneuronal-motoneuronal connections. Fewer corticospinal projections originate from upper motor neurons located in the premotor cortex. Although projections from MI and premotor areas overlap in their termination in the spinal gray matter, several functional differences exist between these two projections. Electrical stimulation of the premotor cortex requires higher stimulus intensities than MI to evoke muscle contractions. It also activates multiple muscles and not individual muscles and proximal movements involving several joints. Lesions of the premotor upper motor neurons affect neither the speed of movement nor the rate of force generated by the muscle contraction. The premotor cortex appears to be more involved with the planning of learned movements than with commanding the execution of movements.

CONTROL OF THE PRIMARY MOTOR CORTEX ACTIVITY

Upper motor neurons in MI command three components of voluntary movements: (1) the speed of movement, (2) the force of muscle contraction, and (3) the direction of movement. Impulse activity in MI upper motor neurons increases several hundred milliseconds before movement initiation, accelerates with the increased force required for the dynamic phase of the movement, and decreases somewhat during any tonic, holding phase of the movement. This activity results from three inputs to MI: (1) cortical-cortical projections from primary (SI) and secondary (SII) somatosensory cortical areas in the parietal lobe posteriorly, (2) the premotor cortex anteriorly, and (3) projections from motor nuclei in the thalamus. The somatosensory inputs provide somatotopically organized proprioceptive (muscle) and exteroceptive (cutaneous) information occurring as the result of the movement. Thus, the hand area of the SI cortex projects to the adjoining hand area of the MI cortex. The premotor cortex is subdivided into a lateral premotor area on the lateral part of the hemisphere and a supplementary motor area (SMA) where the premotor cortex continues onto the medial surface of the hemisphere. Self-initiated movement sequences are organized primarily in the SMA and transmitted to MI for execution. Movement sequences triggered by external somatosensory stimuli and visually guided movement information from the parieto-occipital cortex reach MI through the lateral premotor area. Movements are conceived in the frontal lobe anterior to the premotor cortex. The thalamic motor nuclei (1) provide direct access from the cerebellum to upper motor neurons for controlling rapidly executed highly skilled movements and (2) transmit the output of the basal ganglia to premotor cortical areas.

UPPER MOTOR NEURON SYNDROME

Lesions involving the pyramidal system, especially the pyramidal tract, are common. This is because the pyramidal tract extends through the entire brain and spinal cord, thereby making it susceptible to vascular and traumatic damage at any central nervous system (CNS) level. Moreover, the pyramidal tract contains numerous myelinated nerve fibers that make it susceptible to damage in demyelinating diseases such as multiple sclerosis (MS) and amyotrophic lateral sclerosis (ALS).

A lesion of the upper motor neuron is also called a **supranuclear lesion** because damage occurs in the pathway carrying impulses to the lower motor neuron. A lesion of lower motor neurons is called a **nuclear lesion** when the neuronal cell bodies are involved and an **infranuclear lesion** when the lower motor neuron axons are involved. The principal signs of the upper motor neuron syndrome (as given in the introductory case in this chapter) include the absence of volitional movements (paralysis), increased muscle tone, exaggerated myotatic reflexes, and an extensor plantar response—all of these in the contralateral limbs. A comparison of the upper and lower motor neuron syndromes is in Table 6-1.

CAPSULAR STROKE

The most frequent pyramidal system disorder results from a vascular accident in the internal capsule and is called "capsular stroke," as illustrated in the case at the beginning of this chapter. After interruption of the corticospinal and corticobulbar tracts in the internal capsule, there is paralysis of the contralateral upper and lower limbs and the contralateral lower facial muscles. In some cases, a transient weakness may be seen on the contralateral side of the tongue and soft palate as a result of corticobulbar tract damage.

Immediately after a capsular stroke, volitional movements in the contralateral limbs are absent. With time, movements in the more proximal parts of the limbs recover rather completely, but the recovery of movements in more distal parts is less complete. Rapid individual finger movements such as those used in playing a piano never return. The basis for this partial return of volitional movements is described in Chapter 7.

In addition to the paralysis, the patient has **hypertonia** or increased muscle tone. This is manifested by increased resistance to passive stretch and is especially pronounced in the antigravity muscles, that is, the flexors of the arm and fingers and the extensors of the leg. Severe hypertonia is **spasticity,** and this, accompanied by the loss of volitional movements contralaterally, is called

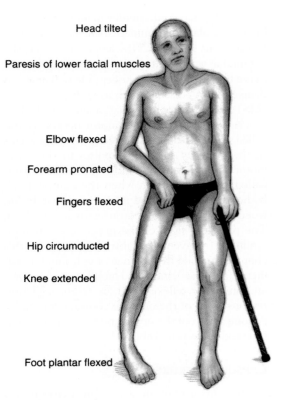

Head tilted

Paresis of lower facial muscles

Elbow flexed

Forearm pronated

Fingers flexed

Hip circumducted

Knee extended

Foot plantar flexed

Figure 6-5   Right spastic hemiplegia. Gait resulting from left capsular lesion.

spastic hemiplegia (Fig. 6-5). A characteristic of the increased resistance seen in spasticity is the **clasp-knife response** (Fig. 6-6). This response consists of a sudden collapse of all resistance while a muscle is being rapidly stretched. The clasp-knife effect is caused by increased activity of the Golgi tendon organs whose Ib afferent fibers are excitatory to spinal interneurons that inhibit the alpha motor neurons responsible for the hypertonia and increased resistance to passive stretch (Fig. 5-13).

In the upper motor neuron syndrome, the myotatic reflexes are most hyperactive or exaggerated in the antigravity muscles, for example, the biceps muscle in the upper limb and the quadriceps muscle in the lower limb. As a result, the biceps and patellar reflexes are exaggerated (Fig. 6-7). Accompanying the severe hyperactive reflexes that occur in spastic hemiplegia is **clonus,** which consists of a rapid series of rhythmic contractions that are elicited by stretching a muscle (Fig. 6-8). Clonus is caused by the hyperactive myotatic reflexes; the brisk contraction of one group of muscles is sufficient to initiate myotatic responses in their antagonists, and so forth.

The most well-known sign associated with the upper motor neuron syndrome is the **extensor plantar** or **Babinski response** (Fig. 6-9). This abnor-

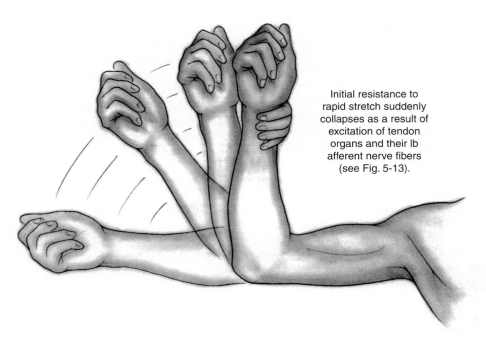

Initial resistance to rapid stretch suddenly collapses as a result of excitation of tendon organs and their Ib afferent nerve fibers (see Fig. 5-13).

Figure 6-6   The clasp-knife response.

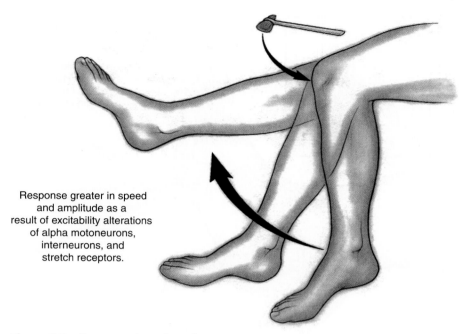

Response greater in speed and amplitude as a result of excitability alterations of alpha motoneurons, interneurons, and stretch receptors.

Figure 6-7   Exaggerated patellar reflex.

On stretching the Achilles tendon, the brisk contraction of the agonists initiates a myotatic reflex in the antagonists and so forth, resulting in repetitive contractions

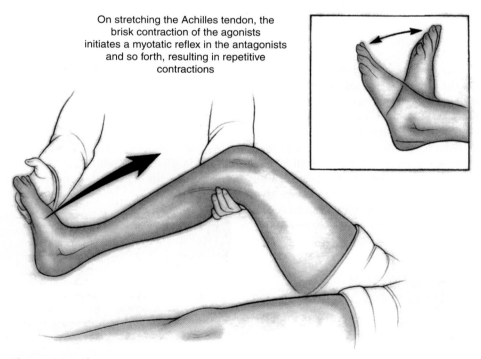

Figure 6-8   Clonus.

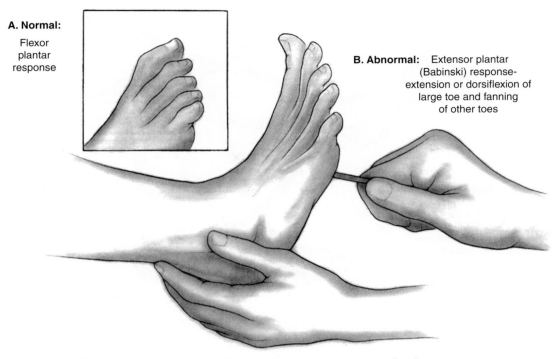

A. Normal:

Flexor plantar response

B. Abnormal: Extensor plantar (Babinski) response-extension or dorsiflexion of large toe and fanning of other toes

Figure 6-9   Plantar responses. **A.** Normal flexor. **B.** Abnormal extensor or Babinski.

mal cutaneous reflex consists of extension or dorsiflexion of the large toe and fanning of the other toes on stroking the lateral aspect of the sole of the foot with a hard, blunt instrument. When the corticospinal system is normal, this stimulus elicits flexion of all the toes—the flexor plantar response. The Babinski sign is a spinal withdrawal reflex that is normally suppressed directly by the cerebral cortex. It is seen in normal infants before the corticospinal tract is fully myelinated and functional; otherwise, it is almost invariably associated with corticospinal tract damage.

PATHOPHYSIOLOGY OF SPASTICITY

Spasticity is characterized by the increase in resistance to velocity-dependent passive stretch in the absence of voluntary movement: the more rapid the stretch, the greater the resistance. This suggests that abnormal stretch reflexes are the underlying basis for hypertonicity. A normal peripheral stimulus may provoke an abnormal response in partially

denervated lower motor neurons by three central mechanisms: (1) an increase in the intrinsic excitability of motor neurons resulting in a lower threshold for firing, (2) increased excitability of lower motor neurons to extrinsic intact descending neuromodulatory pathways, and (3) the plasticity of Ia afferents to reinnervate the synaptic sites vacated by the degenerated corticospinal axons.

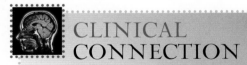

CLINICAL CONNECTION

That Ia afferents play a significant role in the cause of spasticity is suggested by two clinical observations. First, spasticity is abolished by cutting dorsal root afferents from the affected muscles, as is commonly performed as a treatment for cerebral palsy. Second, intrathecal administration to the spinal cord of the drug baclofen, an agonist to the γ-aminobutyric acid B (GABA$_B$) receptor on the terminals of Ia afferents, results in a decrease in the release of neurotransmitter by the primary afferents (presynaptic inhibition).

TABLE 6-1	Comparison of Upper and Lower Motor Neuron Syndromes		
	Upper Motor Neuron or Supranuclear Lesion	**Lower Motor Neuron or Nuclear-Infranuclear Lesion**	
Possible locations	CNS only	CNS	PNS
Common causes	CVA, tumors, trauma, demyelinating diseases (MS, ALS), infectious diseases	CVA, polio, tumor, trauma (ruptured disc, gun shot, etc.)	Trauma, metabolic disorders (alcoholism, diabetes)
Structures involved	Upper motor neurons in cerebral cortex or corticospinal and nuclear tracts	Brainstem or spinal alpha motor neurons or their intramedullary rootlets	Motor fibers in every cerebrospinal nerve except I CN, II CN, and VIII CN
Distribution of abnormalities	Never individual muscles—groups of muscles supplied by motor nuclei below level of lesion Corticonuclear—contralateral lower facial muscles Corticospinal—limb muscles—contralateral if lesion is above decussation, ipsilateral if below	Segmental—limited to muscles innervated by damaged alpha motor neurons or their axons	
Status of voluntary movements	Deficient—paralysis or paresis especially of skilled movements	Deficient—paralysis, final common pathway interrupted	
Character of passive stretch (status of muscle tone)	Increased—particularly in antigravity muscles (flexors of upper limbs, extensors of hip and knee, plantar flexors of foot and toes); clasp-knife response may be present	Decreased—loss of final common pathway produces hypotonicity in affected muscles	
Status of myotatic reflexes	Hyperactive or exaggerated—muscle spindle threshold decreased; clonus may be present	Decreased or absent—efferent limb of reflex interrupted	
Status of cutaneous reflexes	Abnormalities in some—plantar becomes extensor rather than flexor; i.e., extensor plantar or Babinski sign	Decreased or absent—plantar reflex, if present, is of normal flexor type except in infants	
Muscle bulk	Slight atrophy owing to disuse	Pronounced atrophy—70–80%	
Classical description	Spastic paralysis	Flaccid paralysis	

ALS, amyotrophic lateral sclerosis; CN, cranial nerve; CNS, central nervous system; CVA, cerebrovascular accident; MS, multiple sclerosis; PNS, peripheral nervous system.

COMBINED UPPER AND LOWER MOTOR NEURON LESIONS

Lesions that damage the pyramidal tract at certain brainstem levels may also involve the intramedullary rootlets of lower motor neurons. These lesions produce combined upper and lower motor neuron signs. The most common of these lesions involves the rootlets of cranial nerves III, VI, or XII, which in their intramedullary courses become closely related to the pyramidal tract (Figs. 6-1,

6-2, 6-3). Owing to the pyramidal tract damage, contralateral spastic hemiplegia results in all cases. Because the upper motor neuron deficit is manifested contralaterally and the cranial nerve or lower motor neuron deficit is ipsilateral, these conditions are referred to as **alternating hemiplegia** or crossed paralyses. The conditions are indicative of a brainstem lesion.

Combined upper and lower motor neuron lesions also occur in the spinal cord. In such spinal cord lesions, spasticity and the other upper motor neuron lesion phenomena occur below the level of the lesion, whereas flaccid paralysis and the other lower motor neuron lesion phenomena occur at the level of the lesion. Both the upper and lower motor neuron signs occur ipsilaterally.

CLINICAL CONNECTION

When a lesion interrupting the pyramidal tract in the cerebral crus extends medially to include the rootlets of the oculomotor nerve, the contralateral spastic hemiplegia is accompanied by ipsilateral oph-thalmoplegia with the eye turned down and out, ptosis, and mydriasis (Fig. 5-4). This combination of signs is referred to as alternating oculomotor hemiplegia, superior alternating hemiplegia or, more commonly, **Weber syndrome.** When a lesion of the pyramidal tract in the basilar pons extends laterally to include the rootlets of the abducens nerve, the contralateral spastic hemiplegia is accompanied by an ipsilateral esotropia and paralysis of abduction (Fig. 5-7). This is known as the alternating abducens hemiplegia syndrome or middle alternating hemiplegia. When a lesion of the corticospinal tract in the medullary pyramid extends laterally to include the rootlets of the hypoglossal nerve, the contralateral spastic hemiplegia is accompanied by paralysis of the ipsilateral side of the tongue (Fig. 5-10). This is called the alternating hypoglossal hemiplegia syndrome or inferior alternating hemiplegia.

CLINICAL CONNECTION

A patient whose spinal cord has been damaged on one side (hemisection) at C8 and T1 would have spasticity, extensor plantar sign, and so forth in the ipsilateral lower limb, and flaccid paralysis, atrophy, and so forth in the intrinsic muscles of the ipsilateral hand.

SPINAL LESIONS

The pyramidal tracts are frequently damaged in the spinal cord. Such injuries most often occur with fractures or dislocations of cervical or thoracic vertebrae caused by automobile accidents or similar types of impact accidents, although vascular accidents, tumors, and inflammatory diseases may also be causes.

CLINICAL CONNECTION

Dislocations and fractures occur most frequently in the lower cervical region and at the thoracolumbar junction. Such injuries usually compress the spinal cord and cause a variable amount of damage. Damage is manifested by a complete loss or a partial loss of function below the level of injury.

When a partial loss of function follows spinal cord trauma, most frequently the damage involves its central part, thus sparing the periphery. In this case, motor activity (and sensations) associated with the lower sacral segments of the spinal cord remains intact even in the acute stage of injury. This phenomenon is called **sacral sparing.**

CLINICAL CONNECTION

When sacral sparing is present, the injured person's recovery of other spinal cord functions is much more likely than when sacral sparing is absent. The anatomic basis for sacral sparing is the somatotopic localization in the long ascending and descending paths where fibers carrying impulses to or from the sacral segments are located nearer the surface of the spinal cord, whereas those carrying impulses from more rostral levels are located deeper.

When the spinal cord is completely transected, three functional abnormalities immediately occur in the parts of the body supplied by the spinal cord segments below the lesion:

1. All voluntary movements are lost, completely and permanently.
2. All sensations are lost, completely and permanently.
3. All reflexes involving the isolated spinal cord segments are temporarily abolished.

This areflexia is the result of **spinal shock,** characterized by an absence of neural activity as a result of the sudden interruption of all supraspinal control. It persists for 1 to 6 weeks; the average is about 3 weeks. After the shock stage, extensor plantar responses appear initially, followed by heightened reflex activity; eventually the limbs become spastic. Spontaneous and cutaneously provoked spasms may occur; initially these spasms are flexor, but later are both flexor and extensor in nature.

CLINICAL CONNECTION

The level of the transection is determined from the clinical picture. With complete transection at C7 or above, the upper and lower limbs are paralyzed (**quadriplegia**). If the lesion is above C5, respiration is also impaired. Transection at the level of C8 to T1 results in paralysis of the lower limbs (**paraplegia**) and weakness in both hands. Thoracic and lumbar transections also result in paraplegia. In addition to the paralysis and loss of sensations, autonomic dysfunctions occur in spinal cord injuries. In acute cervical lesions, "sympathetic shock" results in **bradycardia,** hypotension, **miosis,** and difficulties with temperature regulation (all of which persist for only a few days). The more permanent autonomic disturbances seen with complete spinal cord transection include incontinence and impotence.

Chapter Review Questions

6-1. Give the anatomic basis for the high susceptibility of injury to the pyramidal tract.

6-2. What are the chief distinctions between upper and lower motor neuron lesions affecting the facial muscles?

6-3. Monosynaptic cortical motoneuronal synapses are associated with what movements?

6-4. Upper motor neurons in MI are activated by inputs from the:
a. premotor cortex
b. primary somatosensory cortex
c. secondary somatosensory cortex
d. thalamic motor nuclei
e. all of the above

6-5. Self-initiated movement sequences originate in what cortical area before transmission to upper motor neurons in MI?

6-6. Spasticity can be ameliorated by what surgical or pharmacotherapeutic procedures?

6-7. What abnormalities result from the lesion, appearing as a cross-hatched area in each section below?

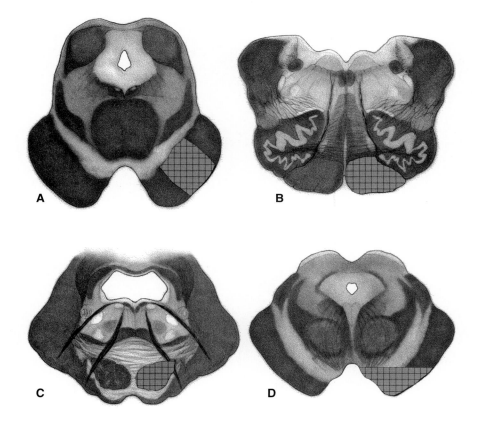

A   B

C   D

Spinal Motor Organization and Brainstem Supraspinal Paths: Postcapsular Lesion Recovery and Decerebrate Posturing

TWO COMATOSE PATIENTS respond differently to sudden startling auditory or painful stimuli. In one patient, the upper and lower limbs extend; in the other, the lower limbs extend and the upper limbs flex.

The organization of complex movements that are controlled by the spinal cord involves the activity of neurons at many levels. The spinal lower motor neurons, which are the final common paths for all voluntary movements of the head, neck, trunk, and limbs, are influenced by the pyramidal system upper motor neurons in the cerebral cortex, as well as by centers in the brainstem and in the spinal cord. These supraspinal centers in the brainstem play a major role in the abnormal posturing that occurs in comatose patients and in the partial recovery of volitional movements after lesions in the internal capsule.

SPINAL MOTOR NEURONS

The spinal alpha motor neurons innervating an individual muscle or a particular group of muscles are arranged in longitudinal columns extending for various distances in a specific part of the anterior horn. The medial cell column extends the entire length of the spinal cord and innervates the paravertebral or axial muscles. The lateral cell column, which is found at the spinal cord enlargements, innervates the muscles of the limbs. Within the lateral cell column further somatotopic organization exists: the proximal limb muscles are represented medially and the distal muscles, laterally (Figs. 5-11, 5-12, 7-1). The most distal muscles (in the fingers and toes) are represented

most dorsolaterally and are limited to the most caudal segments of the cervical and lumbosacral enlargements, respectively.

THE PROPRIOSPINAL SYSTEM OF NEURONS

All movements require the activity of lower motor neurons in more than one spinal cord segment. The number of segments involved in a movement varies. Because axial movements depend on the activity of muscles that extend for great distances along the vertebral column, the paravertebral muscles are innervated by numerous spinal nerves. In contrast, individual finger movements are controlled by the intrinsic muscles of the hand that are innervated by only spinal nerves C8 and T1.

The intersegmental activity required for any particular movement is integrated by the propriospinal system of neurons. The propriospinal

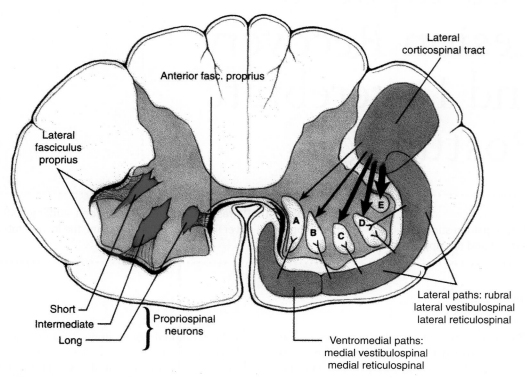

Figure 7-1 Motor organization of a spinal cord segment in the cervical enlargement (A, axial; B, shoulder; C, arm; D, forearm; E, hand; fasc, fasciculus).

system includes three groups of intraspinal neurons whose axons influence homologous areas of the spinal cord gray matter at different levels by traveling through the fasciculi proprii bordering the gray matter (Fig. 7-1):

1. The long propriospinal neurons have axons that ascend and descend in the anterior fasciculus proprius to all levels of the spinal cord. These neurons have a bilateral influence on the more medial motor neurons subserving movements of the axial muscles.

2. The intermediate propriospinal neurons have axons that extend for shorter distances in the ventral part of the lateral fasciculus proprius and influence the motor neurons that innervate the more proximal muscles of the limbs.

3. The short propriospinal neurons are limited to the cervical and lumbosacral enlargements. Their axons travel in the lateral fasciculus proprius and terminate within several segments of their origin. These propriospinal neurons influence the motor neurons that innervate the more distal muscles of the limbs.

BRAINSTEM SUPRASPINAL CENTERS AND THEIR PATHWAYS

The principal brainstem centers that influence spinal motor activity are the vestibular nuclear complex, nuclei in the reticular formation, and the red nuclei.

VESTIBULAR NUCLEI

The vestibular nuclear complex consists of four nuclei (medial, lateral, inferior, and superior) located beneath the vestibular area in the floor and wall of the fourth ventricle in the rostral medulla and caudal pons (Fig. 7-2).

Vestibular nerve fibers carrying input impulses associated with balance and equilibrium synapse in the medial, lateral, and inferior vestibular nuclei. These vestibular nuclei project to the spinal motor nuclei via the lateral and medial vestibulospinal tracts. The lateral vestibulospinal tract, which arises from the lateral vestibular nucleus, strongly facil-

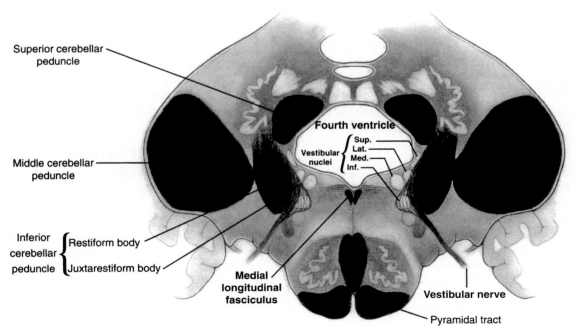

Figure 7-2 Section at the level of the pontomedullary junction showing the relations of the vestibular nerve and nuclei (inf, inferior; lat, lateral; med, medial; sup, superior).

itates the extensor muscles in the ipsilateral limbs. The medial vestibulospinal fibers arise from the medial and inferior vestibular nuclei, descend bilaterally via the **medial longitudinal fasciculus,** and influence muscles of the head, neck, trunk, and proximal parts of the limbs.

RETICULAR NUCLEI

Two regions of the reticular formation project to spinal motor neurons. From the medullary reticular formation arise lateral reticulospinal fibers, and from the pontine reticular formation arise medial reticulospinal fibers.

Although the reticular formation receives input from many sources, it appears that with respect to its role in voluntary movements, the projections from the cerebral cortex are especially important. Both the pontine and medullary groups of reticulospinal neurons are influenced directly by the cerebral cortex via corticoreticular fibers. In addition to the strong cortical input, these reticular nuclei are also influenced by the cerebellum, the vestibular nuclei, and pain fibers ascending from the spinal cord. In general, the pontine reticular neurons facilitate extensor movements and inhibit flexor movements, whereas the medullary reticular neurons inhibit the extensors and facilitate the flexors. The pontine extensor excitatory area is under inhibitory control of higher centers, whereas the medullary inhibitory area is facilitated by the higher centers.

RED NUCLEI

The red nucleus is in the tegmentum of the midbrain at the levels of the superior colliculus and pretectum. Its rostral pole overlaps with the thalamus. Input to the red nucleus comes from two main sources, the cerebral cortex and the cerebellum. Corticorubral fibers arise mainly from the motor cortex, are uncrossed, and are somatotopically organized. Some are collaterals from the corticospinal tract. Cerebellorubral fibers arise chiefly in the contralateral interposed cerebellar nucleus.

The main outputs of the red nucleus are a large rubrobulbar tract and a small, almost indistinct, rubrospinal tract. Both cross immediately after their origin and descend through the brainstem. The red nucleus facilitates flexor movements in the contralateral upper limb, directly through the small rubrospinal tract and indirectly through connections of the rubrobulbar tract with the flexor areas in the medullary reticular formation.

SPINAL CORD ARRANGEMENT OF SUPRASPINAL PATHS

The motor paths descending through the spinal cord from higher centers are divided into three groups: ventromedial, lateral, and cortical (Fig. 7-1). The ventromedial group is located in the anterior funiculus and includes the medial vestibulospinal fibers and medial reticulospinal fibers that chiefly influence the long propriospinal and lower motor neurons in the more medial parts of the anterior horn. The ventromedial group strongly influences movements of the axial muscles.

The lateral group of supraspinal paths is located in the lateral funiculus and includes the rubrospinal tract and any other axons carrying impulses from the red nucleus, as well as other fibers descending in the ventral part of the lateral funiculus (e.g., lateral reticulospinal and lateral vestibulospinal). This group synapses in the central and lateral parts of the anterior horn, strongly influencing proximal and distal muscles of the limbs.

The cortical group consists of the lateral corticospinal tract, which synapses throughout the intermediate zone and in the dorsolateral part of the anterior horn. Many of its fibers terminate directly on lower motor neurons, especially those innervating the most distal muscles of the limbs. In fact, the alpha motor neurons supplying the intrinsic muscles of the hand are not influenced by any other descending path. Thus, the location of supraspinal fibers within the white matter of the spinal cord is closely related to their areas of termination and ultimately to the muscles and movements that they influence.

CLINICAL IMPLICATIONS OF SPINAL MOTOR ORGANIZATION

Spinal cord somatotopic organization holds not only for the alpha motor neurons but also for the gamma motor neurons, the interneuronal pools, the propriospinal neurons, and the terminations of the supraspinal paths. Thus, the most medial part of the anterior horn controls the bilateral axial movements associated with posture. These movements are most strongly influenced by the supraspinal paths located in the ventromedial parts of the spinal cord, chiefly the medial vestibulospinal and reticulospinal tracts. Because postural adjustments of the vertebral column require muscular activity bilaterally and at multiple levels, intersegmental communication is necessary. This occurs through the long propriospinal neurons whose axons pass bilaterally to reach homologous regions in the anterior horn at far rostral and caudal levels. Although movements by the paravertebral muscles can be commanded by the corticospinal tracts, the influence of the cortex is relatively small and occurs only through interneurons.

Movements of proximal limb muscles are represented in the more central and ventral parts of the anterior horn. The motor neurons here are influenced most strongly by the lateral reticulospinal and vestibulospinal tracts and less strongly by the corticospinal tracts. Because these movements are chiefly unilateral and may be limited to a single limb, intersegmental connections are ipsilateral and more limited. These occur through intermediate propriospinal neurons.

Movements of more distal muscles, especially the flexors of the upper limb, are most strongly influenced by the corticospinal and rubral tracts. Intersegmental connections occur via the short propriospinal neurons.

Movements in the most distal parts of the limbs, e.g., the fingers, are under direct control of the cerebral cortex. The alpha motor neurons supplying the intrinsic muscles of the hand are located in the retrodorsolateral cell column of segments C8 and T1, and these motor neurons are innervated solely by large numbers of corticospinal fibers that synapse directly on them.

Therefore, three groups of descending paths regulate movements. The ventromedial group (medial vestibulospinal and reticulospinal tracts) has the strongest influence on the axial muscles. The lateral group (lateral vestibulospinal and reticulospinal tracts) strongly influences the proximal and distal limb muscles. The cortical group weakly reinforces the ventromedial paths for axial movements, more strongly reinforces the lateral paths for proximal and distal limb movements, and is solely responsible for the very skilled movements of the individual fingers.

POSTCAPSULAR LESION RECOVERY

The clinical relevance of the spinal motor organization and the brainstem supraspinal paths is best exemplified in the recovery of function after a pyramidal tract lesion occurs in the internal capsule. The patient readily recovers neck and trunk movements because the dependence of such movements on the pyramidal tract is very meager. The main supraspinal control of neck and trunk movements is via the ventromedial descending paths. Recovery of function occurs more slowly and less completely from the proximal to the distal parts of the limbs because of the increased influence exerted by the corticospinal tract. Nevertheless, because of the strong influences on the proximal and distal limb muscles by the lateral descending paths, some recovery does occur. It is only in the movements that are solely dependent on the corticospinal tract that no recovery occurs. Thus, rapid and independent finger movements are permanently lost.

DECEREBRATE AND DECORTICATE POSTURING

The brainstem motor nuclei and their spinal projections are of limited use in localizing focal lesions. However, their activity (or inactivity) may be used as indicators of the levels of brainstem impairment in comatose patients with brainstem compression, usually caused by herniation.

When brainstem impairment occurs between the levels of the rostral poles of the red nucleus and vestibular nuclei (rostral midbrain to midpons; Fig. 7-3), **decerebrate posturing** occurs (Fig. 7-4). In this phenomenon, as exemplified in the case at the beginning of this chapter, the upper and lower limbs extend when a comatose patient receives an appropriate stimulus (startling painful or auditory stimuli). This extensor posturing is thought to occur because of the impairment of the extensor inhibition normally exerted on the reticular formation by the cerebral cortex. As a result, the spinal extensor motoneurons are driven by extensor facilitation parts of the reticular formation, which are activated by the pathways transmitting impulses elicited by the appropriate noxious stimulus. The lateral vestibular nuclei are also intimately involved. As shown in experimental decerebrate animals, the extensor posturing is greatly reduced when the lateral vestibular nuclei are ablated.

If the impairment of brainstem activity is located more rostrally, that is, above the level of the red nucleus, **decorticate posturing** occurs (Fig. 7-4). In this case, the lower limbs extend but the upper limbs flex when the comatose patient receives an appropriate stimulus. This phenomenon is a manifestation of activity in brainstem flexor facilitation centers such as the red nucleus, which most strongly influence flexion in the upper limbs.

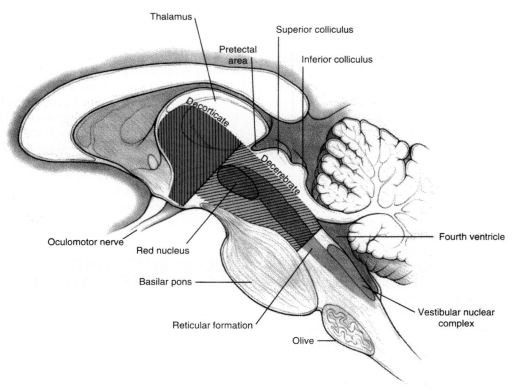

Figure 7-3 Median view of brainstem showing levels of impairment associated with abnormal posturing: rostral to red nucleus—decorticate; midbrain or rostral pons—decerebrate.

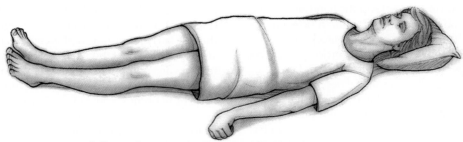

A. Decerebrate : upper and lower limbs extend

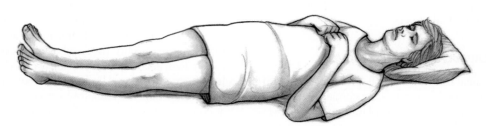

B. Decorticate : upper limbs flex, lower limbs extend

Figure 7-4 Abnormal posturing in comatose state. **A.** Decerebrate (upper and lower limbs extend). **B.** Decorticate (upper limbs flex, lower limbs extend).

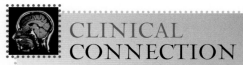

CLINICAL CONNECTION

Decorticate posturing signifies a higher or more rostral level of brainstem impairment than decerebrate posturing. Hence, in comatose patients whose condition alters from decerebrate to decorticate posturing, the prognosis is better than in those patients who pass from decorticate to decerebrate. In the former, brainstem impairment is receding from caudal to rostral levels, whereas in the latter, impairment is proceeding from rostral to caudal levels and may become life-threatening because of the vital respiratory and cardiovascular centers located in the medulla.

Chapter Review Questions

7-1.   What are the anatomic and functional relationships between the locations of spinal lower motor neurons and the brainstem supraspinal paths?

7-2.   Give an explanation for the recovery of function after a lesion of the pyramidal tract by capsular stroke.

7-3.   Locate the level of impairment in each of the comatose patients shown below.

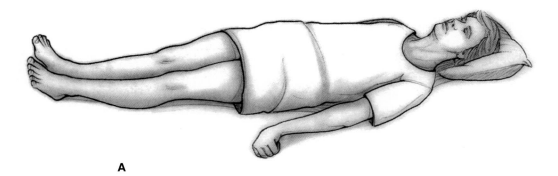

A

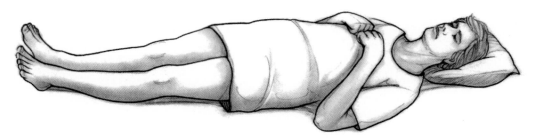

B

8

The Basal Ganglia: Dyskinesia

A 63-YEAR-OLD MAN has been bothered by the shaking of his hands and generalized body stiffness that have become progressively worse during the past 3 years. He moves slowly and deliberately, shuffling his feet as he walks. His shoulders and trunk stoop forward, and his arms hang at his sides. His face remains mask-like with no changes of expression. In both hands, a resting tremor of the pill-rolling type stops only when the patient performs a voluntary movement such as picking up a pencil. Examination reveals a generalized hypertonicity with greatly increased resistance to passive stretch in all directions. Although the patient moves his limbs infrequently, examination reveals no paralysis or sensory disturbances in any part of the body.

The term "basal ganglia" refers to the large, strongly interconnected nuclear masses deep within the cerebral hemispheres, diencephalon, and midbrain that are instrumental in the initiation of voluntary movements and the control of the postural adjustments associated with voluntary movements. Abnormalities of the basal ganglia result in movement disorders such as **Parkinson** and **Huntington diseases.** The basal ganglia are the corpus striatum (in the cerebral hemisphere), the subthalamic nucleus (in the diencephalon), and the substantia nigra (in the midbrain).

CORPUS STRIATUM

The **corpus striatum** is subdivided anatomically into the caudate and lentiform nuclei. These two large nuclear masses are deep within the cerebral hemisphere, with the comma-shaped caudate nucleus located in the wall of the lateral ventricle (Fig. 8-1). The caudate nucleus is divided into three parts: head, body, and tail. The head is the largest part and protrudes into the anterior horn of

the lateral ventricle. Posteriorly, the head tapers, and at the level of the interventricular foramen, it becomes the body. The tail of the caudate nucleus continues from the body and arches downward and forward into the temporal lobe, where it eventually becomes continuous with the amygdaloid nucleus (Fig. 8-2A).

The lentiform nucleus is wedge-shaped and consists of several segments that form the putamen and the globus pallidus (Figs. 8-2B, 8-3, 8-4). The putamen is in the most lateral position and is located between the external capsule and globus pallidus. The globus pallidus is located between the putamen and the internal capsule and is divided into lateral (outer) and medial (inner) segments.

The lentiform nucleus is separated from the thalamus by the posterior limb of the internal capsule (Figs. 8-2 through 8-5), and superiorly it is separated from the head of the caudate nucleus by the **anterior limb of the internal capsule.** Inferiorly, the putamen fuses with the caudate nucleus by thin strands of gray matter that span the anterior limb of the internal capsule (Figs. 8-2B, 8-5). In brain slices, the alternate strands of gray and

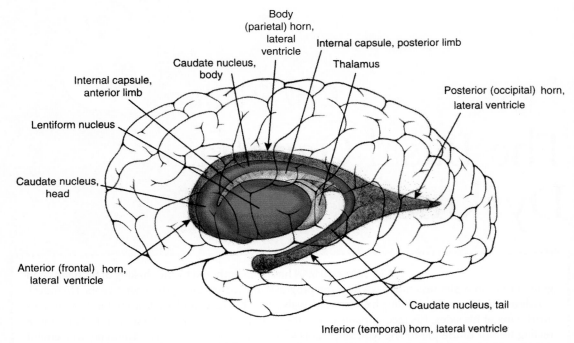

Figure 8-1   Lateral view of the position of the corpus striatum and its relations in the left cerebral hemisphere.

white matter provide the striated appearance for which the corpus striatum was named.

Because of numerous morphologic and physiologic similarities, the caudate nucleus and putamen are referred to as the striatum. The striatum is formed predominately by medium-size spiny neurons of two functional types depending on which dopaminergic receptor they have (D1 or D2) and to which segment of the pallidum they project. The globus pallidus, however, is morphologically and physiologically dissimilar from the rest of the corpus striatum. It is referred to as the pallidum. As a result, the corpus striatum consists of the caudate nucleus, the putamen, and the globus pallidus structurally, but the striatum and pallidum functionally (Fig. 8-6).

SUBTHALAMIC NUCLEUS

The subthalamic nucleus is the largest nuclear mass in the subthalamus, the wedge-shaped subdivision of the diencephalon located ventral to the thalamus and lateral to the hypothalamus. The subthalamus contains three nuclei: (1) the zona incerta dorsolaterally, (2) the prerubral field dorsomedially, and (3) the subthalamic nucleus

ventrally (Fig. 8-4). The subthalamic nucleus appears as a prominent biconvex structure nestled in the arm of the most rostral part of the cerebral crus, often referred to as the peduncular part of the internal capsule.

SUBSTANTIA NIGRA

The substantia nigra is the largest nuclear mass of the midbrain (Fig. 8-7), extending throughout its length and even overlapping with the subthalamus rostrally (Fig. 8-4). It consists of two parts: a more dorsal **compact part** and a more ventral **reticular part.** The compact part contains neurons filled with **melanin,** which accounts for the black color of the substantia nigra. The reticular part intermingles with the fiber bundles of the cerebral crus and extends more rostrally than does the compact part (Fig. 8-4). Reticular nigra neurons are morphologically, physiologically, and functionally identical to medial pallidal neurons. Indeed, the reticular nigra is actually continuous with the medial pallidum by way of strands of neurons scattered through the most rostral part of the cerebral crus and its continuation with the internal capsule (Fig. 8-4).

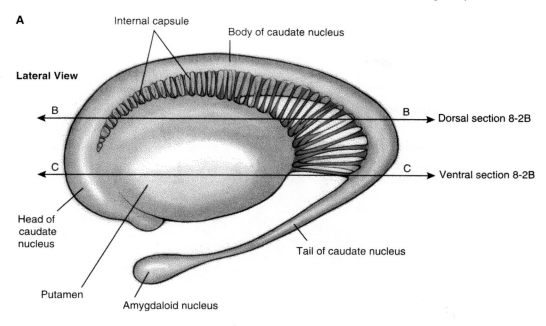

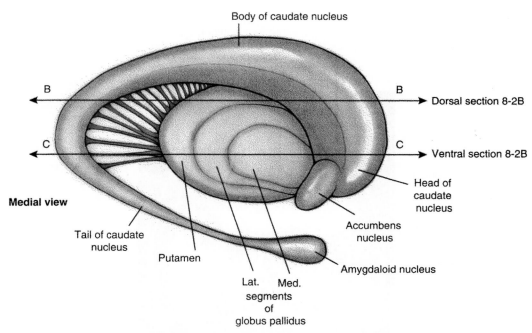

Figure 8-2   A. Left lateral and right medial views of the corpus striatum and amygdaloid nucleus. Horizontal lines B-B and C-C indicate levels of B and C. (*continued*)

B

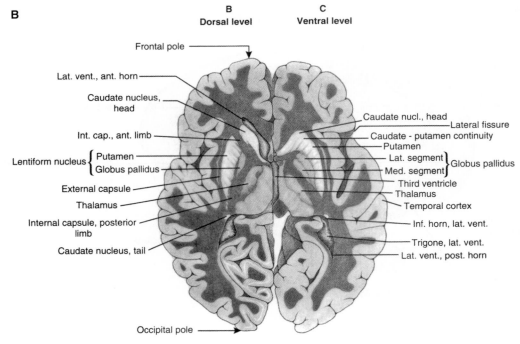

B
Dorsal level

C
Ventral level

Frontal pole

Lat. vent., ant. horn

Caudate nucleus, head

Int. cap., ant. limb

Lentiform nucleus { Putamen
Globus pallidus

External capsule

Thalamus

Internal capsule, posterior limb

Caudate nucleus, tail

Caudate nucl., head
Lateral fissure
Caudate - putamen continuity
Putamen
Lat. segment } Globus pallidus
Med. segment
Third ventricle
Thalamus
Temporal cortex
Inf. horn, lat. vent.
Trigone, lat. vent.
Lat. vent., post. horn

Occipital pole

Figure 8-2 (*Continued*)   **B.** Horizontal section through dorsal level of corpus striatum **C.** Horizontal section through ventral level of corpus striatum (ant, anterior; cap, capsule; inf, inferior; int, internal; lat, lateral; med, medial; nucl, nucleus; post, posterior; vent, ventricle).

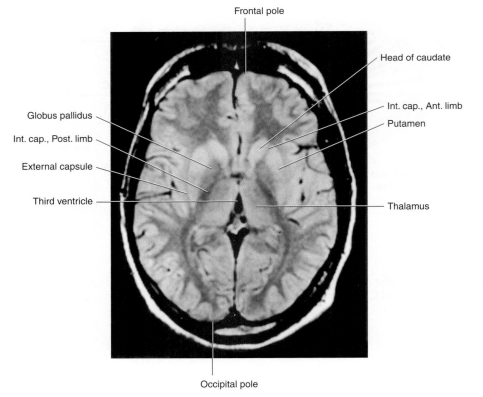

Frontal pole

Head of caudate

Int. cap., Ant. limb

Putamen

Globus pallidus

Int. cap., Post. limb

External capsule

Third ventricle

Thalamus

Occipital pole

Figure 8-3   Horizontal (axial) magnetic resonance image similar to level in Fig. 8-2C (ant, anterior; cap, capsule; int, internal; post, posterior).

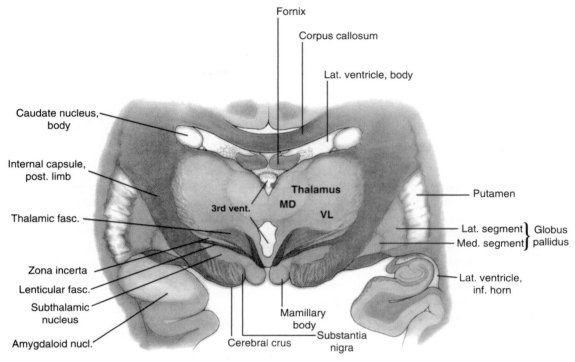

Figure 8-4 Coronal section at the level of the subthalamus and mamillary bodies (fasc, fasciculus; inf, inferior; lat, lateral; MD, mediodorsal; med, medial; nucl, nucleus; post, posterior; vent, ventricle; VL, ventral lateral).

CONNECTIONS OF THE BASAL GANGLIA

OVERVIEW

The basal ganglia link with the thalamus and cerebral cortex through a number of segregated topographically organized parallel circuits that subserve different functions. The **sensorimotor** circuit emphasized in this chapter focuses on pathways through the basal ganglia that regulate voluntary movements through thalamocortical projections to premotor, supplementary motor and primary motor areas of the cortex. The description

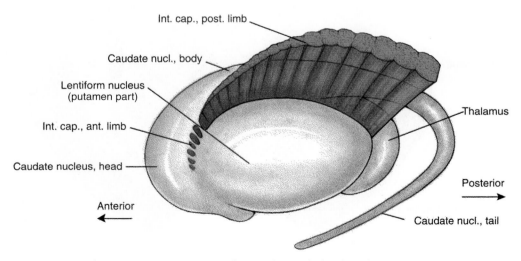

Figure 8-5 Relation of corpus striatum and internal capsule, left lateral view (ant, anterior; cap, capsule; int, internal; nucl, nucleus; post, posterior).

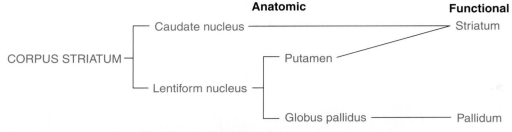

Figure 8-6 Anatomic and functional subdivisions of corpus striatum.

of parallel circuits important for eye movements and nonmotor behaviors such as mood and cognition are not included in this chapter.

The connections of the basal ganglia (Fig. 8-8A) are extremely complex and for description purposes are divided into:

1. Input from sources outside the basal ganglia;
2. Interconnections between the nuclear masses that form the basal ganglia;
3. Output from the basal ganglia to motor centers elsewhere in the brain.

INPUT

The basal ganglia receive input mainly from the cerebral cortex (Fig. 8-8A). Virtually all areas of the cerebral cortex project in an orderly manner to the striatum. These corticostriate projections reach the caudate nucleus and putamen directly from the adjacent white matter, most via the anterior limb of the internal capsule. Corticostriatal projections from motor, premotor, and somatosensory areas of the cerebral cortex project somatotopically to the putamen. A thalamic input to the striatum arises in the intralaminar nuclei. A direct cortical projection also passes from the motor and premotor areas to the subthalamic nucleus.

INTERCONNECTIONS

The most important connections between individual nuclei of the basal ganglia are:

1. Reciprocal connections between the striatum and substantia nigra;

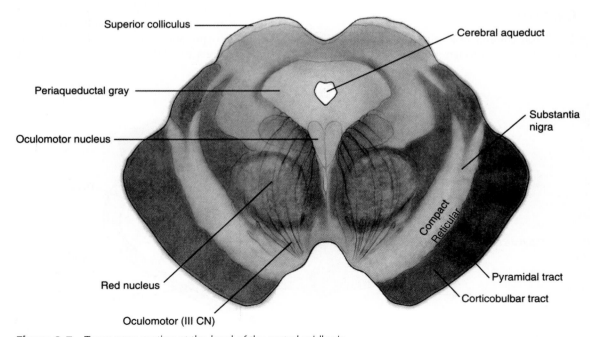

Figure 8-7 Transverse section at the level of the rostral midbrain.

A

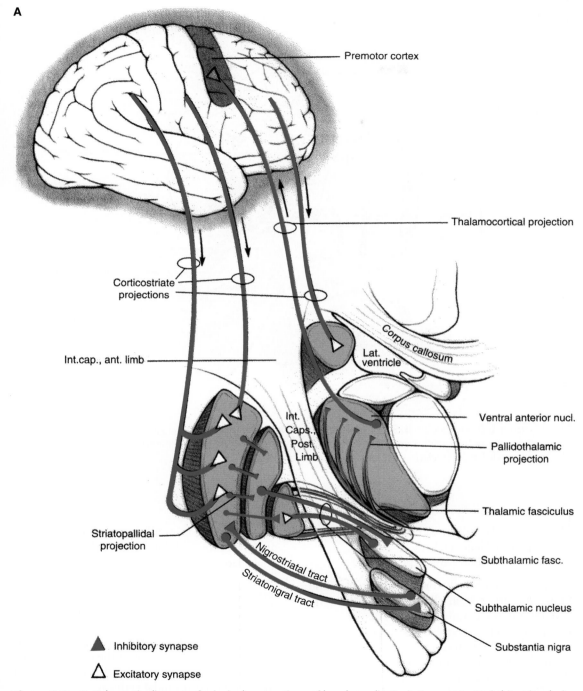

Figure 8-8   A. Schematic diagram of principal connections of basal ganglia. Excitatory synapses (white triangles); inhibitory synapses (blue triangles). (*continued*)

B

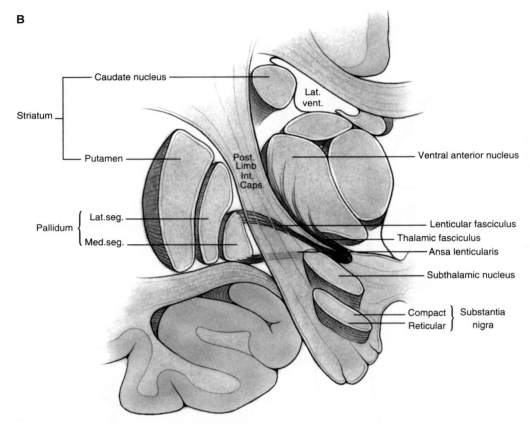

Figure 8-8 (*Continued*)   **B.** Schematic diagram of principal output of basal ganglia. Position of pallidothalamic projections (ant, anterior; caps, capsule; fasc, fasciculus; int, internal; lat, lateral; med, medial; nucl, nucleus; post, posterior; vent, ventricle).

2. Reciprocal connections between the pallidum and subthalamic nucleus;
3. A massive striatopallidal projection.

A topographically organized striatonigral projection arises from all parts of the striatum and terminates mainly in the reticular nigra. From the compact nigra arises the nigrostriatal projection, which terminates in the caudate nucleus and putamen in a manner reciprocal to the striatonigral projections.

The pallidum and subthalamic nucleus are interconnected by the subthalamic fasciculus, a small bundle that intersects with the internal capsule, where it separates these two nuclei. The pallidosubthalamic fibers arise chiefly from the lateral segment of the globus pallidus, whereas the subthalamopallidal fibers project chiefly to the medial pallidal segment (Fig. 8-8A).

Extending from all parts of the striatum to all parts of the pallidum are abundant striatopallidal fibers. Striatopallidal projections can be either direct or indirect. Medium spiny neurons with D1 receptors project to the medial pallidum, whereas striatal neurons with D2 receptors project to the lateral pallidal segment. The corticostriate and striatopallidal projections are topographically organized; hence, specific areas of the cerebral cortex influence specific parts of the globus pallidus via the corticostriatopallidal pathway.

OUTPUT

The chief output nucleus of the basal ganglia is the medial pallidum, which exerts a strong influence on the thalamus. Pallidothalamic fibers arise from the medial segment and are gathered in two bundles—the **lenticular fasciculus** and the **ansa lenticularis.** The lenticular fasciculus arises from the dorsal surface of the medial pallidum (Fig. 8-8B), passes medially initially through the posterior limb of the internal capsule, and then passes through the subthalamus where it is located between the subthalamic nucleus and zona incerta (Fig. 8-4). The ansa lenticularis arises from the ventral surface of the medial pallidum (Fig. 8-8B) and loops anterior to the internal capsule to enter the subthalamus. Both bundles join and travel in the **thalamic fasciculus** (Figs. 8-4, 8-8) chiefly to the ventral anterior nucleus. From this nucleus, the pallidal influences are carried via thalamocortical projections to the premotor area of the cerebral cortex which, in turn, projects to the motor cortex and its upper motor neurons. Thus, ultimately the basal ganglia influence movements through the pyramidal system.

In addition to these conspicuous pallidothalamic connections, there are fewer projections from the reticular nigra also directed to the thalamus.

These nigrothalamic fibers also terminate chiefly in the ventral anterior nucleus and appear to be mainly concerned with head and eye movements.

FUNCTIONAL CONSIDERATIONS

Knowledge is gradually being revealed about the physiologic influences of the various parts of the basal ganglia and also that of the principal neurotransmitters (Fig. 8-9). Cortical influences on the striatum and subthalamic nucleus are excitatory, with **glutamate** acting as the neurotransmitter. The dopaminergic nigrostriatal connection appears to have facilitatory effects on striatal neurons with D1 receptors and depressant effects on others with predominately D2 receptors. Striatal output to the reticular nigra and to the pallidum is inhibitory, with **γ-aminobutyric acid (GABA)** as the neurotransmitter. Excitatory impulses reach the subthalamic nucleus from the cerebral cortex and reach the pallidum from the subthalamic nucleus, with

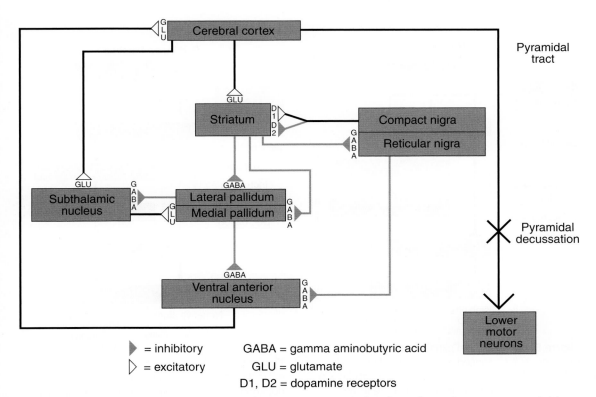

Figure 8-9 Principal physiologic circuitry and neurotransmitters in basal ganglia. Excitatory synapses (white triangles); inhibitory synapses (blue triangles).

glutamate being the neurotransmitter in both cases. The pallidum and the reticular nigra inhibit the ventral anterior thalamic nucleus, with GABA as the neurotransmitter. The ventral anterior nucleus activates the premotor cortex with glutamate as the neurotransmitter.

MOVEMENT PROGRAMS ARE ENABLED OR INHIBITED BY THE BASAL GANGLIA

Tonically active pallidothalamic and nigrothalamic projections inhibit thalamic neurons, thereby preventing activation of neurons in the cerebral cortex. This inhibition is differentially modulated by parallel activity in the direct and indirect pathways from the striatum to the medial pallidum (Fig. 8-10). Through the direct pathway, cortical excitation of striatal neurons and subsequent inhibition of medial pallidal neurons result in *disinhibition* of thalamic neurons, permitting activation of cortical neurons. Conversely, cortical activation of the indirect pathway results in striatal inhibition of lateral pallidal neurons, leading to disinhibition of subthalamic

neurons, increased activation of medial pallidal neurons, increased inhibition of thalamic neurons, and, hence, inactivation of cortical neurons.

Dopamine differentially affects the activity in the direct and indirect pathways by activation of the D1 and D2 receptors. Striatal neurons in the direct pathway have D1 receptors that facilitate activity in this circuit, whereas striatal neurons in the indirect pathway have D2 receptors that decrease activity in the circuit. The direct and indirect pathways work in parallel to regulate movements. Areas of the frontal cortex identify a desired movement program. Cortical activation of the direct pathway in due course disinhibits thalamic neurons required for specific movement program activation, thereby enabling the initiation of the desired movement by the cortex. Concurrent activation of the indirect pathway will lead to inhibition of different thalamic neurons involved in competing movement programs. In summary, the direct and indirect pathways through the basal ganglia enable the cortical initiation of desired voluntary movements by the selective disinhibition of some thalamocortical projection neurons and selective inhibition of other thalamocortical projection neurons.

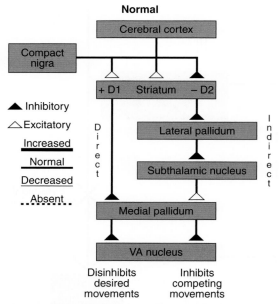

Figure 8-10   The basal ganglia control voluntary movements by balanced activity in the direct and indirect pathways to the medial pallidum, resulting in selective disinhibition of desired movements and inhibition of undesired movements in different ventral anterior (VA) neurons.

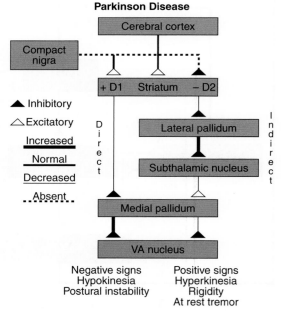

Figure 8-11   Alterations in activity in the direct and indirect pathways resulting from the loss of striatal dopamine lead to decreased ventral anterior (VA) disinhibition, resulting in hypokinesia, and decreased VA inhibition, resulting in hyperkinesia.

MANIFESTATIONS OF BASAL GANGLIA DISORDERS

The abnormalities associated with malfunctions of the basal ganglia are the result of an imbalance in activity in the direct and indirect pathways as a result of the loss of control normally exerted on the striatum by the substantia nigra or on the pallidum by the striatum and subthalamic nucleus. In primates, and particularly in humans, the cerebral cortex is the "supreme" motor center. In humans, the cerebral cortex receives the sensory input, and its association areas generate the will to move. The striatum relieves the cortex from sequencing all the specific movement programs necessary for a desired action and the concomitant suppression of conflicting movements. The striatum permits and controls movement through the chief efferent nucleus of the basal ganglia, the medial pallidum, which projects to the premotor cortex via the ventral anterior nucleus of the motor thalamus. The premotor cortex programs complex voluntary movements through connections with the motor cortex and its upper motor neurons. Honing of striatal and pallidal output occurs through reciprocal connections with the substantia nigra and the subthalamic nucleus, respectively.

Abnormalities of the basal ganglia result in **negative** and **positive signs** (Figs. 8-11 to 8-13). The negative signs are actions the patient wants to perform but cannot; the positive signs are spontaneous actions the patient does not want to perform but cannot prevent. The negative signs occur because the abnormal neurons can no longer elicit an activity. The positive signs occur because of the loss of control or the release of other parts of the motor system, thereby producing an abnormal pattern of movement.

NEGATIVE SIGNS

Negative signs of basal ganglia disease (Fig. 8-11) include **akinesia, bradykinesia,** and abnormal postural adjustments. Akinesia refers to the hesitancy in starting a movement and bradykinesia to the slowness with which the movement is executed. Neither occurs because of paresis or paralysis; these signs do not exist in basal ganglia disorders. Abnormal postural adjustments take the form of head and trunk flexion and the incapacity to make appropriate adjustments when falling or tilting, or when attempting to stand after sitting or reclining. A form of abnormal postural adjustments is seen in dystonia, in which unusual fixed postures

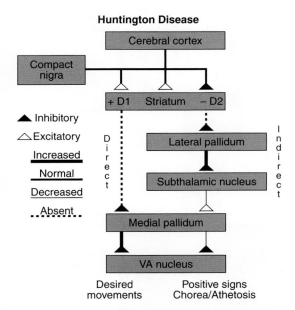

Figure 8-12 Degeneration of striatal neurons alters the balance of activity in the direct and indirect pathways, resulting in loss of ventral anterior (VA) inhibition of undesired movements being superimposed on normal desired movements.

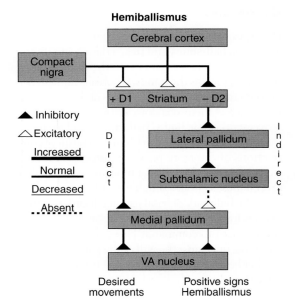

Figure 8-13 Damage to the subthalamic nucleus alters activity in the indirect pathway leading to loss of ventral anterior (VA) inhibition and undesired movements being superimposed on desired movements.

occur spontaneously. Such abnormalities occur with bilateral lesions of the globus pallidus in which the patient is unable to keep the head and trunk upright: the neck is flexed so that the chin rests on the chest, and when the patient is walking, the body bends at the waist so that the trunk is almost horizontal.

POSITIVE SIGNS

Positive signs of basal ganglia disease (Fig. 8-11) include alterations in muscle tone and various forms of **dyskinesia.** Both are manifestations of the "release" phenomena, the loss of pallidal inhibition of thalamic neurons. Alterations in muscle tone in basal ganglia disorders usually take the form of hypertonicity. In severe cases, there is **rigidity** in which the tone in all of the muscles acting on a joint is increased. In such cases, the increased resistance to passive stretch is bidirectional and occurs throughout the range of the movement. It is described as **lead-pipe rigidity.** If severe tremor is present, the resistance to passive stretch exhibits intermittent jerkiness with a ratchetlike characteristic. The frequency of the jerks corresponds to the frequency of the tremors. The hypertonicity in this case is termed **cogwheel rigidity.**

DYSKINESIAS

Dyskinesias take the form of tremors, **chorea, athetosis, ballismus,** and **tics.** Tremors are rhythmic or oscillatory movements in the distal parts of the limbs, such as the hands. Chorea is rapid, jerky movements in the more distal parts of the limbs and in the face. Athetosis is slow, writhing, or snakelike movements of the limbs. Ballismus is violent flinging movements of the entire limb as a result of contractions of the more proximal muscles. Tics are stereotypical and repetitive movements involving several muscle groups simultaneously.

The hallmark of basal ganglia disorders is that various forms of dyskinesia occur "at rest," i.e., in the absence of a command. These abnormal movements occur against the will of the patient and can neither be prevented from starting nor interrupted once they do start.

PARKINSON DISEASE

The combination of tremor, rigidity, akinesia, bradykinesia, and abnormal postural adjustments

occurs in Parkinson disease, also called **paralysis agitans,** the best-known basal ganglia disease and the disease described in the case at the beginning of this chapter. The tremor consists of rhythmic movements in the thumbs and fingers at the rate of three to six per second that resemble pill-rolling movements and diminish during voluntary movement. The rigidity is more prominent in the advanced stages of the disease. The akinesia and bradykinesia are so severe that movements are initiated and carried out very slowly; in fact, the patient appears almost paralyzed. The akinesia accompanied by the tremor was the basis of the term "paralysis agitans." Characteristically, the parkinsonian patient has a mask-like facial expression and, when attempting to walk, is stooped over (Fig. 8-14), shuffles the feet, does not swing the arms and, on gaining momentum, is unable to stop and falls if not caught. In advanced stages, handwriting becomes small and speech is reduced to a whisper.

Parkinson disease is associated with degeneration of the dopamine neurons in the substantia

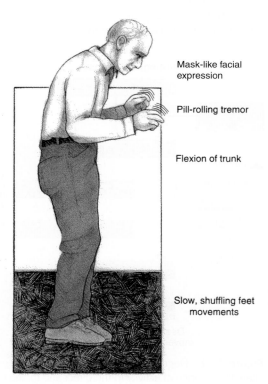

Mask-like facial expression

Pill-rolling tremor

Flexion of trunk

Slow, shuffling feet movements

Figure 8-14   Parkinson disease posture. Mask-like fascial expression, pill-rolling tremor, trunk flexed, slow-shuffling gait.

nigra. The resulting dopamine deficiency in the striatum is treated by the administration of levo-dopa (Dopar, Procter & Gamble, Norwich, NY), a dopamine precursor that can be transported through the blood-brain barrier. Surgical procedures such as bilateral ablations of the medial pallidum or, currently and more successfully, deep brain stimulation after implantation of self-stimulating electrodes into the subthalamic nuclei are being used to treat severe tremors in advanced parkinsonian patients. Both procedures interrupt the abnormal basal ganglia output that results in the severe tremors.

HUNTINGTON DISEASE

The most well-known disease associated with the striatum is Huntington chorea (Fig. 8-15). This progressive disorder is acquired by inheriting a dominant gene and is caused by degeneration of striatal neurons. Neuronal degeneration may also occur in the cerebral cortex; such patients suffer progressive dementia. Athetosis may also occur in Huntington disease. In fact, athetosis and chorea,

or intermediate forms of the two (choreoathetosis), are frequently encountered. Athetosis has been associated primarily with abnormalities in the striatum, although pathologic changes in the pallidum have also been found. The gene associated with Huntington disease has recently been identified.

LESIONS OF THE SUBTHALAMIC NUCLEUS

A contralateral hemiballismus is associated with abnormalities of the subthalamic nucleus. Such abnormalities are usually vascular in nature, and it is fortunate that these extremely violent conditions are most often of short duration. If they are long-lasting and cannot be controlled by medication, the motor parts of the thalamus (ventral anterior and ventral lateral nuclei) may be ablated cryosurgically as a last resort. This procedure was also the treatment of choice of severe Parkinson disease before the advent of levodopa. In both cases, the motor thalamus is ablated, interrupting the abnormal influence of the basal ganglia on the motor areas of the cortex.

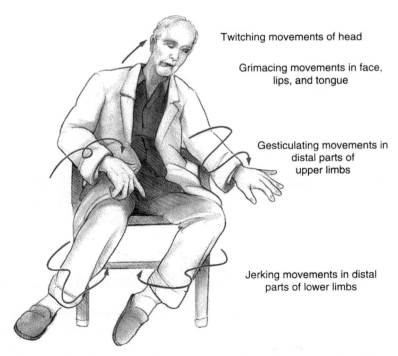

Twitching movements of head

Grimacing movements in face, lips, and tongue

Gesticulating movements in distal parts of upper limbs

Jerking movements in distal parts of lower limbs

Figure 8-15 Huntington chorea posture. Jerking of head, smacking of lips and tongue, gesticulation of distal parts of upper and lower limbs.

TARDIVE DYSKINESIA

Tardive dyskinesia is a basal ganglia disorder that involves the face, lips, and tongue and is manifested by involuntary chewing movements accompanied by smacking of the lips and tongue. It is often seen in workers exposed to manganese and in patients who have undergone long-term treatment with drugs such as chlorpromazine. This disorder is thought to result from a hypersensitivity to dopamine and its agonists.

CEREBRAL PALSY

Cerebral palsy is a nonprogressive neonatal central nervous system disorder that affects the motor system and sometimes impairs mental function. The cortical neurons giving rise to the pyramidal tract and the basal ganglia are most often involved, the cerebellum much less frequently. Hence, spasticity or dyskinesia is seen commonly, and **ataxia** is found only occasionally. Lesions may be found in the cerebral cortex, hemispheric white matter, striatum, and thalamus and rarely in the cerebellar cortex or white matter. According to the National Institute of Neurological Disorders and Stroke, congenital cerebral palsy is present at birth and can be attributed to infections during pregnancy, Rh incompatibility leading to jaundice, or severe oxygen shortage or trauma to the head during labor and delivery. Birth complications including asphyxia are estimated to account for about 6% of congenital cerebral palsy cases. About 10 to 20% of cerebral palsy children acquire the disorder after birth as a result of brain damage after infections, such as meningitis or encephalitis, or head injury, most often from a motor vehicle accident, a fall, or child abuse.

HYPERKINESIA AND SUBTHALAMIC NUCLEUS

The **hyperkinetic disorders** exemplified by chorea, athetosis, ballismus, and tics appear to result from impairment of the strong excitatory influence exerted by the subthalamic nucleus on the medial pallidum (Figs. 8-11 to 8-13). This impairment may occur because of damage to the nucleus itself, as seen in ballismus. More commonly, however, it occurs because of decreased activity in the indirect pathway from the striatum to the lateral pallidum which, in turn, inhibits the subthalamic nucleus. In both cases, the ultimate effect is a decrease in the inhibition exerted on the motor thalamus by the medial pallidum. Hence, the connections between the motor thalamus and the motor areas of the cortex are hyperactive.

HYPOKINESIA AND DOPAMINE

In Parkinson disease, the akinesia, bradykinesia, and impaired postural reflexes, sometimes referred to as **hypokinetic disorders,** result from decreased dopamine in the striatum (Fig. 8-11). This deficiency apparently causes increased activity of striatal inhibitory connections to the inhibitory pallidosubthalamic circuit, and decreased activity of striatal inhibition of the pallidal and perhaps nigral projections to the motor thalamus. In both cases, the ultimate effect is increased inhibition of the motor thalamus. Hence, the connections between the motor thalamus and motor areas of the cortex are underactive. Because decreased dopamine in the striatum results in decreased activity of other striatal inhibitory neurons, the hyperkinetic disorder of rigidity also occurs in Parkinson disease.

COGNITION

In addition to their well-known roles in the initiation and control of voluntary movements, parts of the basal ganglia appear to be intimately involved in the cognitive aspects of behavior. The two components of the striatum may subserve different functions. It appears that the putamen may be more associated with motor activity, whereas the caudate nucleus may be associated with cognitive functions. Although both exert their influence through the pallidum mainly to the ventral anterior nucleus, those parts of the ventral anterior nucleus that project to the premotor cortex are influenced by the putamen. However, those parts of the ventral anterior nucleus and other thalamic nuclei that project to the prefrontal cortex appear to be influenced by the caudate nucleus. Therefore, the striatum likely receives input from all parts of the cerebral cortex, thereby accessing what is going on and programming what needs to be done next.

Chapter Review Questions

8-1. What are the anatomic and functional subdivisions of the corpus striatum?

8-2. Medium spiny neurons in the striatum are distinguished functionally by what type of receptors?

8-3. What is the chief input to the basal ganglia?

8-4. What characterizes the physiologic effects of activation of the direct pathway on thalamic ventral anterior neurons?

8-5. Activation of the indirect pathway is responsible for what component of intended movements?

8-6. Output of the basal ganglia indirectly regulates activity of upper motor neurons in the primary motor cortex chiefly through what connections?

8-7. Lead-pipe rigidity is characterized by:

 a. co-contraction of agonist and antagonist muscles

 b. selective activation of antigravity muscle groups

 c. increased excitability of gamma motor neurons

 d. selective activation of brainstem motor centers

 e. all of the above

8-8. What are the cardinal manifestations of basal ganglia disorders?

8-9. Movement disorders resulting from pathology in the basal ganglia are manifested chiefly by what motor command pathway?

8-10. What structures are involved and what abnormalities result from the lesion or lesions in each section below?

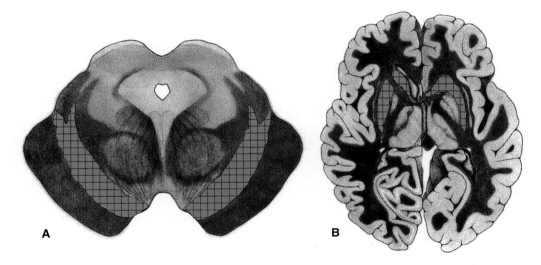

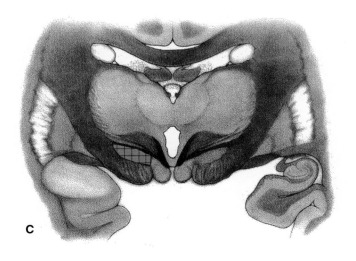

CHAPTER 9

The Cerebellum: Ataxia

A 56-YEAR-OLD WOMAN, who was a heavy cigarette smoker for 35 years, is experiencing difficulties in walking and in using her right arm. Both symptoms became progressively worse during a period of 4 months. Examination shows an intention tremor and dysmetria in her right upper and lower limbs while she performs the finger-to-nose and heel-to-shin tests. In addition, she has difficulty with heel-to-toe walking and tends to veer toward the right. She is unable to supinate and pronate her right arm repetitively even for a short time.

The cerebellum is the large, bilaterally symmetric "little brain" in the posterior cranial fossa. Through its afferent and efferent connections, the cerebellum influences the timing and force of contractions of voluntary muscles that result in smooth, coordinated movements.

Three is the key number associated with the cerebellum. The cerebellum is divided sagittally into three areas and horizontally into three lobes. The cerebellum is connected to the brainstem by three pairs of peduncles, its cortex is composed of three layers, its output occurs through three nuclei, and three cerebellar syndromes can be identified.

ANATOMIC SUBDIVISIONS

The surface of the cerebellum is thrown into numerous parallel folds, the folia, oriented in the transverse plane, i.e., in an ear-to-ear direction. Folia sharing a common stem of white matter form a lobule. Ten lobules form the cerebellar cortex. In the sagittal plane, the cerebellum consists of a median part, the **vermis,** and lateral expansions of the vermis, the hemispheres (Fig. 9-1). Each hemisphere is divided into paravermal or intermediate and lateral parts. The lateral hemisphere is largest in the posterior lobe.

In the transverse plane, two major fissures separate the lobules into the three lobes of the cerebellum (Fig. 9-1). Each lobe is named anatomically, phylogenetically, and functionally (Fig. 9-2). The small **flocculonodular lobe** is most inferior and lies posterior to the posterolateral fissure. The flocculonodular lobe is phylogenetically the most ancient part of the cerebellum, and it receives its major input from the vestibular apparatus; hence, it is referred to as the **archicerebellum** or the **vestibulocerebellum.** The **anterior lobe** is most superior and lies anterior to the primary fissure. It appeared somewhat later in evolution than the vestibulocerebellum, and its main input is from the limbs via their spinal connections; hence, the anterior lobe is called the **paleocerebellum** or the **spinocerebellum.** Between the posterolateral and primary fissures is the largest part of the cerebellum, the **posterior lobe.** It is the newest part and has very strong connections with the cerebral cortex; hence, it is called the **neocerebellum** or the **cerebrocerebellum.**

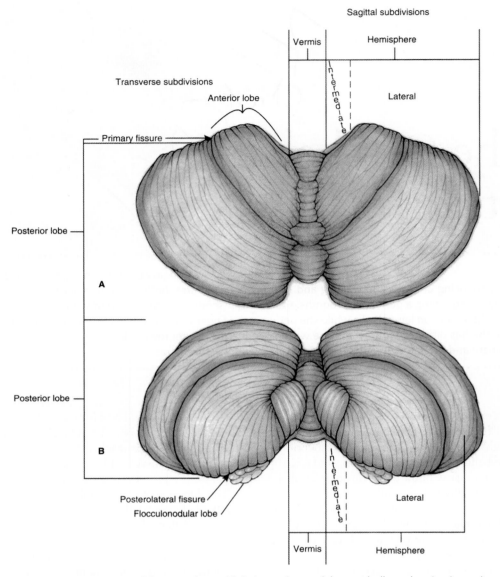

Figure 9-1   Drawings of the superior and inferior surfaces of the cerebellum showing its sagittal and transverse subdivisions. **A.** Superior surface; **B.** Inferior surface.

Anatomic	Phylogenetic	Functional
Anterior lobe	Paleocerebellum	Spinal cerebellum
Primary fissure		
Posterior lobe	Neocerebellum	Cerebral cerebellum
Posterolateral fissure		
Flocculonodular lobe	Archicerebellum	Vestibular cerebellum

Figure 9-2   Anatomic, phylogenetic, and functional subdivisions of the cerebellum.

CEREBELLAR PEDUNCLES

Three pairs of cerebellar peduncles, containing input and output fibers, connect the cerebellum and brainstem (Figs. 9-3, 9-4). The **inferior cerebellar peduncle** arches dorsally from the dorsolateral surface of the medulla. Its composition is chiefly input fibers, although it does contain some output fibers. It consists of a large lateral part, the restiform body, and a small medial part, the juxtarestiform body.

The **middle cerebellar peduncle,** or brachium pontis, is the largest peduncle and connects the basilar part of the pons to the cerebellum. Its fibers are entirely input.

The **superior cerebellar peduncle,** or brachium conjunctivum, connects the cerebellum to the midbrain. Although it contains a limited number of input fibers, its most abundant and most important components are output fibers.

CEREBELLAR CORTEX

HISTOLOGY

The cytoarchitecture of the cerebellar cortex is of uniform structure throughout. Each **folium** is composed of an internal part consisting of white matter, and an external part that forms the cortical gray matter (Fig. 9-5). The cortex has three layers, which from external to internal are:

1. The **molecular layer,** characterized by few neurons;
2. The **Purkinje cell layer,** a single row of huge neurons unique to the cerebellum;
3. The **granular layer,** composed of numerous densely packed, small **granule cells.**

The molecular layer contains chiefly the massive dendritic trees of the **Purkinje neurons** interspersed with stellate and basket neurons and a profusion of axons oriented parallel to the surface of the cerebellum. The **stellate neurons** are found in the superficial part of the molecular layer, the **basket cells** in the deep part. In addition to myriad granule cells in the internal cortical layer, the cell bodies of the **Golgi neurons** are also located here.

The cerebellar cortex receives information from many parts of the nervous system, both central and peripheral. Hence, the cerebellum has numerous afferent connections; in fact, it is said to have 40 times as many afferent fibers as efferent. The cerebellar cortex is dissimilar to the

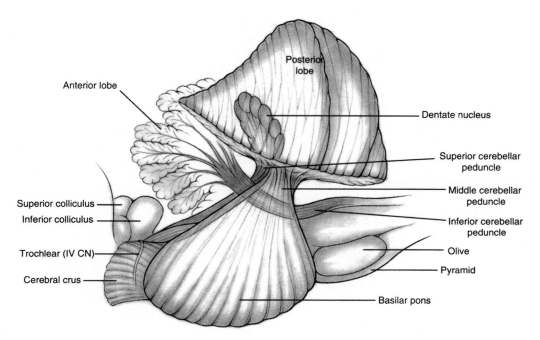

Figure 9-3 Three-dimensional drawing of the relation of cerebellar peduncles (left lateral view of dissected specimen; CN, cranial nerve).

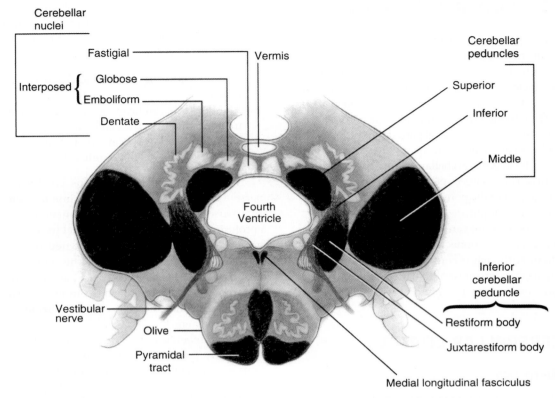

Figure 9-4   Relation of cerebellar peduncles in transverse section at pontomedullary junction.

cerebral cortex in many ways, the most important of which are:

1. None of its activity contributes directly to consciousness.
2. Its hemispheres possess ipsilateral representation of the body parts, whereas the motor areas of the cerebral hemispheres possess contralateral representation.

CIRCUITRY OF THE CEREBELLAR CORTEX

There are two major types of input fibers to the cerebellar cortex: climbing and mossy. The **climbing fibers** arise from the olivocerebellar afferents from the inferior olivary nucleus. The inferior olivary complex consists of the large convoluted principal or main nucleus (Fig. 9-4) and two accessory nuclei, the dorsal and medial.

The massive olivocerebellar projections pass medially, decussate, sweep through the opposite inferior olivary nucleus and medullary tegmentum, and enter the cerebellum through the infe-

rior cerebellar peduncle. The **mossy fibers** arise from all of the other cerebellar afferent fibers, which are described later in this chapter.

On entering the cerebellar cortex, the climbing fibers pass through the granule cell and Purkinje cell layers, and a single olivocerebellar axon will climb onto the larger dendritic branches of a Purkinje cell (Fig. 9-5) where it makes multiple excitatory glutamatergic synapses. Climbing fiber activation of Purkinje cells is so powerful that when an olivocerebellar axon fires it always evokes in the Purkinje cell an atypical action potential called a **complex spike** (Fig. 9-6). This complex spike is characterized by an initial spike followed by a voltage-gated calcium conductance, resulting in a prolonged depolarization on which are superimposed secondary smaller amplitude spikes.

Unlike the climbing fibers, mossy fibers branch repeatedly in the cerebellar white matter and even after entering the granule cell layer. Each mossy fiber has as many as 50 terminals called **rosettes,** which are large and lobulated, synapse with dendrites of about 20 granule cells, and are also in con-

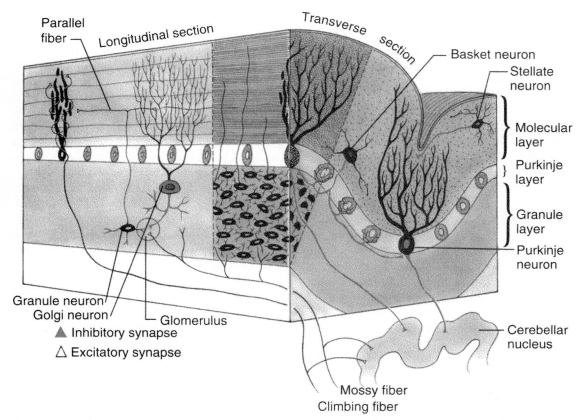

Figure 9-5 Functional histology of cerebellar cortex in a folium sectioned in the transverse and longitudinal planes. Blue synapses inhibitory; white synapses excitatory.

tact with axons of Golgi neurons. Surrounded by a glial cell layer this entire mass is called a **glomerulus.** Mossy fibers are glutamatergic and excite granule cells.

The granule cells give rise to axons that enter the molecular layer and bifurcate, forming the parallel fibers. These parallel fibers synapse on spines on the Purkinje cell dendrites, as well as the dendrites of the stellate, basket, and Golgi neurons. As a parallel fiber courses orthogonally through the Purkinje cell dendritic trees, it will synapse only once on each Purkinje cell. Many parallel fibers firing synchronously are necessary to activate a Purkinje cell and evoke a typical action potential called a **simple spike** (Fig. 9-6).

Granule cells are the *only* excitatory neurons in the cerebellar cortex, and are glutamatergic. All other cortical neurons are γ-aminobutyric acid (GABA)-ergic and inhibitory. The stellate and basket neurons inhibit the Purkinje neurons, and the Golgi neurons inhibit the granule cells. The Purkinje neurons, the sole output neurons of the

cerebellar cortex, inhibit the neurons in the cerebellar nuclei, which give rise to the output fibers of the cerebellum. Because the neurons of the cerebellar nuclei are excited by collateral branches of the climbing and mossy fibers, the output of the cerebellar nuclei is regulated and fine-tuned by cortical inhibitory impulses from the Purkinje neurons.

NEURONAL ACTIVITY IN THE CEREBELLAR CORTEX

Purkinje cells are the only output neurons in the cortex and their complex and simple spike activities have been recorded during movements (Fig. 9-6). In the resting state, complex spike activity is very low (1 to 3 Hz) and random, whereas simple spike activity is relatively high (50 Hz). Simple spike activity increases on sensory input and during movements, thereby encoding the degree and extent of the peripheral stimulus or movement parameters. In contrast, the low firing frequency of complex spikes cannot transmit significant information about

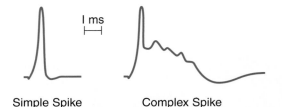

Simple Spike   Complex Spike

Figure 9-6 Simple spike evoked in a Purkinje cell after mossy fiber activation of granule cells and resultant parallel fiber excitation of the neuron. Complex spike recorded in Purkinje neurons in response to activation of olivocerebellar climbing fiber afferents.

sensory stimuli or movements. Olivocerebellar evoked complex spikes can affect Purkinje cell simple spike activity to parallel fiber input. The inferior olive and olivocerebellar afferents appear to signal errors in movements, and complex spikes may be instructional to Purkinje cells needed for learning a new motor task. Behavioral studies have shown that the acquisition of a new movement is correlated with an increase of complex spike activity and a suppression of simple spike activity. As the movement becomes coordinated, complex spike activity returns to normal, but simple spike activity remains depressed. This change in synaptic efficacy of some parallel fiber inputs is called **long-term depression (LTD)** and involves a decrease in Purkinje cell responsiveness to those parallel fibers that were selectively active 100 to 200 milliseconds after the climbing fiber–evoked complex spike.

CLINICAL CONNECTION

Although the precise function of the inferior olivary complex is unknown, unilateral lesions of this structure in experimental animals result in abnormalities similar to destruction of the contralateral half of the cerebellum. In humans, olivary lesions virtually always include the adjacent pyramid whose injury overshadows the cerebellar signs. An exception occurs in cases of olivocerebellar degeneration, a disorder that usually begins at 40 to 50 years of age, in which atrophy of the inferior olive results in progressive ataxia of the upper and lower limbs. In addition to the gait ataxia and intention tremor, dysarthria may develop. Focal lesions of olivocerebellar projections affect the patient's ability to learn new motor tasks.

CEREBELLAR NUCLEI

The cerebellum influences motor centers at various levels almost exclusively through the cerebellar nuclei. These paired neuronal masses, embedded in the medullary white matter near the roof of the fourth ventricle, are, from medial to lateral, the fastigial, interposed (composed of globose and emboliform parts), and dentate (Fig. 9-4). Cells in each nucleus receive excitatory impulses from collateral branches of the mossy and climbing fibers and inhibitory impulses from Purkinje cells in topographically defined parts of the cerebellar cortex. Purkinje neurons in the vermis and flocculonodular lobe project to the fastigial nuclei (Fig. 9-7), whereas those in the intermediate parts of the hemisphere project to the interposed nuclei. Those in the lateral parts of the hemispheres project to the dentate nuclei. The cerebellar nuclei have descending and ascending efferent projections that excite motor centers in the brainstem and thalamus. Generally the midline vermis and fastigial nuclei control head, trunk, and proximal limb movements bilaterally, whereas the hemisphere and interposed and dentate nuclei control progressively more distal limb movements ipsilaterally.

Neuronal activity in the vermis and fastigial nuclei is correlated with posture, gait, and eye movements. Activity in the hemisphere and interposed and dentate nuclei is mainly correlated with multijoint movements of the limbs. Unitary activity in the paravermis and interposed nuclei is temporally correlated with somatosensory feedback during a movement and especially during the firing of antagonist muscles and therefore is involved with correcting ongoing movements. Activity in the lateral hemispheres and particularly the dentate nuclei precedes by about 100 milliseconds activity in the motor cortex and the onset of movement.

POSTERIOR LOBE

The lateral parts of the cerebellar hemispheres are chiefly concerned with the learning and storage of all of the sequential components of skilled movements. The major input to the lateral parts of the cerebellar hemispheres originates in the association areas of the cerebral cortex where the desire to perform a volitional movement occurs, and the major output of the cerebellar hemisphere is directed to the motor cortex where skilled movements are rep-

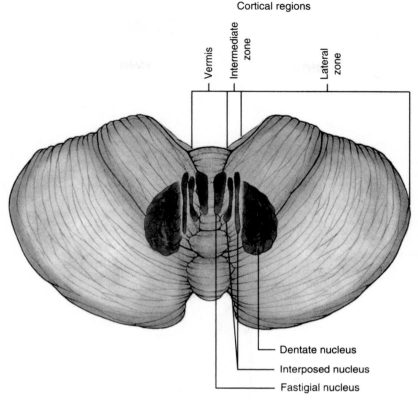

Figure 9-7 Input relations of cerebellar cortex to cerebellar nuclei. The cortical area anatomically related to each nucleus is the principal source of Purkinje neuron input to the nucleus.

resented. As has been described previously, activity in this part of the cerebellum and in its nucleus, the dentate, precedes the activity in the motor cortex that ultimately commands a particular movement.

CONNECTIONS OF THE POSTERIOR LOBE

The posterior lobe, by far the largest of the cerebellar lobes, has massive reciprocal connections with the cerebral cortex (Fig. 9-8). It receives by far the largest group of cerebellar mossy fiber afferents, the corticopontocerebellar projections. Most of the corticopontine fibers arise from the sensorimotor, premotor, and posterior parietal parts of the cerebral cortex, although the association areas of all the lobes contribute heavily. The corticopontine fibers reach the ipsilateral pontine nuclei by coursing through the internal capsule and cerebral crus (Fig. 9-9). The pontine nuclei give rise to the transverse pontine fibers which, after crossing and proceeding through the contralateral basilar

pons, form the massive middle cerebellar peduncles that project chiefly to the posterior lobe.

Axons from Purkinje neurons in the lateral parts of the posterior lobe project to the dentate nucleus. Dentatofugal fibers pass to the contralateral ventral lateral nucleus of the thalamus, from whence there is a thalamocortical projection to the motor cortex. The dentatofugal fibers pass rostrally in the superior cerebellar peduncle. This prominent bundle arises mainly from the dentate nucleus, although it also contains a considerable number of fibers from the interposed nucleus and a small contribution from the fastigial nucleus. The superior cerebellar peduncle courses initially in the roof of the fourth ventricle (Fig. 9-9), then moves into the ventricular wall and, in the rostral pons, enters the tegmentum. At the level of the inferior colliculus, it decussates before continuing rostrally through the red nucleus and the prerubral field in the dorsomedial part of the subthalamus. Here, it is joined by pallidothalamic fibers, and the

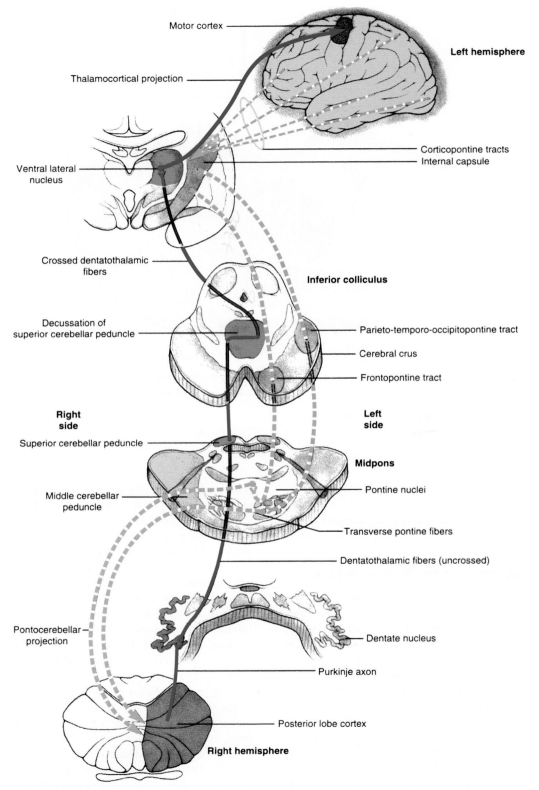

Figure 9-8   Schematic diagram showing posterior lobe circuitry. Input (broken lines); output (solid lines).

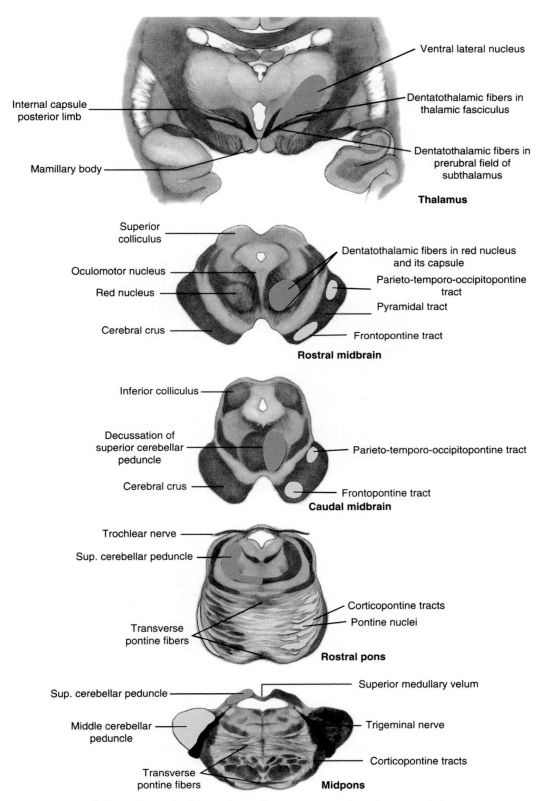

Figure 9-9   Relations of posterior lobe pathways in transverse sections (sup, superior).

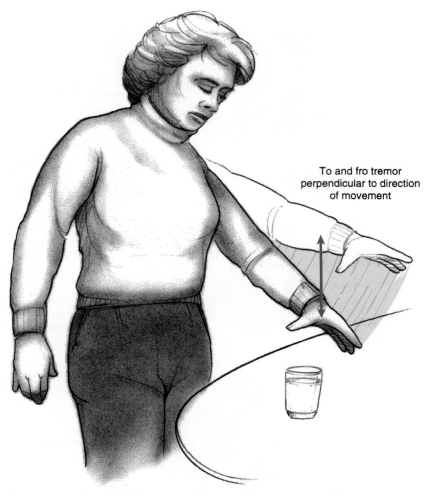

To and fro tremor
perpendicular to direction
of movement

Figure 9-10 Posterior lobe syndrome: Intention tremor. To and fro movements perpendicular to intended direction of movement.

two groups of fibers form the thalamic fasciculus, which passes to the motor thalamus.

POSTERIOR LOBE SYNDROME

The neocerebellar or **posterior lobe syndrome,** commonly resulting from cerebrovascular accidents, tumors, trauma, or degenerative diseases, is manifested by a loss of coordination of voluntary movements (ataxia) and decreased muscle tone, the latter being most prominent in acute lesions. The ataxic patient is unable to direct the limb to a target without its progression being interrupted by a swaying to and fro that is perpendicular to the direction of the movement (Fig. 9-10). This is referred to as **intention tremor** because it occurs only when a volitional movement is being performed; it is not present at rest.

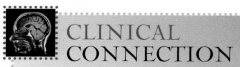

CLINICAL CONNECTION

Various degrees of intention tremor occur with neocerebellar damage, but the most severe tremors are associated with damage to the dentatothalamic tract that occurs in multiple sclerosis (MS) or midbrain infarctions.

Other manifestations of posterior lobe lesions, as described in the case at the beginning of this chapter, are **dysmetria,** in which the patient overshoots or undershoots when attempting to touch a target, and **dysdiadochokinesia,** the inability to perform rapid alternating movements such as repetitive hand pronation and supination. In unilateral lesions, ataxia is found ipsilaterally; in bilateral lesions both sides are involved. Speech, too, may be affected; the normal rhythm and flow of words is disrupted, and words are slurred or broken into their individual syllables. The patient may attempt to compensate by breaking words into syllables and uttering them with great force (explosive speech).

PATHOPHYSIOLOGY OF LIMB ATAXIA

Ataxia is characterized by abnormalities in the timing, range, force, speed, and sequencing of muscle contractions and resultant movements. These abnormalities are best demonstrated in electromyographic recordings from muscles in the affected limbs, thereby revealing the underlying basis for the ataxic movements. Normal, rapid single-joint movements are characterized by an initial accelerated movement by contraction of the agonist muscle, decelerated by an appropriately timed contraction of the antagonist muscle, and then finally completed by a second small burst of activity in the agonist (reciprocal contractions). After damage to the lateral cerebellum, dentate nucleus, or its efferent projections, contraction of the agonist is not followed by timely reciprocal contraction of the antagonist muscle, resulting in the delayed slowing of the movement and overshooting the target. In a simple single-joint movement, the inability to control the force of agonist muscle contraction and the timing of reciprocal antagonist contraction can be demonstrated in the upper limb of patients when flexion of the forearm is restrained by the examiner. An unexpected release of the forearm results in patients striking themselves. This is called **rebound phenomenon.**

In complex movements, such as reaching, delayed antagonist activity occurs across multiple joints, resulting in oscillations of agonist-antagonist contractions. These desynchronized contractions result in abnormalities in controlling the range of movements (hypometric-undershooting or hypermetric-overshooting of the target) (Fig. 9-11). Intention tremor is a manifestation of the altered agonist-antagonist contractions.

The speed of movement is also affected as characterized in a simple movement by the inability to coordinate alternating repetitive movements (dysdiadochokinesia). Complex multijoint movements must be broken down into elementary components that are slower because the movements at each joint must be successively adjusted under visual control.

ANTERIOR LOBE

The vermal and paravermal parts of the anterior lobe chiefly maintain coordination of limb movements while the movements are being executed and, hence, the anterior lobe has strong connections with the spinal cord (Fig. 9-12). In the anterior lobe, lower limb representation is largest and located anteriorly, whereas the upper limb and then the head are represented posteriorly.

CONNECTIONS OF THE ANTERIOR LOBE

Through the spinal cord and, to a certain extent, the brainstem, the cerebellum receives voluminous information from general sensory receptors throughout the body. Much of this information is from muscular, joint, and cutaneous **mechanoreceptors** that project monosynaptically via the spinocerebellar, cuneocerebellar, and trigeminocerebellar tracts to the vermal and paravermal parts of the anterior lobe chiefly.

Discrete proprioceptive information, chiefly from muscle spindles and tendon organs of individual lower limb muscles, and exteroceptive information from small cutaneous receptive fields reach the cerebellum through the dorsal spinocerebellar

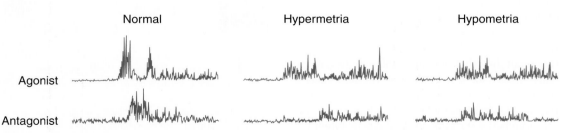

Figure 9-11   Rectified electromyographic records illustrating the temporal pattern of agonist and antagonist activation during movement in a normal patient and a patient with a posterior lobe syndrome.

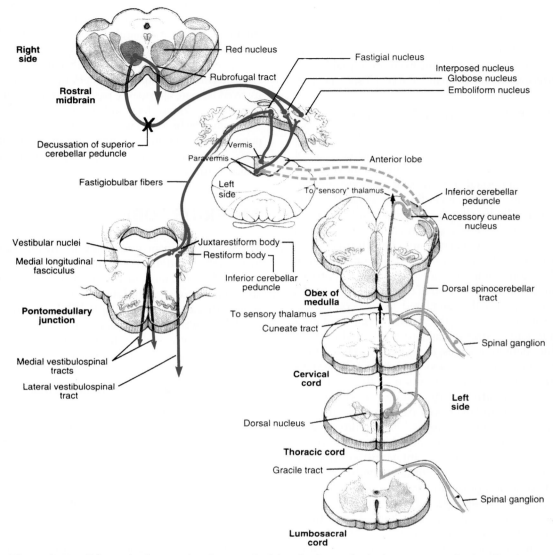

Figure 9-12 Schematic diagram showing anterior lobe circuitry to the brainstem. Input (broken lines); output (solid lines).

tract. This tract arises from the dorsal nucleus of Clarke (nucleus thoracicus), which forms a column of neurons in the medial part of lamina VII from spinal cord levels C8 to L2. Neurons in the dorsal nucleus receive either proprioceptive or exteroceptive input directly from collateral branches of primary afferent axons ascending in the lumbosacral parts of the gracile tract. The axons of the dorsal nucleus of Clarke ascend ipsilaterally as the dorsal spinocerebellar tract and enter the cerebellum via the inferior cerebellar peduncle (Fig. 9-13).

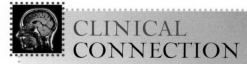

CLINICAL CONNECTION

The dorsal spinocerebellar tract may be damaged in demyelinating diseases such as MS and Friedreich ataxia as well as in lateral medullary or inferior cerebellar peduncle lesions. When the tract is damaged, cerebellar input from the ipsilateral lower limb is impaired. As a result, ipsilateral lower limb ataxia occurs.

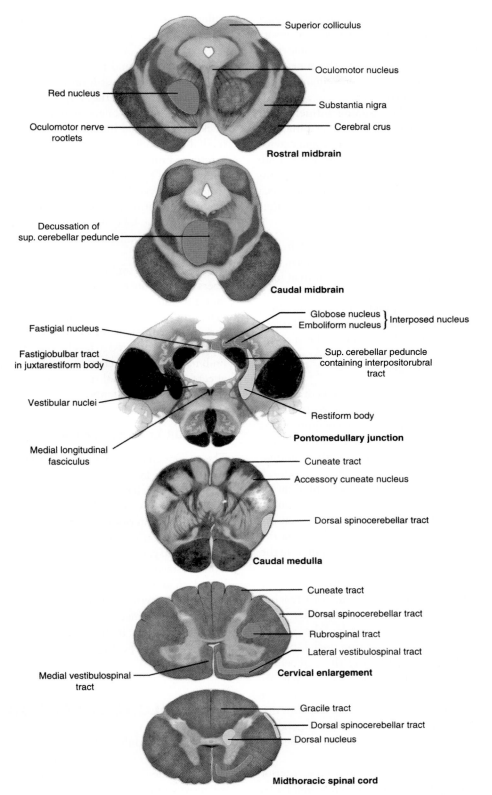

Figure 9-13 Relation of anterior lobe pathways in transverse sections (sup, superior).

Equivalent types of information from the upper limb ascend in the cuneate tract to the accessory cuneate nucleus. Its neurons, which resemble those of the Clarke column, give rise to the cuneocerebellar tract that also enters the cerebellum through the inferior cerebellar peduncle.

Information of the ongoing influences of the descending motor pathways on the spinal gray matter and convergent proprioceptive and exteroceptive information from the entire lower limb reach the cerebellum through the ventral spinocerebellar tract. This tract differs from the dorsal spinocerebellar tract not only because of its different function, but also because it:

1. Originates from neurons scattered in the intermediate zone and anterior horn, and along the border of the anterior horn at lumbar levels;
2. Decussates in the spinal cord and, therefore, carries impulses from the contralateral side;
3. Enters the cerebellum through the superior cerebellar peduncle and decussates to its original (ipsilateral) side.

The medical importance of the ventral spinocerebellar tract rivals that of the rostral spinocerebellar tract, which arises from neurons in the intermediate zone of the cervical enlargement and carries exteroceptive and proprioceptive information from the upper limbs.

Trigeminocerebellar fibers carry information from the temporomandibular joint, masticatory and external ocular muscles, and so forth. Sensory information also reaches the cerebellum via the reticular formation, which receives input from the spinal cord and brainstem.

Information pertaining to activity in the motor cortex and its pyramidal tract neurons reaches the anterior lobe via the pontine nuclei. This information comes from collaterals of the pyramidal tract fibers. From the pontine nuclei, pontocerebellar fibers cross and enter the cerebellum through the contralateral middle cerebellar peduncle to reach the lateral parts of the anterior lobe. Through these connections, the anterior lobe receives information about the impending influence of the corticospinal fibers on an ongoing movement.

Axons from Purkinje neurons in the anterior lobe, especially its vermal and paravermal parts,

influence the fastigial nuclei, interposed nuclei, and the lateral vestibular nucleus. Through the fastigial nucleus and its connections with the vestibular nuclei and reticular formation, which occur via the juxtarestiform part of the inferior cerebellar peduncle, the vermis of the anterior lobe has a strong, bilateral influence on head, neck, and proximal limb muscles via the ventromedial descending motor paths. Through the interposed nucleus and its connections with the contralateral red nucleus and reticular formation, which occur via the superior cerebellar peduncle and its decussation (Fig. 9-9), the paravermal part of the anterior lobe influences the more distal muscles of the limbs via the lateral descending motor paths.

The fastigial and interposed nuclei also send fibers via the superior cerebellar peduncle to the motor thalamus which, in turn, projects to the primary motor cortex. Through such connections the fastigial nucleus affects components of the pyramidal tract related to head, neck, and proximal limb movements, whereas the interposed nucleus affects those pyramidal tract components related to distal limb movements.

ANTERIOR LOBE SYNDROME

The most common lesions of the anterior lobe result from the malnutrition accompanying chronic alcoholism, which results in damage to the Purkinje neurons initially those located more anteriorly. Patients with **anterior lobe syndrome** suffer the loss of coordination chiefly in the lower limbs; they have marked gait instability (Fig. 9-14) and walk as if drunk, staggering and reeling in a somewhat stiff-legged manner. Sliding the heel of one foot smoothly down the shin of the other leg (the heel-shin test) is extremely difficult, if not impossible, for the patient to do. If the degeneration progresses posteriorly, the upper limbs and speech may also be affected.

FLOCCULONODULAR LOBE

The flocculonodular lobe, or vestibular part of the cerebellum, is responsible for coordination of the muscles associated with equilibrium and eye movements.

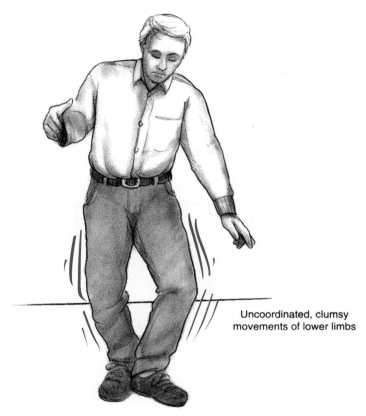

Figure 9-14   Anterior lobe syndrome: Gait ataxia. Clumsy movements of lower limbs.

CONNECTIONS OF THE FLOCCULONODULAR LOBE

Direct and indirect impulses from the vestibular apparatus in the inner ear carry information about position and movements of the head. The direct vestibulocerebellar impulses reach the cerebellum via central projections of the vestibular nerve without synapsing (Fig. 9-15). The indirect vestibulocerebellar impulses come from the vestibular nuclei. Both groups enter the cerebellum in the medial part of the inferior cerebellar peduncle, the juxtarestiform body (Fig. 9-3), and pass chiefly to the flocculonodular lobe and the adjacent parts of the vermis.

Axons from Purkinje neurons in the flocculonodular lobe influence the vestibular nuclei and the adjacent reticular formation indirectly through the fastigial nuclei and directly from the Purkinje cells. The fastigiobulbar projections as well as the direct flocculonodular projections reach the vestibular nuclei through the juxtarestiform body.

Vestibulospinal projections and vestibulo-ocular projections then descend and ascend in the medial longitudinal fasciculus (MLF) to reach the motor neurons innervating the axial muscles and the external ocular muscles, respectively.

FLOCCULONODULAR LOBE SYNDROME

Lesions of the flocculonodular lobe and posterior vermis cause disturbances of balance manifested chiefly by a lack of coordination of the paraxial muscles, a condition referred to as **truncal ataxia** (Fig. 9-16). The patient has no control over the axial muscles and, hence, attempts to walk on a wide base with the trunk constantly reeling and swaying. In severe cases, it is impossible for the patient to sit or stand without falling. This condition is most often seen in young children with **medulloblastomas** arising in the roof of the fourth ventricle, although it may be encountered in older children and adults with other types of tumors in the same region.

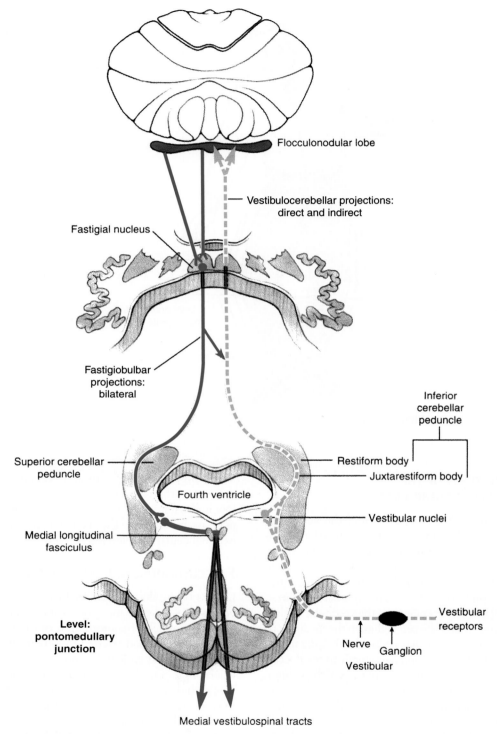

Figure 9-15 Schematic diagram of flocculonodular lobe circuitry. Input (broken lines); output (solid lines).

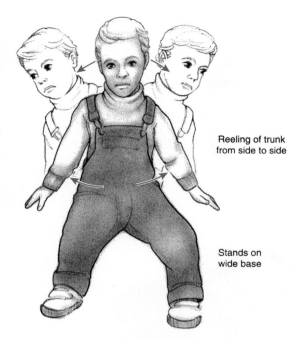

Reeling of trunk from side to side

Stands on wide base

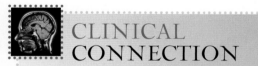

Figure 9-16   Flocculonodular lobe syndrome: Truncal ataxia. Standing on wide base and reeling from side to side.

CLINICAL CONNECTION

The long-standing view that the cerebellum is solely a motor control structure is changing on the basis of functional imaging studies that indicate the cerebellum is also involved in autonomic, cognitive, and complex behavioral activities. The lateral and inferior areas of the cerebellar posterior lobe and parts of the dentate nucleus appear to be involved with planning, verbal fluency and language, attention, and behavior. These cerebellar cognitive areas receive input, via the pons, from frontal, parietal, and occipital association areas and project back to these cortical areas through the thalamus. A "cerebellar cognitive affective syndrome" is receiving increasing attention to explain higher order dysfunction after cerebellar lesions.

Chapter Review Questions

9-1.   Name the cerebellar peduncles and give the principal components of each.

9-2.   Activation of olivocerebellar climbing fibers evokes what type of response in Purkinje cells?

9-3.   What neuron(s) is(are) excitatory in the cerebellar cortex?

a. Purkinje cells
b. basket cells
c. stellate cells
d. Golgi cells
e. granule cells

9-4.   Long-term synaptic depression refers to what phenomena in the cerebellar cortex?

9-5.   Name the cerebellar nuclei and give their chief excitatory and inhibitory inputs.

9-6.   What is the relationship among the three sagittal zones of the cerebellum and the cerebellar nuclei?

9-7.   Give the cardinal manifestations of the three cerebellar syndromes.

9-8.   Impulse activity in the lateral hemisphere and dentate nucleus generally (a) precedes, (b) occurs coincident with, or (c) follows a voluntary movement?

9-9.   Past-pointing would be characterized by what observation in electromyographic recordings from antagonist and agonist muscle pairs?

9-10.   Information processing in the anterior lobe cortex chiefly compares what two types of information and pathways?

9-11.   Can a patient with a midline medulloblastoma perform a normal skilled movement?

9-12.   What abnormalities result from a lesion of (1) the inferior cerebellar peduncle and, (2) the red nucleus?

9-13.   What structures are involved and what abnormalities result from the lesions appearing as cross-hatched areas in the sections on the next page?

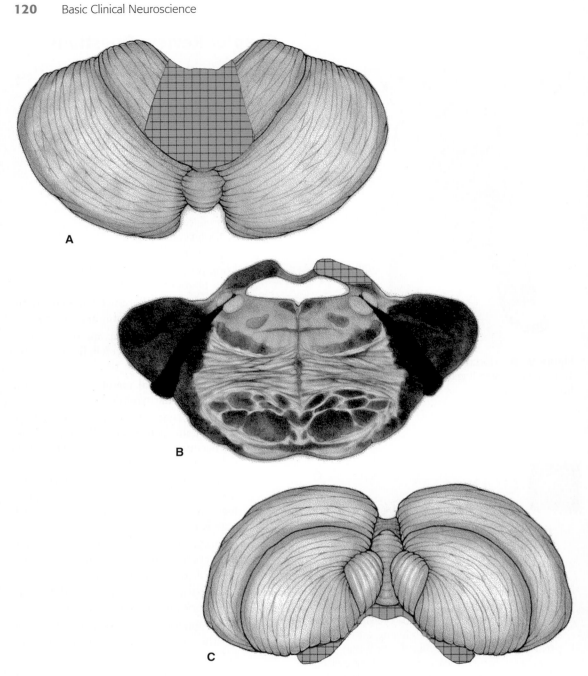

A

B

C

The Ocular Motor System: Gaze Disorders

A PATIENT COMPLAINS of double vision whenever looking toward the right side. Examination shows that on attempting to gaze to the right, the right eye abducts normally but the left eye fails to adduct. Both gaze to the left and convergence for near vision are normal.

Our sense of vision depends on intact visual pathways that transmit information from receptors in the eyes to the brain. For normal vision to occur, the eyes must move in such a way that an object in the visual field is focused precisely on the visual receptors in the binocular zone of each eye. Otherwise, double vision (diplopia) occurs. Eye movements are controlled by complex and well-organized central nervous system connections involving centers in the brainstem and cerebral cortex.

TYPES OF EYE MOVEMENTS

Eye movements are of two types: vergence and conjugate. Vergence movements occur when eyes shift between distant and near objects. When the shift is from distant to near objects, the eyes converge; when from near to distant, they diverge. Conjugate movements occur when the eyes move in the same direction, i.e., to the right, left, up, or down.

Two main types of conjugate movements are **saccadic** and **smooth pursuit.** Saccadic movements are voluntary when vision is being moved rapidly from one target to another, such as searching for something in the horizon or reading a printed page. Saccadic may also be reflex, as in nystagmus and rapid eye movement sleep. Smooth pursuits are reflex movements that keep an image of a moving target fixed on the retinae.

Other types of conjugate movements are **optokinetic** and **vestibulo-ocular.** Optokinetic movements keep a visual field that is moving past the eyes fixed on the retinae as long as possible and then quickly refixate on the upcoming visual field, e.g., viewing the passing landscape in a moving vehicle or viewing a rotating drum with vertical stripes. Vestibulo-ocular movements keep targets fixed on the retinae during brief movements of the head and will be described with the vestibular system (Chapter 13).

OCULAR MOTOR NUCLEI

The movement of each eye is controlled by the coordinated action of six muscles: four recti (superior, medial, lateral, and inferior) and two obliques (superior and inferior). The muscles are innervated by three cranial nerves: the oculomotor, trochlear, and abducens. The clinical testing of the individual muscles is given in Figure 10-1.

121

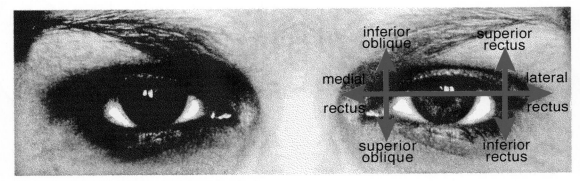

Figure 10-1   Clinical testing of extraocular muscles.

The six pairs of external ocular muscles responsible for keeping both eyes focused on the same object are controlled by gaze centers, highly specialized groups of neurons in the brainstem and cerebral cortex.

BRAINSTEM GAZE CENTERS

There are three centers in the brainstem that control eye movements. The horizontal gaze center is in the pons, and the vertical gaze and vergence centers are in the midbrain.

HORIZONTAL CENTER

The **horizontal gaze center** is located in the paramedian pontine reticular formation (PPRF). The center on each side is responsible for conjugate movements toward that side; hence, a unilateral lesion results in paralysis of gaze toward the ipsilateral side. From each center, nerve impulses pass to the ipsilateral abducens nucleus and, via the con-

tralateral medial longitudinal fasciculus (MLF), to the lower motor neurons in the oculomotor nucleus innervating the medial rectus muscle (Fig. 10-2). In this way, the lateral rectus muscle of the ipsilateral eye and the medial rectus muscle of the contralateral eye contract simultaneously. The connection to the oculomotor nucleus occurs via interneurons in the abducens nucleus whose axons cross and ascend in the contralateral MLF.

VERTICAL CENTER

The **vertical gaze center** is in the accessory oculomotor nuclei at the rostral end of the MLF in the midbrain. This gaze center is bilateral and there are interconnections via the posterior commissure. Upward movements are represented more dorsally, downward more ventrally.

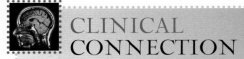

CLINICAL CONNECTION

Vertical gaze disorders, most commonly upward gaze paralysis, often result from pressure being exerted on the rostral midbrain by a pineal gland tumor or dilation of the rostral part of the cerebral aqueduct. In such cases, paralysis of convergence may also occur.

CLINICAL CONNECTION

Clinical evidence supports the contralateral MLF route to the oculomotor nucleus. A unilateral lesion of the MLF rostral to the abducens nucleus results in paralysis of adduction in the eye ipsilateral to the lesion when the patient attempts to gaze toward the opposite side. The affected eye does adduct during convergence; hence, the medial rectus muscle and its innervation are functional. This phenomenon is referred to as **internuclear ophthalmoplegia** and is represented in the clinical case at the beginning of this chapter. If present bilaterally, it is almost invariably associated with multiple sclerosis.

VERGENCE CENTER

A brainstem center controlling convergence and divergence of the eyes, as when directing vision from far to near or near to far objects, is also located in the rostral midbrain near the oculomotor nuclei.

CORTICAL GAZE CENTERS

Within the cerebral cortex are several centers associated with eye movements. The most well known

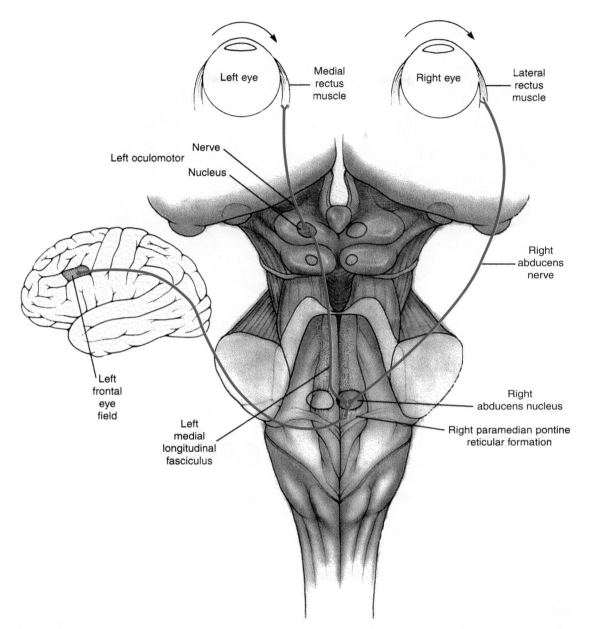

Figure 10-2 Schematic drawing of dorsal view of brainstem showing pathways for voluntary gaze to the right.

are the **frontal eye field,** the **parietal and temporal eye fields,** and the **occipital eye field.**

FRONTAL EYE FIELD

The chief center in the cerebral cortex for voluntary eye movements is located primarily in the posterior part of the middle frontal gyrus and is called the frontal eye field (Fig. 10-3). Stimulation of this area results in aversive eye movements in the form of **saccades.** The frontal eye field projects to the vertical

and horizontal gaze centers (Fig. 10-2) and to the superior colliculus.

Lesions affecting horizontal gaze and the resulting abnormalities are given in Figure 10-4.

PARIETAL AND TEMPORAL EYE FIELDS

Areas in the posterior parts of the parietal and temporal lobes (Fig. 10-3) also influence eye movements. The superior parietal lobule affects saccadic movements through reciprocal connections with

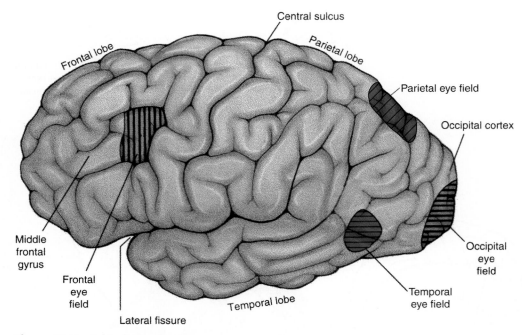

Figure 10-3   Cortical gaze centers.

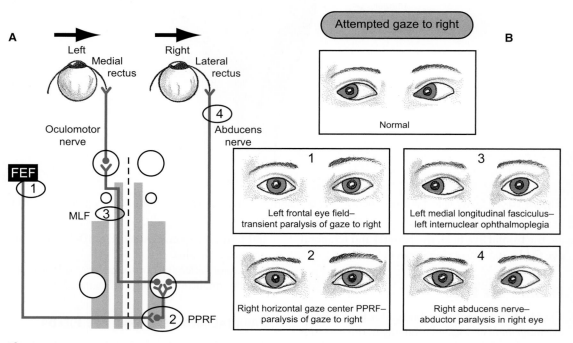

Figure 10-4   Lesions affecting horizontal gaze. **A.** Pathways and locations of lesions. **B.** Abnormalities with attempted gaze to the right (FEF, frontal eye field; MLF, medial longitudinal fasciculus; PPRF, paramedian pontine reticular formation).

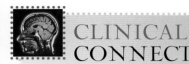

CLINICAL CONNECTION

Because of the tonic influence of each frontal eye field on the contralateral horizontal gaze center, acute lesions of the frontal eye field result in conjugate deviation of the eyes toward the side of the lesion and paralysis of voluntary gaze toward the contralateral side (Fig. 10-4). An irritative lesion such as occurs in a focal seizure results in deviation of the eyes to the contralateral side. Such abnormalities are transient because of the bilateralism of these cortical connections with the brainstem gaze centers.

the frontal eye field and projections to the superior colliculus.

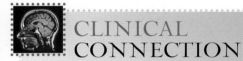

CLINICAL CONNECTION

The superior parietal lobule plays a role in visual attention, which is closely related to saccadic eye movements. Patients with lesions in this area neglect objects on the opposite side and have difficulty in making eye movements toward that side.

An area in the posterior part of the lateral surface of the temporal lobes appears to be the chief cortical center associated with smooth pursuit movements, although the superior parietal lobule and frontal eye field may also be involved. This area receives input from the visual cortex and sends impulses to dorsolateral pontine nuclei, which then make connections with the vestibular nuclei via the vestibulocerebellum (Fig. 10-5). Lesions in the temporal eye field or in the dorsolateral pontine nuclei result in the loss of smooth pursuit when targets are moving toward the side of the lesion.

The temporal eye field is also associated with optokinetic movements. An example of these movements occurs in an individual in a moving vehicle watching an object in the passing landscape. The eyes will automatically follow the particular object in the landscape until it disappears from view, at which time the eyes move rapidly in the opposite direction and fix on a new object in the landscape. A similar phenomenon occurs when vision is directed at vertical black and white

stripes on a slowly rotating drum. The eyes will fix on a particular stripe, follow it until it disappears from view, and then move rapidly in the opposite direction to fix on a new stripe on the drum. These slow drifting and fast return movements are referred to as **optokinetic nystagmus.**

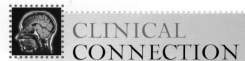

CLINICAL CONNECTION

An absence or decrease in optokinetic nystagmus results from lesions of subcortical or cortical structures involved in the visual motion pathway which includes the visual cortex and posterior temporal areas (see Chapter 14). The absence or decrease is manifested only when an object is rotating toward the side of the lesion.

OCCIPITAL EYE FIELD

The primary visual and visual association areas in the occipital cortex form the occipital eye field, which controls vergence movements. Convergence occurs when vision is directed from a far to a near target. This phenomenon is called the **near response** and includes simultaneous contraction of the medial rectus muscles, accommodation of the lenses, and constriction of the pupils. Occipitofugal fibers pass to the vergence centers adjacent to the oculomotor nuclei, which then project to the oculomotor nuclear complex. Somatic oculomotor neurons innervate the medial rectus muscles, and visceromotor (parasympathetic) oculomotor neurons influence via postganglionic fibers from the ciliary ganglia the ciliary muscles for the accommodation of the lens and the pupillary constrictor muscles. Divergence occurs via connections to the abducens nuclei, which are made through the reticular formation, not the MLF, because divergence is not impaired by MLF lesions.

SUPERIOR COLLICULUS

The superior colliculus consists of alternating gray and white layers that are subdivided into superficial, intermediate, and deep layers. The superficial layers receive input directly from the retina and cortical visual association areas (Fig. 10-6). The frontal eye field projects to the

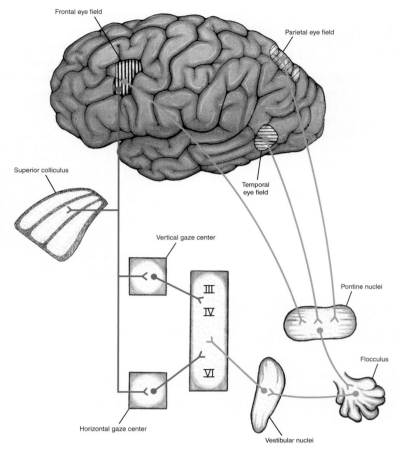

Figure 10-5   Schematic of saccadic and smooth pursuit paths. Saccadic = dark blue; smooth pursuit = light blue.

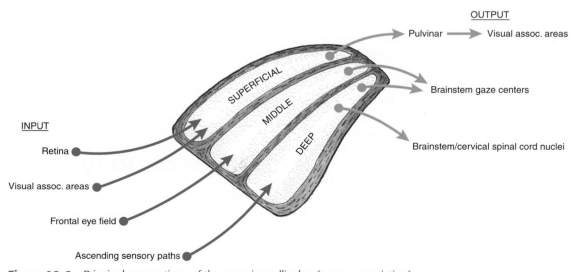

Figure 10-6   Principal connections of the superior colliculus (assoc, association).

intermediate layers, and sensory paths ascending through the brainstem, especially the pain and auditory paths, project to the deep layers. Output from the superior colliculus ascends to visual association areas via the pulvinar and descends into the brainstem and spinal cord. The latter are responsible for reflex turning of the head and eyes in response to startling pain or auditory stimuli.

The role of the superior colliculus in the control of ordinary eye movements is not entirely clear. Because of the input it receives from the retina and cortical eye fields and its output to the brainstem gaze centers, this structure undoubtedly plays a role as a visuomotor integration center especially concerned with reflex ocular motor movements. Lesions of the superior colliculi do not result in major eye movement abnormalities owing to the diversity of the connections between the cortical and brainstem gaze centers. For instance, the frontal eye fields project bilaterally to the brainstem gaze centers via (1) corticonuclear paths that travel with the corticospinal tracts to the levels of the gaze centers, where the fibers then enter the tegmentum to reach these centers, and (2) a transtegmental route that descends through the tegmentum of the midbrain and pons. Thus, focal lesions in the brainstem interrupt only a small portion of the total input to the gaze centers.

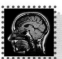

CLINICAL CONNECTION

Programming of eye movements appears to occur not only in the cerebral cortex and brainstem but also in the basal ganglia. Input reaches the head of the caudate nucleus via corticostriate projections from the frontal eye field, prefrontal cortex, and the posterior parietal cortex. Outputs chiefly from the substantia nigra (reticular part) pass to the ventral anterior nuclei and medial dorsal thalamic nuclei, which, in turn, directly influence the frontal eye field and adjacent parts of the prefrontal cortex. In basal ganglia disorders such as Parkinson disease, normal spontaneous ocular movements are lacking or seldom occur. This phenomenon, along with slightly widened palpebral fissures and infrequent blinking, gives the eyes a staring appearance.

Cerebellar coordination of eye movements occurs via connections of the flocculonodular lobe and fastigial nuclei with the vestibular nuclei. Vestibulo-ocular connections then carry the cerebellar influences to the nuclei of the ocular motor nerves. Unilateral cerebellar lesions result in a conspicuous nystagmus, especially when the eyes are directed toward the side of the lesion.

Chapter Review Questions

Locate the lesion in each of the following:

10-1.   Attempted gaze to the left results in:

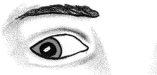
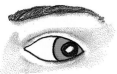

10-2.   Attempted gaze to the right results in:

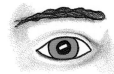
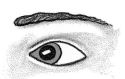

10-3.   Attempted gaze to the left results in:

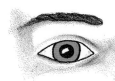
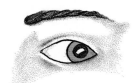

10-4.   Attempted gaze to the right results in:

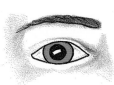
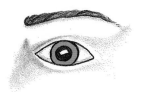

11

The Somatosensory System: Anesthesia and Analgesia

THE FOLLOWING THREE SETS of neurologic symptoms are indicative of lesions involving the somatosensory pathways at three different levels in the central nervous system (CNS):

1. The first patient has loss of general sensations below the umbilicus, such that on the right side only the touch, pressure, and proprioceptive senses are lost whereas on the left side only the pain and temperature senses are lost.
2. The second patient has loss of pinprick and temperature sensations on the left side in the limbs, trunk, neck, and back of the head and on the right side on the face and anterior part of the scalp.
3. The third patient has total left hemianesthesia, that is, loss of pinprick, temperature, touch, pressure, and proprioceptive senses on the left side of the entire body.

All sensations arising from skin, connective tissues, voluntary muscles, periosteum, teeth, and so forth belong to the general somatic sensory system, more commonly referred to as the **somatosensory system.**

GENERAL SENSES

The general senses include light touch or tactile discrimination and sensations of pressure or deep touch, vibration, proprioception, pain, and temperature. The somatosensory pathways consist of three neurons: the first neuron is in the sensory ganglia, the second is in the spinal cord or brainstem or both, and the third is in the thalamus.

LIGHT TOUCH

Light touch is also called tactile sense and refers to the awareness and precise location of very delicate mechanical stimuli such as stroking the hairs on

129

the skin or, in hairless areas, stroking the skin with a wisp of cotton or a feather. Light touch includes three other phenomena: **two-point sense, stereognosis,** and **graphesthesia.** Two-point sense is the ability to distinguish stimulation by one or two points applied to the skin. The minimal distance between the two points that can be felt separately varies considerably on different parts of the body. Two points can be distinguished as close as 1 mm on the tip of the tongue and 2 to 4 mm on the finger tips, whereas on the dorsum of the hand two points closer than 20 to 30 mm cannot be distinguished from one another. Stereognosis is the ability to recognize objects by touch alone, using the object's size, shape, texture, weight, and so forth. Graphesthesia is the ability to recognize numbers or letters drawn on the skin. Both stereognosis and graphesthesia require intact light touch pathways and memory; in other words, the objects, numbers, or letters must be known to the individual being tested.

PRESSURE

The perception of pressure involves stimuli applied to subcutaneous structures. Pressure sense is tested by firmly pressing on the skin with a blunt object and by squeezing subcutaneous structures and muscles. Pressure sensations are often referred to as deep touch.

VIBRATION SENSE

When the shaft of an oscillating high-frequency (256 vibrations per second) tuning fork is gently applied to the skin overlying bony prominences, vibrations in the subcutaneous tissues are perceived. **Vibration sense,** therefore, requires intact pathways from deep structures such as subcutaneous connective tissue, periosteum, and muscle.

When an oscillating low-frequency (128 vibrations per second) tuning fork is used, the sensation is described as "flutter" or fine vibrations in the skin itself. Flutter sensations are associated with the light touch pathways.

PROPRIOCEPTION: LIMB POSITION AND MOTION SENSE

Limb position or posture sense is the awareness of the position of the skeletal parts of the body. Motion sense is the awareness of active or passive movements of the skeletal parts of the body. Motion sense can be tested by passively flexing and extending individual fingers and toes, the hand and foot, the forearm and leg, and so on. With eyes closed, the subject should be able to recognize the direction, speed, and range of the movement. Position sense can be tested by passively moving a limb or one of its parts to a certain position and having the subject move the opposite limb to the same position. A patient who can stand with the feet together and the eyes open, but who sways and falls when the eyes are closed, has the **Romberg sign,** which indicates an absence of position sense in the lower limbs (see Chapter 13).

PAIN

There are two types of pain or nociceptive (*noci* means noxious) sensations: fast and slow. **Fast pain** is of the sharp, pricking type and is well localized. The ability to feel fast pain is tested by alternately touching the tip and head of a safety pin to the surface of the skin. The patient should be able to readily distinguish the sharpness of the tip of the pin from the dullness of the head. **Slow pain** is of the dull, burning type and is diffuse rather than localized. It results from tissue injury.

TEMPERATURE

Temperature sensations range from cold to hot and can be tested by touching the skin with test tubes filled with either cold or warm water.

PERIPHERAL COMPONENTS

The peripheral fibers of the somatosensory system are the branches of unipolar neurons in the dorsal root (spinal) ganglia and the homologous ganglia of the trigeminal, facial, glossopharyngeal, and vagus nerves. These are the first neurons in the paths and, hence, are referred to as the primary somatosensory neurons or first-order neurons. Each possesses only one process, the axon, which bifurcates into a peripheral branch and a central branch. The central branch enters the dorsal root of the spinal nerve or the sensory root of the appropriate cranial nerve, and passes to the spinal cord or brainstem, respectively. The peripheral branch enters the spinal or cranial nerve and eventually terminates at a somatosensory receptor that responds to a specific type of stimulus.

Somatosensory Receptors

Tactile, temperature, and nociceptive stimulation to the body surface activates specialized exteroceptors, and position and movement of the limbs activate proprioceptors. Bare or encapsulated sensory nerve endings transduce the physical stimulus into electrical receptor potentials that encode stimulus strength and duration into action potentials conducted by the primary afferent axons to the CNS. The cutaneous area over which a receptor is activated is called a receptive field. The size of receptive fields for the same receptor types varies in different parts of the body, generally being smallest at the tips of the fingers and perioral areas and largest on the back. The principal somatosensory receptors and their functions are given in Table 11-1.

Tactile Receptors

Tactile stimulation activates encapsulated **mechanoreceptors** by stretching the receptor membrane and opening ionic channels, leading to the receptor's depolarization and the resultant generation of action potentials in the primary afferent axons. Mechanoreceptors can be slowly adapting and fire continuously throughout the stimulus, signaling the pressure and shape of the object touching the skin. Rapid-adapting mechanoreceptors signal the onset and cessation of a stimulus and are important for sensing movement of an object across the skin.

Tactile information is propagated by the largest and fastest conducting myelinated axons.

Five different mechanoreceptors differ morphologically by their structure and location in the skin (Fig. 11-1), and physiologically by the relative sizes of their receptive fields and most importantly by the types of functional information they encode. Discrete tactile stimulation is detected by **Merkel discs** and **Meissner corpuscles** located in superficial layers predominately in glabrous skin. Merkel discs are encapsulated by a single epithelial cell whereas Meissners corpuscles are encapsulated by many flattened epithelial cells. Merkel discs have the smallest receptive fields and most importantly signal discrete indentations of the skin. Merkel discs also provide information about the curvature of objects. Meissner corpuscles are responsive to abrupt changes in the shape of the edges of objects or irregularities on the surface of objects. In hairy skin, sensory axons are incorporated in the hair follicle. Displacements of adjacent hairs activate different **hair follicle receptors,** providing additional information to the brain about discrete tactile stimulation.

Pacinian corpuscles and **Ruffini endings** are buried in the subcutaneous tissue and sense displacements of wide areas of the skin. Pacinian corpuscles have relatively large receptive fields compared with other mechanoreceptors but are the most sensitive mechanoreceptors because they are capable of detecting high-frequency stimulation (vibration). Ruffini endings sense stretching of the skin and provide information about the shapes of objects.

TABLE 11-1   Classification of Somatosensory Receptors

Category	Name	Function
Mechanoreceptors	Meissner corpuscles	Tactile: shapes/surfaces
	Merkel discs	Tactile: indentations
	Hair follicle receptors	Tactile (in hairy skin)
	Ruffini endings	Stretching and shapes
	Pacinian corpuscles	Vibrations
	Muscle spindles	Proprioception
Nociceptors	Aδ mechanical (encapsulated)	Pinprick
	C-polymodal (free nerve ending)	Tissue damage
Thermoreceptors	Free nerve endings	Cold or warmth

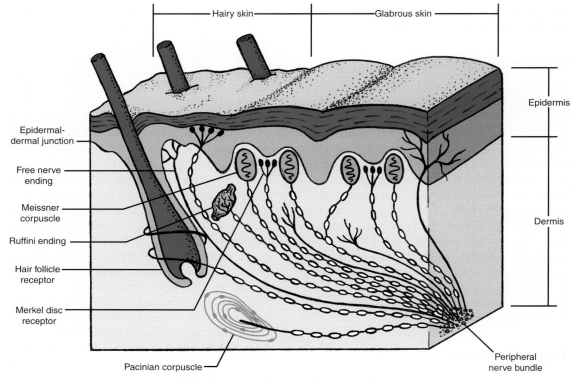

Figure 11-1 Drawings of the different types of somatosensory receptors.

TEMPERATURE RECEPTORS

Cold, cool, warm, and hot sensations below and above normal skin temperature (34°C) are sensed by **thermoreceptors.** Cold receptors fire most vigorously about 10°C below normal skin temperature whereas warmth receptors signal at their highest frequency 10°C above normal skin temperature. Warmth receptors are not activated by temperatures above 50°C. Temperatures at 50°C or higher are perceived as pain.

PAIN RECEPTORS

Nociceptors signal painful or noxious stimuli. **Mechanical nociceptors,** which are associated with fast pain, are free nerve endings activated by sharp or pinprick type stimuli. Their firing rate increases proportionally to the intensity of the potentially destructive stimulus, and the signal is propagated rapidly to the CNS by myelinated (Aδ) afferents. **Thermal nociceptors** signal noxious heat (above 45°C) or cold (below 5°C) temperatures. **Polymodal nociceptors** respond to any destructive mechanical, thermal, or chemical stim-

uli resulting from tissue damage and are the underlying basis for the sensation of slow, burning type of pain. Thermal and the burning pain sensations are conducted slowly along unmyelinated (C) primary afferent axons.

SOMATOSENSORY NERVE FIBERS

The nerve fibers conducting general sensations vary in their sizes or diameters and in their conduction velocities. In general, the larger the fiber, the faster the conduction velocity. The velocity at which a nerve fiber conducts impulses is important because the faster the conduction, the quicker the impulses reach the CNS where a response can be elicited. The nerve fibers conducting tactile, pressure, vibration, and proprioceptive sensations are larger and faster conducting than those nerve fibers conducting pain and temperature impulses.

Nerve fibers are classified in two ways, by conduction velocity and by diameter. Nerve fibers are classified according to conduction velocity as type A, B, or C, with A indicating the fastest conduction velocity and C the slowest. Nerve fibers are classified according to diameter into groups I, II,

TABLE 11-2   Classification of Somatosensory Nerve Fibers

Numerical Class	Myelinated	Diameter (μm)	Conduction Velocity (m/s)	Letter Class	Types of Sensations
I	Yes	12–20	75–120	Aα	Limb position and motion
II	Yes	6–12	30–75	Aβ	Tactile, pressure, vibration
III	Yes	1–6	5–30	Aδ	Fast pain, cold
IV	No	<1.5	0.5–2	C	Slow pain, warmth

III, and IV. Groups I, II, and III consist of myelinated fibers of decreasing size, whereas group IV consists of unmyelinated fibers. The classifications of the various types of somatosensory fibers are given in Table 11-2.

There is a positive correlation between the intensity of a stimulus and the number and frequency of propagated action potentials. Strong stimuli generate larger receptor potentials, which are coded as a greater number and higher frequency of action potentials. The duration of a stimulus is signaled by axons innervating slow-adapting mechanoreceptors. Even then **adaptation** occurs with a constant stimulus of relatively long duration.

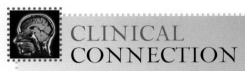

CLINICAL CONNECTION

The differences in the size and conduction velocity of the larger touch fibers and smaller pain fibers in peripheral nerves allow the selective electrical stimulation of one group and not the other. This phenomenon is the basis for the selective stimulation of the larger touch fibers by **transcutaneous electrical nerve stimulation (TENS),** a current clinical treatment for the relief of some forms of chronic pain.

DERMATOMES

The area of skin supplied by the somatosensory fibers from a single spinal nerve is called a **dermatome** (Fig. 11-2). Although there is overlap among the dermatomes, they are very useful in localizing the levels of lesions. The dermatomes essential to know for neuroanatomy problem solving are C2, back of the head; C5, tip of the shoulder; C6, thumb; C7, middle finger; C8, small finger; T4 or T5, nipple; T10, umbilicus; L1, inguinal ligament;

L4 or L5, big toe; S1, small toe; and S5, perianal region.

SPINAL TACTILE, VIBRATION, AND PROPRIOCEPTION PATHWAYS

A series of three neurons transmits the touch system impulses from the mechanoreceptors in the periphery to the cerebral cortex, where these sensations are perceived (Figs. 11-3, 11-4).

FIRST-ORDER NEURONS

The larger, fast-conducting unipolar neurons in the dorsal root or spinal ganglia are the primary touch, vibration, and proprioception neurons. The central branches enter the spinal cord through the more medial parts of the dorsal roots (Fig. 2-4) and are funneled medially into the dorsal funiculus or column, where they immediately turn and ascend. As the entering touch and proprioception fibers turn to ascend, they give branches that enter the spinal gray matter for reflex and pain modulation purposes. (The role of muscle spindle afferent fibers in the myotatic reflex is described in Chapter 5, and the role of touch afferent fibers in pain modulation is described later in this chapter.) Those entering below midthoracic levels form the gracile tract, and those entering above midthoracic levels form the cuneate tract. In the cervical segments of the spinal cord, the two tracts are partially separated by the posterior intermediate septum.

Because new fibers are added to the dorsal columns at their lateral surfaces, a precise somatotopic localization exists, i.e., fibers conducting impulses from the sacral dermatomes are most medial, whereas those from the lumbar, thoracic, and cervical dermatomes are located progressively more

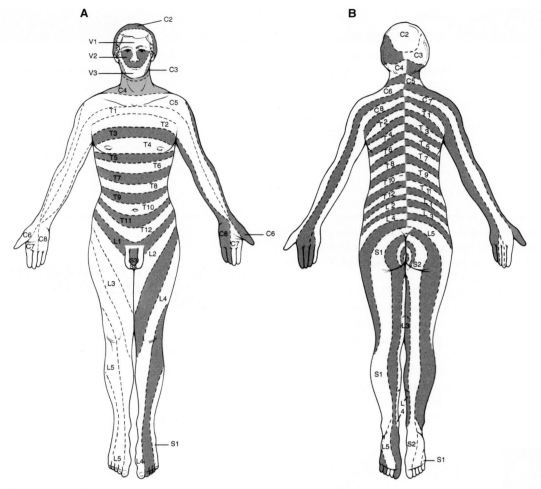

Figure 11-2 Dermatomes. **A.** Anterior surface. **B.** Posterior surface.

laterally. Some shifting occurs in the rostral half of the spinal cord because the sacral fibers here occupy most of the dorsal part of the dorsal column and hence tend to be spared when the central part of the spinal cord is damaged.

> ## CLINICAL CONNECTION
>
> Because the gracile and cuneate tracts ascend to the brain without crossing, their unilateral interruption at any level of the spinal cord results in the loss of the tactile, pressure, vibration, and proprioceptive sensations in the dermatomes on the ipsilateral (same) side below the level of the lesion.

SECOND-ORDER NEURONS

The axons of the gracile and cuneate tracts terminate on the secondary somatosensory neurons located in the gracile and cuneate nuclei, the dorsal column nuclei, within the caudal medulla. Axons from the dorsal column nuclei form small bundles of myelinated fibers termed **internal arcuate fibers** (Figs. 11-3 to 11-5), which pass anteromedially as they arch toward the midline. The axons from the dorsal column nuclei cross the midline as the "sensory decussation" and immediately begin to ascend in a large bundle located next to the midline, the **medial lemniscus.**

The tactile and proprioceptive senses are somewhat segregated in the dorsal columns and their nuclei. The tactile fibers are positioned more dorsally in the dorsal columns and synapse in the

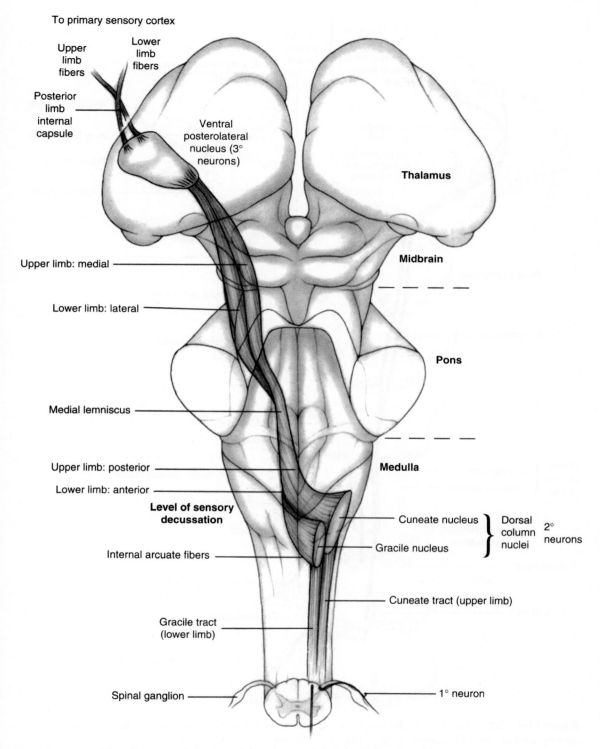

Figure 11-3   Three-dimensional drawing of dorsal view of dorsal column-medial lemniscus system (1°, primary or first-order; 2°, secondary or second-order; 3°, tertiary or third-order).

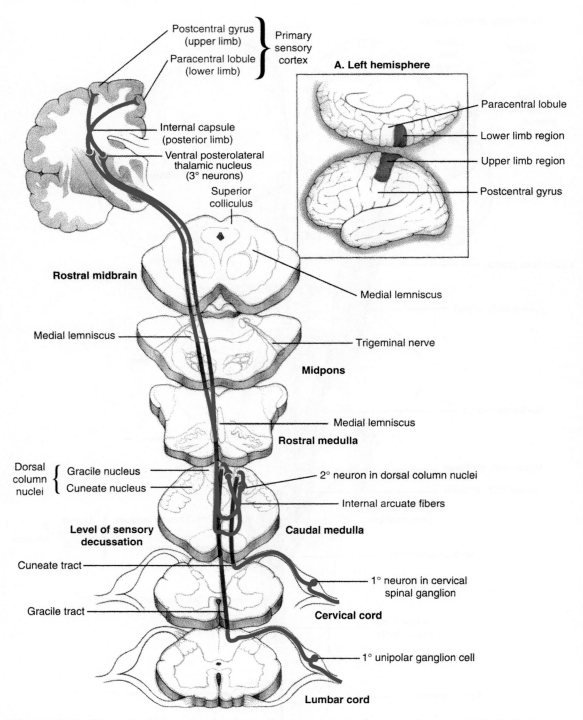

Figure 11-4 Schematic diagram showing the touch system pathway from spinal nerves. **A.** Distribution in primary sensory cortex (1°, primary or first-order; 2°, secondary or second-order).

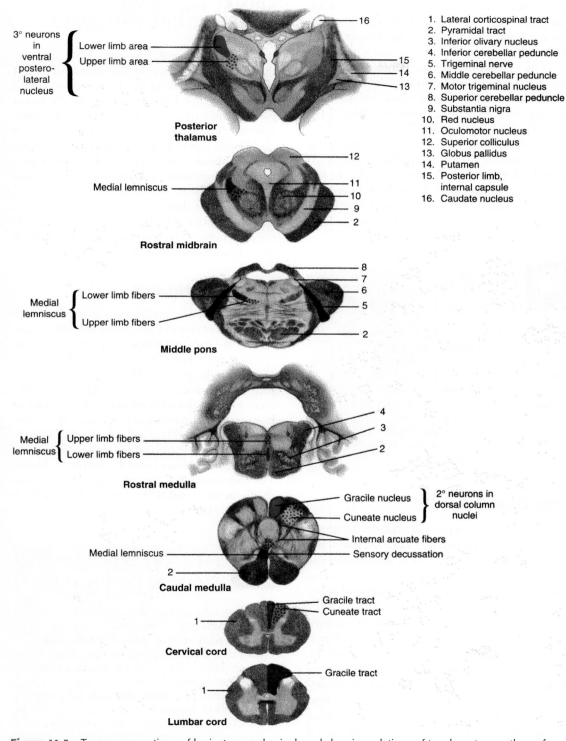

Figure 11-5   Transverse sections of brainstem and spinal cord showing relations of touch system pathway from spinal nerves (2°, secondary or second-order; 3°, tertiary or third-order).

more caudal parts of the dorsal column nuclei. The proprioceptive fibers are more ventral in the dorsal columns and synapse more rostrally in the nuclei.

The medial lemniscus borders the midline in the medulla and contains axons from the gracile nucleus in its anterior half and from the cuneate nucleus in its posterior half (Figs. 11-3 to 11-5). Thus, in the medulla, the medial lemniscus contains impulses from the contralateral lower limb anteriorly and from the contralateral upper limb posteriorly. In the pons, the medial lemniscus gradually shifts laterally and becomes oriented horizontally. At this point, the lower limb is represented laterally and the upper limb medially.

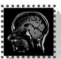

CLINICAL CONNECTION

The level of the dorsal column nuclei and sensory decussation is of medical significance because a unilateral lesion that interrupts the impulses before they decussate, that is, a lesion in the dorsal columns or their nuclei, results in losses of the tactile, vibration, and proprioceptive senses on the ipsilateral side below the level of the lesion. However, a unilateral lesion beyond the sensory decussation, that is, a lesion in the medial lemniscus or subsequent structures in the path, results in the loss of these sensations contralaterally.

THIRD-ORDER NEURONS

The medial lemniscus passes without interruption to the ventral posterolateral (VPL) nucleus of the thalamus. The VPL nucleus is somatotopically organized, so that the contralateral lower limb is represented laterally and the contralateral upper limb medially.

Axons from tertiary somatosensory neurons within the VPL nucleus pass laterally as thalamocortical fibers and enter the posterior limb of the internal capsule where they are located in its more posterior part. They terminate in the primary somatosensory (SI) cortex, which is located in the postcentral gyrus and the adjacent posterior part of the paracentral lobule. The contralateral upper limb is represented approximately in the dorsal half of the postcentral gyrus, and the contralateral lower limb is represented in the posterior part of the paracentral lobule (Fig. 11-4).

SPINAL PAIN AND TEMPERATURE PATHWAYS

Recent anatomic and clinical evidence indicates that the fast and slow pain paths are dissimilar. It is now thought that the fast pain associated with pinprick is carried by a phylogenetically newer pathway often referred to as the **neospinothalamic system.** Slow pain, however, is transmitted by phylogenetically older neurons that form the **paleospinothalamic** and **spinoreticulothalamic systems.** The anatomic differences in these systems are described later.

A series of three neurons transmits fast pain and temperature impulses from the receptors in the periphery to the cerebral cortex where these sensations are perceived (Figs. 11-6, 11-7).

FIRST-ORDER NEURONS

The smaller, slower conducting unipolar neurons in the dorsal root or spinal ganglia are the primary neurons for the pain and temperature impulses carried by the spinal nerves. The central branches of their axons enter the spinal cord through the more lateral parts of the dorsal rootlets (Fig. 2-4), which funnel them into the **dorsolateral fasciculus** or **tract of Lissauer.** On entering this tract, each axon bifurcates into an ascending and a descending branch. These branches extend for one or two segments and give off collateral branches along their entire length. The collaterals enter the gray matter and synapse chiefly in the dorsal horn (laminae I through VI; Figs. 11-7, 11-8).

CLINICAL CONNECTION

The entrance and termination of primary pain fibers in the dorsal horn form the anatomic basis for the relief of pain in neurosurgical destruction of the **dorsal root entry zone (DREZ).** This procedure is especially useful in cases of chronic pain resulting from avulsion of spinal nerves from the cord and in cancer-related pain syndromes.

In some cases of **dorsal rhizotomy,** that is, cutting the dorsal roots to relieve chronic pain, the pain persists. In such cases, the persisting pain can be relieved by a second operation that removes the spinal ganglia. The obvious explanation for this phenomenon is the entrance of pain fibers via the ventral roots. Such aberrant routes have been shown to exist in humans.

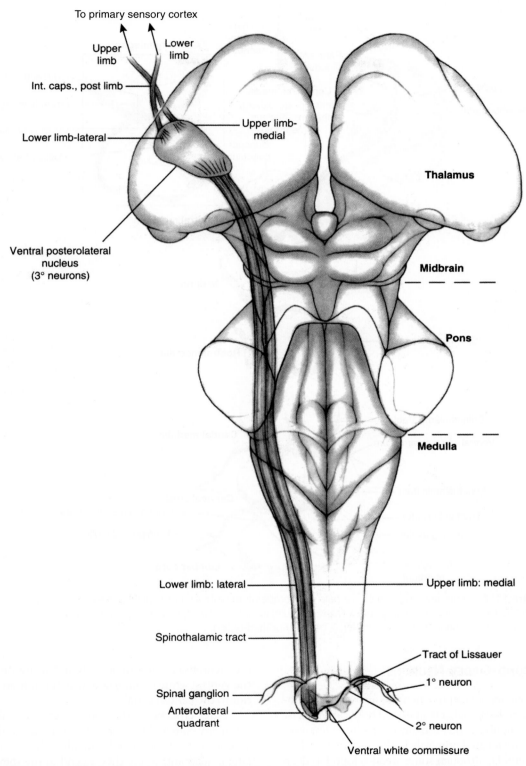

Figure 11-6 Three-dimensional drawing of dorsal view of spinothalamic system (caps, capsule; int, internal; post, posterior; SI, primary somatosensory; 1°, primary or first-order; 2°, secondary or second-order; 3°, tertiary or third-order).

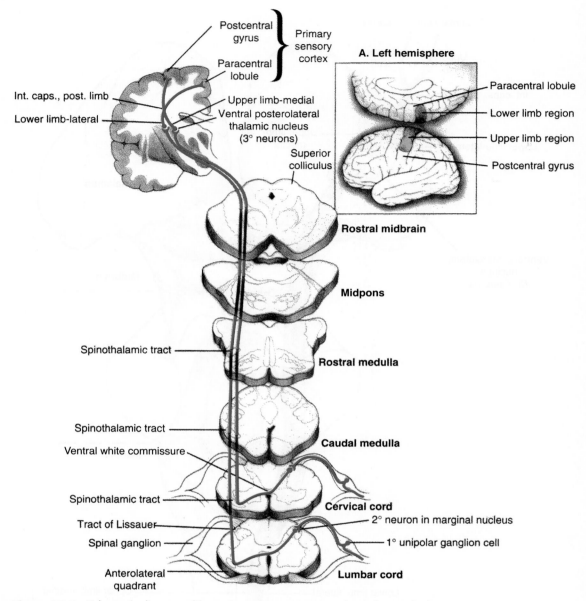

Figure 11-7 Schematic diagram of fast pain and temperature pathway from spinal nerves. **A.** Distribution in primary sensory cortex (caps, capsule; int, internal; post, posterior; 1°, primary or first-order; 2°, secondary or second-order; 3°, tertiary or third-order).

SECOND-ORDER NEURONS

Secondary nociceptive neurons are widely distributed in the spinal gray matter. Those carrying fast pain impulses, and probably temperature impulses also, are located primarily in the marginal nucleus (lamina I), although some are also found as deep as the proper sensory nucleus (laminae IV and V). The axons from the secondary pain and tempera-

ture neurons pass ventromedially and decussate in the ventral white commissure, which is just anterior to the central canal.

After crossing to the contralateral side, the secondary pain and temperature axons pass to the anterior part of the lateral funiculus, the anterolateral quadrant, where they ascend in the spinothalamic tract. Because fibers are added to this tract at its medial surface, somatotopic localization

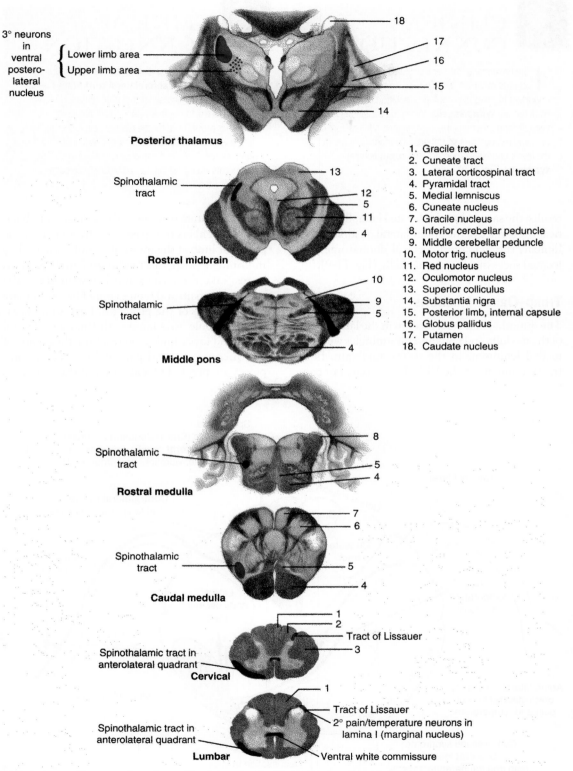

3° neurons in ventral postero-lateral nucleus
{ Lower limb area
  Upper limb area }

18
17
16
15
14

Posterior thalamus

Spinothalamic tract
13
12
5
11
4

Rostral midbrain

Spinothalamic tract
10
9
5
4

Middle pons

Spinothalamic tract
8
5
4

Rostral medulla

Spinothalamic tract
7
6
5
4

Caudal medulla

1
2
Tract of Lissauer
3
Spinothalamic tract in anterolateral quadrant
Cervical

1
Tract of Lissauer
2° pain/temperature neurons in lamina I (marginal nucleus)
Spinothalamic tract in anterolateral quadrant
Lumbar
Ventral white commissure

1. Gracile tract
2. Cuneate tract
3. Lateral corticospinal tract
4. Pyramidal tract
5. Medial lemniscus
6. Cuneate nucleus
7. Gracile nucleus
8. Inferior cerebellar peduncle
9. Middle cerebellar peduncle
10. Motor trig. nucleus
11. Red nucleus
12. Oculomotor nucleus
13. Superior colliculus
14. Substantia nigra
15. Posterior limb, internal capsule
16. Globus pallidus
17. Putamen
18. Caudate nucleus

Figure 11-8 Transverse sections of brainstem and spinal cord showing relations of fast pain and temperature pathway from spinal nerves (trig, trigeminal; 2°, secondary or second-order; 3°, tertiary or third-order).

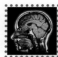

results: the sacral fibers are located laterally, that is, near the surface of the anterolateral quadrant. The lumbar, thoracic, and cervical dermatomes are located successively most medially (Fig. 11-9).

THIRD-ORDER NEURONS

The spinothalamic tract ascends in the lateral parts of the medulla and pons and intermingles with the medial lemniscus in the rostral midbrain. Both tracts terminate in the VPL. The tertiary fast pain

and temperature neurons in the VPL give off thalamocortical fibers that pass laterally and enter the posterior limb of the internal capsule, where they intermingle with the tactile and limb position axons. Like the tertiary touch system fibers, the tertiary fast pain and temperature fibers terminate in those parts of the postcentral gyrus and paracentral lobule associated with the contralateral upper and lower limbs. On reaching these parts of the SI cortex, the fast pain and temperature impulses are precisely localized, and the sharpness

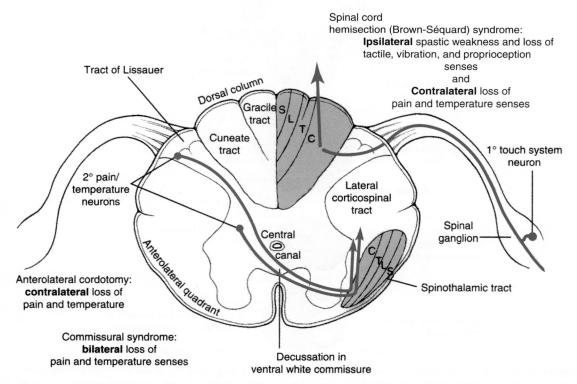

Figure 11-9. Spinal cord somatosensory and motor pathways and their clinical syndromes (C, cervical; L, lumbar; S, sacral; T, thoracic; 1°, primary or first-order; 2°, secondary or second-order).

and intensity of the pinprick stimuli and the warmth or coldness of the temperature sensations are perceived.

CLINICAL SIGNIFICANCE OF SPINAL SOMATOSENSORY PATHWAYS

Within the spinal cord, the somatosensory paths are located in the dorsal columns and the anterolateral quadrants. Axons in the dorsal columns transmit the tactile, pressure, vibration, and proprioception impulses (Table 11-3). The more medial gracile tract conducts these types of discriminative impulses from the spinal nerves below midthoracic levels (Fig. 11-9), i.e., chiefly from the lower limb. The more lateral cuneate tract conducts the discriminative impulses from the spinal nerves above midthoracic levels, i.e., chiefly from the upper limb. The axons of both of these dorsal column tracts arise from large, first-order neurons in the dorsal root or spinal ganglia on the same side. Hence, a unilateral lesion of the dorsal column results in an ipsilateral loss of tactile, pressure, vibration, and proprioception in the parts of the body supplied by the spinal nerves below the level of the lesion.

The anterolateral quadrants contain the spinothalamic tracts that transmit pain and temperature impulses (Table 11-3). The axons of the

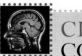

CLINICAL CONNECTION

Severe degeneration of the dorsal columns accompanied by loss of the discriminative touch, vibratory, and proprioceptive senses commonly occurs in **tabes dorsalis,** a syndrome resulting from syphilitic infection of the large-diameter axons and their ganglion cells. The dorsal column degeneration and sensory losses also occur in cases of pernicious anemia. Degeneration of the more medial parts of the gracile tract, i.e., the sacral and lower lumbar portions, occurs in lesions involving the dorsal roots in the cauda equina.

spinothalamic tract arise from second-order neurons in the contralateral dorsal horn. As a result, the spinothalamic tract transmits pain and temperature impulses from the opposite side.

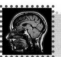

CLINICAL CONNECTION

The **Brown-Séquard** syndrome results from a lesion involving either the right or left half of the spinal cord. The cardinal manifestation of this spinal cord hemisection is alternating somatosensory loss below the level of the lesion. The touch, vibration, and proprioceptive senses are lost on the same side, and pain and temperature senses are lost on the opposite side (Fig. 11-9).

TABLE 11-3   Comparison of Dorsal Columns and Anterolateral Quadrants of Spinal Cord

	Dorsal Columns	Anterolateral Quadrants
Sensory components	Tactile, vibration, and proprioception	Pain and temperature
Major tracts	Gracile and cuneate	Spinothalamic
Origins of tracts	Ipsilateral spinal ganglia Below midthoracic: gracile Above midthoracic: cuneate	Contralateral dorsal horn at all levels
Results of damage	Ipsilateral loss—tactile, vibration, and proprioception	Contralateral loss—pain and temperature
Medical importance	Hemisected cord (Brown-Séquard syndrome): below level of lesion Contralateral pain and temperature Ipsilateral tactile, vibration, and proprioception Also, ipsilateral lower limb spastic paralysis, Babinski sign, and so forth (because of lateral corticospinal tract interruption)	

GENERAL SENSATIONS FROM THE HEAD

General sensations from the face, anterior scalp, orbit, oral and nasal cavities, sinuses, teeth, and supratentorial dura are conducted chiefly in the trigeminal nerve. The facial, glossopharyngeal, and vagus nerves contain small numbers of somatosensory fibers that are distributed to the external ear, the posterior part of the tongue, and the tonsillar region. The primary somatosensory neurons are unipolar ganglion cells in the trigeminal ganglion of cranial nerve (CN) V, the geniculate ganglion of CN VII, the superior (petrosal) ganglion of CN IX, and the superior (jugular) ganglion of CN X. The central connections of all the cranial nerve somatosensory fibers are made with the trigeminal sensory nuclei.

TRIGEMINAL SENSORY NUCLEI

A continuous nuclear column related to somatosensory impulses extends from the level of the superior colliculus caudad through the brainstem and the entire spinal cord. At spinal levels, this nuclear column is represented by the dorsal horn laminae and nuclei that conduct pain and temperature sensations. In the brainstem, this nuclear column is represented by the sensory trigeminal nuclei (Fig. 11-10).

At midpontine levels, where the trigeminal nerve enters, the principal trigeminal nucleus is located. Extending caudally from this nucleus is the spinal trigeminal nucleus, which becomes continuous with the dorsal horn of the spinal cord. The spinal trigeminal nucleus consists of three parts: oral, interpolar, and caudal. The oral and interpolar parts are chiefly associated with trigeminal reflexes related to blinking, lacrimation, and salivation. The caudal part is associated primarily with pain and temperature impulses from the face.

The primary neurons for proprioceptive reflexes from the muscles of mastication, teeth, periodontal membrane, and the external ocular muscles form the mesencephalic trigeminal nucleus. This nucleus extends rostrally from the principal trigeminal nucleus to the level of the superior colliculus as a slender column of unipolar ganglion-like cells located in the lateral part of the periaqueductal gray matter. Accompanying it is the mesencephalic trigeminal tract, formed by the axons of this nucleus, which emerge from the brainstem in the motor root of the trigeminal nerve. The central connections of the mesencephalic trigeminal nucleus are primarily with the motor trigeminal nucleus and form monosynaptic reflexes associated with control of the force of bite and chewing.

CRANIAL TOUCH AND PROPRIOCEPTION PATHWAYS

Touch impulses from mechanoreceptors in the head are conducted centrally, chiefly in the trigeminal nerve. Central connections are made with trigeminal nuclei, and the impulses ascend via the trigeminothalamic system. Three neurons transmit the impulses from the receptor to the cerebral cortex (Figs. 11-10, 11-11).

FIRST-ORDER NEURONS

The primary trigeminal touch system neurons are large unipolar cells in the trigeminal (CN V) ganglion. The central branches of their axons approach the pons in the sensory root of the trigeminal nerve and pass dorsomedially toward the pontine tegmentum (Fig. 11-12A).

SECOND-ORDER NEURONS

The primary trigeminal touch system axons terminate on secondary neurons in the principal trigeminal nucleus. Axons from most of these secondary somatosensory neurons cross at midpontine levels and ascend in the contralateral trigeminothalamic tract, sometimes called the ventral trigeminal tract. A small number of axons that ascend ipsilaterally from the second-order neurons in the principal trigeminal nucleus form the dorsal trigeminal tract. The clinical significance of this tract is not known.

THIRD-ORDER NEURONS

The secondary trigeminothalamic fibers terminate in the ventral posteromedial (VPM) nucleus. Within the VPM the oral cavity is represented medially and facial structures laterally. Tertiary trigeminal touch system neurons in the VPM send thalamocortical axons via the posterior limb of the internal capsule to the ventral part of the postcentral gyrus, the SI cortex face area, where the type of sensation and its precise localization are perceived.

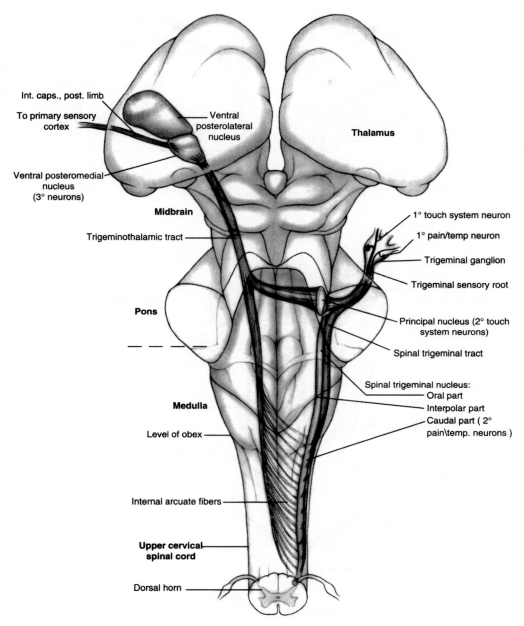

Int. caps., post. limb

To primary sensory
cortex

Ventral
posterolateral
nucleus

Thalamus

Ventral posteromedial
nucleus
(3° neurons)

Midbrain

Trigeminothalamic tract

1° touch system neuron

1° pain/temp neuron

Trigeminal ganglion

Trigeminal sensory root

Pons

Principal nucleus (2° touch
system neurons)

Spinal trigeminal tract

Spinal trigeminal nucleus:
Oral part
Interpolar part
Caudal part (2°
pain\temp. neurons)

Medulla

Level of obex

Internal arcuate fibers

**Upper cervical
spinal cord**

Dorsal horn

Figure 11-10   Three-dimensional drawing of a dorsal view of somatosensory pathways from cranial nerves (caps, capsule; int, internal; post, posterior; temp, temperature; 1°, primary or first-order; 2°, secondary or second-order; 3°, tertiary or third-order).

CRANIAL PAIN AND TEMPERATURE PATHWAYS

A series of three neurons transmit fast pain and temperature impulses from the cranial nerve nociceptors and thermoreceptors to the cerebral cortex where they are perceived (Figs. 11-10, 11-11).

FIRST-ORDER NEURONS

Smaller unipolar neurons in the trigeminal ganglion transmit pain and temperature impulses. The central branches of the axons of these unipolar trigeminal ganglion cells enter the pons via the sensory root of the trigeminal nerve and pass

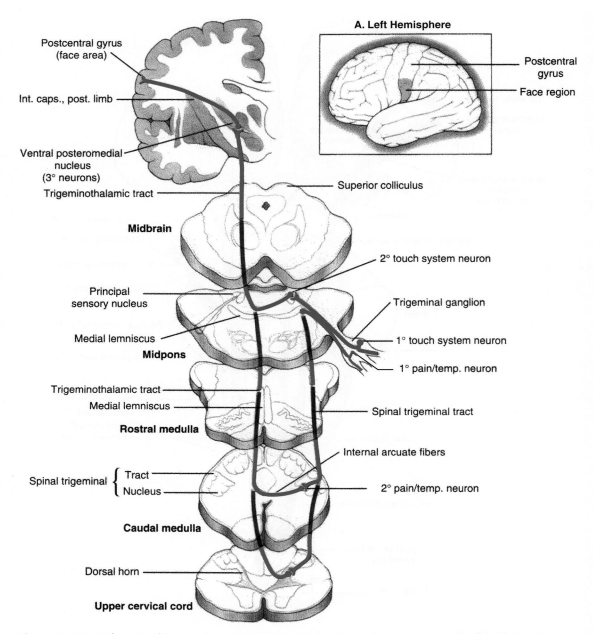

Figure 11-11 Schematic diagram of somatosensory pathways from cranial nerves. **A.** Distribution in primary sensory cortex (caps, capsule; int, internal; post, posterior; temp, temperature; 1°, primary or first-order; 2°, secondary or second-order; 3°, tertiary or third-order).

dorsomedial at the junction of the middle cerebellar peduncle and basilar part of the pons (Fig. 11-12B). On reaching the pontine tegmentum, they form a conspicuous bundle, the spinal trigeminal tract, which descends through the pons and medulla and intermingles with the dorsolateral tract of Lissauer in the upper cervical segments of the spinal cord.

Pain and temperature impulses from the facial, glossopharyngeal, and vagus nerves have as their primary neurons small unipolar cells in their respective ganglia, namely, the geniculate of CN VII, the superior (petrosal) of CN IX, and the superior (jugular) of CN X. The central branches of their axons enter the brainstem with their respective nerves and join the spinal trigeminal tract.

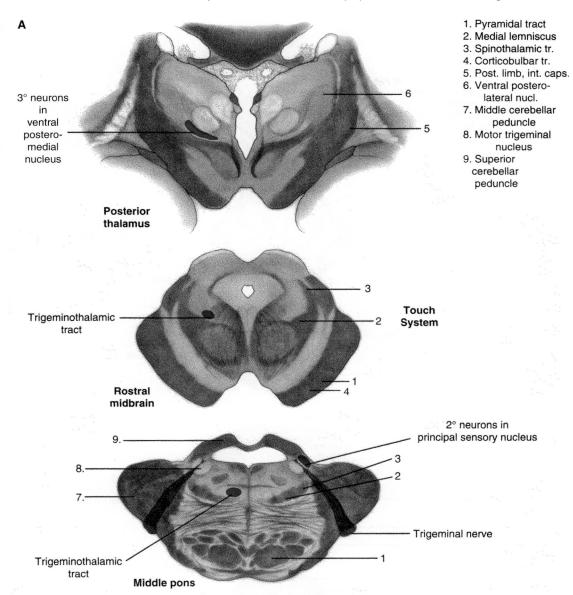

A

3° neurons in ventral postero-medial nucleus

Posterior thalamus

1. Pyramidal tract
2. Medial lemniscus
3. Spinothalamic tr.
4. Corticobulbar tr.
5. Post. limb, int. caps.
6. Ventral postero-lateral nucl.
7. Middle cerebellar peduncle
8. Motor trigeminal nucleus
9. Superior cerebellar peduncle

Trigeminothalamic tract

Touch System

Rostral midbrain

2° neurons in principal sensory nucleus

Trigeminal nerve

Trigeminothalamic tract

Middle pons

Figure 11-12 Transverse sections of brainstem showing relations of somatosensory pathways from cranial nerves. **A.** Touch system. (*continued*)

SECOND-ORDER NEURONS

The primary pain and temperature fibers descending in the spinal trigeminal tract terminate in the caudal part of the spinal trigeminal nucleus. This caudal subnucleus extends from the level of the obex to the spinal cord, where it becomes continuous with the dorsal horn. Interruption of the spinal trigeminal tract anywhere from its origin in the midpons inferiorly to the level of the obex results in complete loss of pain and temperature sensations on the ipsilateral side of the face and anterior scalp.

Second-order pain and temperature neurons in the caudal part of the spinal trigeminal nucleus and the adjacent reticular formation give rise to axons that cross the midline and ascend in the trigeminothalamic tract. This tract is located in the reticular formation near the upper limb part of the medial lemniscus at medullary, pontine, and midbrain levels and is sometimes called the ventral trigeminal tract.

B

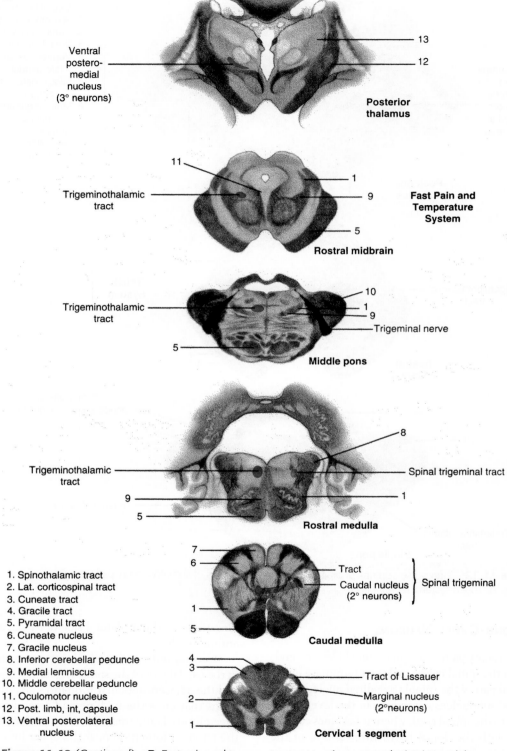

Ventral postero-medial nucleus (3° neurons)

13

12

Posterior thalamus

11

Trigeminothalamic tract

1

9

5

Fast Pain and Temperature System

Rostral midbrain

10

Trigeminothalamic tract

1

9

Trigeminal nerve

5

Middle pons

8

Trigeminothalamic tract

Spinal trigeminal tract

9

1

5

Rostral medulla

7

6

Tract

Caudal nucleus (2° neurons)

} Spinal trigeminal

1

5

Caudal medulla

1. Spinothalamic tract
2. Lat. corticospinal tract
3. Cuneate tract
4. Gracile tract
5. Pyramidal tract
6. Cuneate nucleus
7. Gracile nucleus
8. Inferior cerebellar peduncle
9. Medial lemniscus
10. Middle cerebellar peduncle
11. Oculomotor nucleus
12. Post. limb, int, capsule
13. Ventral posterolateral nucleus

4

3

Tract of Lissauer

2

Marginal nucleus (2°neurons)

1

Cervical 1 segment

Figure 11-12 (*Continued*) **B.** Fast pain and temperature system (caps, capsule; int, internal; lat, lateral; nucl, nucleus; post, posterior; tr, tract; 1°, primary or first-order; 2°, secondary or second-order; 3°, tertiary or third-order).

CLINICAL CONNECTION

Spinal trigeminal tractotomy has been used for the relief of the spontaneous, excruciating pain that occurs in cases of **trigeminal neuralgia** or **tic douloureux.** The advantage of surgically transecting the tract in the medulla at the level of the obex is that the facial pain is alleviated and the **corneal reflex** is spared. In the absence of the corneal reflex, which moistens and cleanses the cornea, infection and ulceration of the cornea may occur. The corneal reflex comprises an afferent limb, the trigeminal nerve, and an efferent limb, the facial nerve. This reflex is elicited when the cornea is touched with a wisp of cotton, thereby stimulating nociceptors whose cell bodies are in the trigeminal ganglion. The afferent corneal reflex impulses descend as pain fibers in the spinal trigeminal tract which, at levels rostral to the obex, give collateral branches that synapse in the oral or interpolar part of the spinal trigeminal nucleus. Connections are then made, via the reticular formation, with the facial nuclei bilaterally. The efferent limb consists of the facial nerve fibers that supply the orbicularis oculi muscles. A small unilateral lesion in the lateral parts of the medulla or caudal half of the pons at any level may interrupt the spinal trigeminal and spinothalamic tracts. In such cases, the patient loses pain and temperature sensations on the ipsilateral side in the face and on the contralateral side in the limbs, trunk, neck, and back of the head.

CLINICAL CONNECTION

Caudal to midpontine levels, the trigeminothalamic tract is almost exclusively conducting pain and temperature impulses from the contralateral side of the face. At more rostral levels, the trigeminothalamic tract conducts all types of somatosensory impulses from the contralateral face.

THIRD-ORDER NEURONS

The secondary fast pain and temperature axons in the trigeminothalamic tract terminate in the VPM nucleus. Tertiary VPM neurons send thalamocortical axons via the posterior limb of the internal capsule to the facial region of the SI cortex, which is located in the ventral part of the postcentral gyrus.

PHYSIOLOGY OF SOMATOSENSATIONS

SURROUND INHIBITION

Somatosensory information about tactile, temperature, and nociceptive input remains functionally segregated in the ascending somatosensory pathways and in the relay through spinal cord, brainstem, and thalamic nuclei before being integrated in the cerebral cortex. Maintaining the resolution of somatosensory transmission in the successive relay nuclei is accomplished by surround inhibition. For example, stimulation of two spatially adjacent areas of the tip of the finger activates separate and overlapping populations of relay neurons. Relay neurons receiving convergent two-point tactile input are subsequently inhibited, thereby maintaining the spatial fidelity of the two stimuli. This phenomenon of surround inhibition is the basis for two-point discrimination.

SOMATOSENSORY CORTICAL PROCESSING

Exteroceptive and proprioceptive information reaches the SI cortex largely unaltered as it is transmitted through the brainstem and thalamus. Processing of somatosensory information occurs within vertical columns of SI cortical neurons. All neurons in a column respond to stimulation of a unique peripheral receptive field. Adjacent columns are activated by different sensory stimuli from spatially contiguous receptive fields, thereby forming the sensory homunculus, for example, the composite of all mechanoreceptor inputs from the distal tip of one digit. The highest resolution of somatosensory input occurs in the most anterior part of the postcentral gyrus in the depth of the central sulcus. In progressively more posterior parts of the SI cortex, the individual receptive fields become functionally integrated. In the associational superior parietal cortex posterior to the SI cortex, somatosensory information converges with other sensory modalities and is an important area for helping to guide voluntary movements.

CLINICAL IMPLICATIONS OF SOMATOSENSORY PATHWAYS

A synopsis of the somatosensory CNS paths (Fig. 11-13) and the somatosensory abnormalities resulting from unilateral lesions at various levels

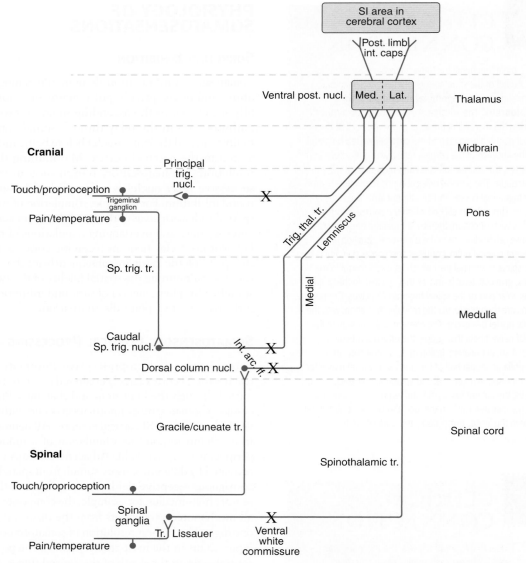

Figure 11-13   Synopsis of somatosensory paths (arc, arcuate; caps, capsule; ff, fibers; int, internal; lat, lateral; med, medial; nucl, nucleus; post, posterior; SI, primary somatosensory; sp, spinal; thal, thalamic; tr, tract; trig, trigeminal).

(Fig. 11-14) are exemplified by the case histories at the beginning of this chapter.

In the first patient, an alternating somatosensory loss is located below the umbilicus: touch, pressure, and limb position of the right side and pain and temperature on the left side. These losses result from interruption of the dorsal column and anterolateral quadrant, respectively, on the right side at the T10 spinal cord level. Only in the spinal cord can a unilateral lesion result in this alternating somatosensory loss.

The second patient has loss of pinprick and temperature sensations on the left side in the limbs, trunk, neck, and back of the head, and on the right side in the face and anterior part of the scalp. These losses result from interruption of the spinothalamic tract and spinal trigeminal tract, respectively, on the right side at some level between midpons and the obex in the medulla. Only in the lateral parts of the caudal pons and rostral medulla can a unilateral lesion result in an alternating pain and temperature loss.

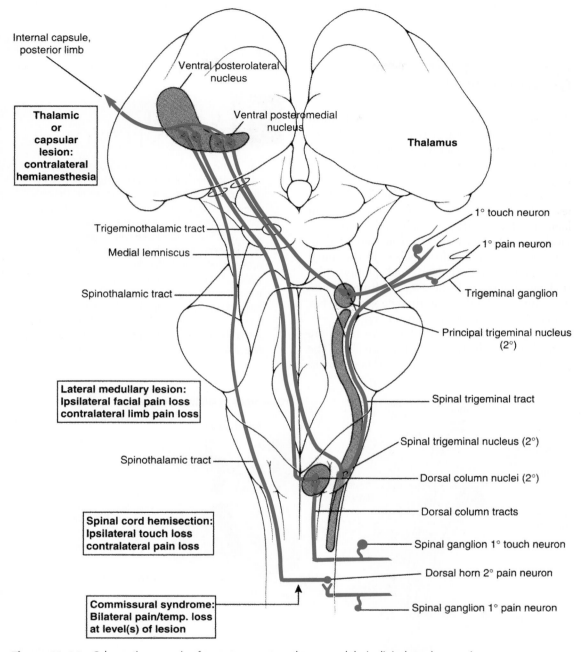

Figure 11-14 Schematic synopsis of somatosensory pathways and their clinical syndromes (temp, temperature; 1°, primary or first-order; 2°, secondary or second-order; 3°, tertiary or third-order).

In the third patient, left hemianesthesia (excluding slow pain) manifests as a result of interruption of the somatosensory structures on the right side. The spinal and trigeminal somatosensory systems intermingle with each other in the forebrain paths. Thus, the paths are together in the ventral posterior thalamic nucleus. As a result, a unilateral lesion in this structure results in a contralateral hemianesthesia. Likewise, a capsular lesion involving the posterior limb will result in contralateral hemianesthesia, but this will be accompanied by contralateral spastic hemiplegia as a result of involvement of the adjacent pyramidal tract.

CENTRAL CONNECTIONS OF SLOW PAIN

Slow pain from spinal nerves is transmitted within the CNS by the phylogenetically older and more diffuse pathways commonly referred to as the paleospinothalamic and spinoreticulothalamic systems (Fig. 11-15).

Most paleospinothalamic neuronal cell bodies are in lamina V. Most nociceptive neurons in laminae VII and VIII, especially in the upper cervical segments, give rise to the spinoreticulothalamic system of slow pain impulses. In the spinal cord, the paleospinothalamic and spinoreticulothalamic tracts are located in the anterolateral quadrants, where they intermingle with the fast pain fibers of the neospinothalamic system.

In the brainstem, the slow pain fibers are located more medially than the fast pain fibers. The paleospinothalamic fibers have collateral axons

that synapse in the medullary reticular formation where they overlap with the synapses of large numbers of spinoreticular fibers. These two inputs to the reticular formation form a massive multisynaptic reticulothalamic system that chiefly projects noci-

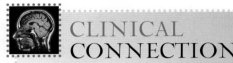

CLINICAL CONNECTION

The immediate result of anterolateral cordotomy is complete loss of all pain (and temperature) senses contralaterally and below the level of the lesion. This complete loss occurs because both the fast and the slow pain fibers are located in the anterolateral quadrants of the spinal cord. Such is not the case in the brainstem where the fast pain fibers ascend in the spinothalamic tract, which is located laterally, whereas the slow pain fibers ascend more medially. Therefore, interruption of the spinothalamic tract in the brainstem results in decreased sensitivity and localization of fast pain, i.e., pinprick (and temperature sense), but not the loss of slow pain. In fact, discrete lesions in the spinothalamic tract in the brainstem may result in agonizing intractable chronic pain of the so-called thalamic type.

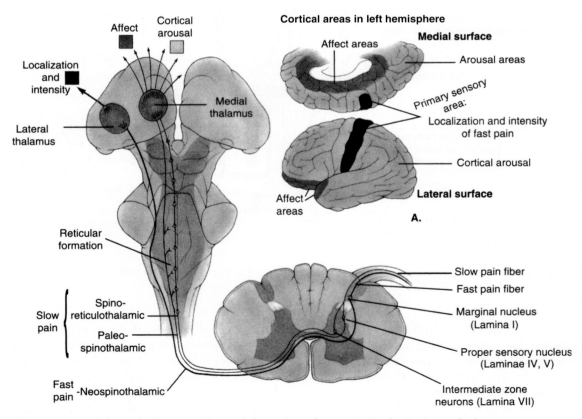

Figure 11-15   Schematic diagram of fast and slow pain pathways. **A.** Distribution in cerebral cortex.

ceptive impulses to more medial parts of the thalamus, which then project to widespread regions of the cerebral cortex.

There is no perception of the pain associated with tissue damage in the SI cortex. The perception of slow pain in other cortical areas accounts for the awareness of pain in contralateral parts of the body in patients with internal capsule or SI cortex damage. Although specific nociceptive functions cannot be located in the cerebral cortex, other than the SI area where the localization and intensity of fast pain occur, the function of other cortical areas can be postulated on the basis of their thalamocortical connections. Thus, it appears that:

1. Intralaminar nuclear connections to widespread cortical areas play a role in cortical arousal and attention.
2. Medial nuclear projections to parts of the limbic system, such as the orbitofrontal cortex and the anterior parts of the cingulate gyrus and insula, are responsible for the affective responses to pain (anguish, depression, fear, anger).

In general, therefore, the cortical areas receiving nociceptive impulses from the lateral part of the thalamus perceive the sensory discriminative aspects of pain, whereas those areas receiving nociceptive impulses from the medial part of the thalamus are for the arousal, attention, affective, and motivational aspects of pain. The peripheral ner-

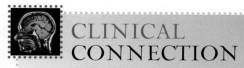

vous system (PNS) and CNS structures and their functional roles in fast and slow pain systems are summarized in Table 11-4. Although information on the central connections and paths of cranial slow pain is meager, it is reasonable to assume that they are similar to those of the paleospinothalamic and spinoreticulothalamic systems, i.e., reticular formation to medial thalamus and then to widespread areas of the cerebral cortex.

PAIN MODULATION

The anatomic features of exogenous and endogenous modulation of the spinal pain paths are fairly well known. In both cases, the interneurons that form the substantia gelatinosa (lamina II) and more ventral laminae (III, IV, and V) of the dorsal horn play a key role (Fig. 11-16). These interneurons act on secondary slow pain neurons and, through their action, the excitability of the sec-

TABLE 11-4 Summary of Spinal Pain Paths

		Fast Pain	Slow Pain
PNS	Nociceptors Nerve fibers	Aδ mechanical Small myelinated (5–30 m/s)	C-polymodal (tissue damage) Unmyelinated (0.5–2 m/s)

CNS	Tracts:
	  Origins
		Neospinothalamic:
		  Marginal nucleus (L I)
		  Proper nucleus (L V)
			Paleospinothalamic:
			  Proper nucleus (L V)
			  Intermediate zone (L VII)
			Spinoreticulothalamic:
			  Intermediate zone (L VII)
			  Anterior horn (L VIII)

	Thalamic terminations	Lateral thalamus (VPL)	Medial thalamus Hypothalamus
	Cortical terminations	SI area	Frontal lobe Limbic lobe
	Functions	Localization and sharpness	Cortical arousal Affect

CNS, central nervous system; L, lamina; PNS, peripheral nervous system; SI, primary somatosensory; VPL, ventral posterolateral.

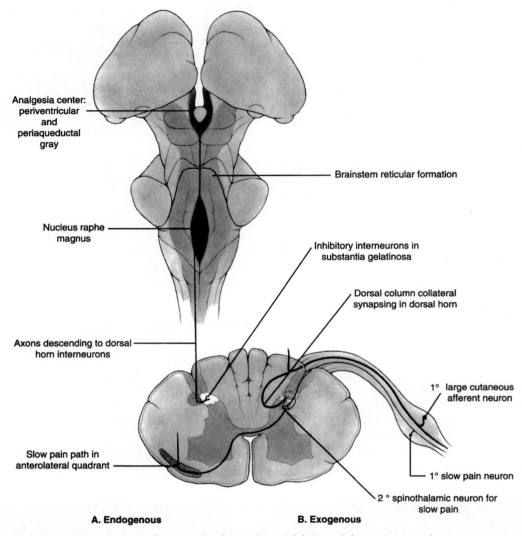

Figure 11-16   Schematic diagram of pathways for modulation of slow pain. **A.** Endogenous; **B.** Exogenous (1°, primary or first-order; 2°, secondary or second-order).

ondary slow pain neurons can be altered to prevent the transmission of pain impulses to higher centers.

EXOGENOUS CONTROL

Large cutaneous afferent nerve fibers conducting touch impulses are able to modulate pain through massive connections with substantia gelatinosa and other dorsal horn neurons. These connections occur via branches of the touch fibers ascending in the dorsal columns. This phenomenon is the basis for the clinical control of chronic pain by TENS. The treatment produces selective activation of the larger cutaneous touch fibers that result in **analgesia**

as a result of activation of the spinal interneurons that inhibit the secondary slow pain neurons.

ENDOGENOUS CONTROL

Groups of neurons in the periaqueductal gray of the rostral midbrain and the periventricular gray of the adjacent diencephalon, on electrical or neural stimulation or the administration of opiates, produce analgesia. Such modulation of pain occurs through connections of this analgesia center with neurons of the nucleus raphe magnus and other reticular formation neurons near the pontomedullary junction. Axons descend from these reticular formation nuclei to the region of the substantia gelatinosa and secondary spinal pain neurons and inhibit the transmission of ascending pain impulses.

This endogenous pain modulation system is used clinically for the relief of some types of chronic pain. The procedure involves the surgical implantation of a stimulating electrode into the analgesia center. The stimulation is controlled by the patient through the use of a battery-powered stimulation unit. The duration of the chronic pain relief is extremely variable but, through this procedure, the patient can obtain relief as often as necessary.

Chapter Review Questions

11-1.   What are the three tactile mechanoreceptors and which is most sensitive?

11-2.   How is the intensity of a cutaneous stimulus transmitted from the receptor into the CNS?

11-3.   A receptive field defines what physiologic aspect of a somatosensory receptor?

11-4.   How is a mechanical stimulus transduced to an electrical signal by an encapsulated mechanoreceptor?

11-5.   What is sensory adaptation?

11-6.   What is the functional importance of surround inhibition in the transmission of somatosensory information?

11-7.   How do the fast and slow pain pathways differ in the forebrain?

11-8.   What is the basis for the relief of pain by transcutaneous electric nerve stimulation (TENS)?

11-9.   Name and locate the general somatic sensory losses anticipated as a result of the following:

a. rupture of disc into left intervertebral foramen between LV5 and SV1
b. left hemisection of spinal cord at T10
c. ventral white commissure from T2 to T4
d. left lateral third of medulla at the obex
e. right medial third of medulla near the pontomedullary junction
f. left ventral posterior nucleus
g. right paracentral lobule

CHAPTER 12

The Auditory System: Deafness

> **A MIDDLE-AGED WOMAN** complains of dizziness, loss of hearing in the left ear, and a sagging of the left side of the face, all of which have gradually become more severe during the past 6 months.

The paths conveying auditory impulses are organized in such a manner that nerve impulses must pass through at least four neurons to reach the cerebral cortex: the first neuron is in a ganglion of cranial nerve (CN) VIII, the second is in the caudal brainstem, the third is in the rostral brainstem, and the fourth is in the thalamus. Unlike other sensory systems, the central auditory paths have bilateral representation of sounds, i.e., input from both ears reaches the auditory cortex in both hemispheres.

THE EAR

The ear, a vestibulocochlear organ concerned with hearing and equilibrium, consists of three parts: external, middle, and internal (Fig. 12-1). The external ear includes the auricle or pinna, the external acoustic meatus, and the tympanic membrane (eardrum). The auricle gathers the sound waves, and the external acoustic meatus amplifies and directs the waves to the tympanic membrane. The tympanic membrane, the partition between the external and middle parts of the ear, is set into vibration by the sound waves.

The middle ear, or tympanic cavity, is an air-filled space in the temporal bone. The middle ear contains three **auditory ossicles** and two small muscles. The malleus, incus, and stapes are the auditory ossicles. The malleus is attached to the inter-nal surface of the tympanic membrane and to the incus. The incus articulates with the stapes. The vibrations of the tympanic membrane are transferred to the malleus and then conducted through the incus and stapes to the internal ear. Sound vibrations can also be conducted to the internal ear by the temporal bone. This phenomenon, **bone conduction,** is far less efficient than the conduction via the ossicles in the middle ear.

Movements of the ossicles may be dampened reflexly by the two small muscles in the middle ear. The tensor tympani muscle, innervated by the trigeminal nerve, is attached to the malleus. This tensor muscle dampens low tones by pulling the malleus internally, thereby increasing the tension on the tympanic membrane. The stapedius muscle, innervated by the facial nerve, is attached to the stapes. This muscle decreases sound intensity by pulling the stapes away from the opening into the internal ear.

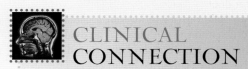

CLINICAL CONNECTION

A lesion of the facial nerve proximal to its branches to the stapedius muscle results in hyperacusis, abnormally loud sounds in the affected ear.

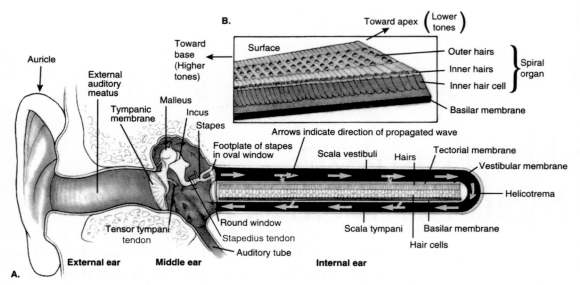

Figure 12-1   Principal parts of the auditory apparatus. **A.** The external, middle, and internal parts of the ear. **B.** Surface and side view of the basilar membrane and spiral organ, which increases in width from base to apex.

The internal ear is located in the temporal bone and consists of fluid-filled spaces that form the bony and membranous labyrinths. The **bony labyrinth** contains **perilymph** and consists of vestibular parts that are described in Chapter 13 and an auditory part, the **cochlea.** The **membranous labyrinth** is located within the bony labyrinth and is composed of a series of connecting ducts filled with **endolymph.**

The cochlea, so named because it is shaped like the shell of a snail, consists of three fluid-filled spaces: scala vestibuli, scala tympani, and cochlear duct (Fig. 12-2). The scalae vestibuli and tympani, partially enclosed in bone, are parts of the bony labyrinth, contain perilymph, and are continuous with each other at the helicotrema (Fig. 12-1). The cochlear duct is part of the membranous labyrinth and, therefore, contains endolymph. The **vestibular,** or **Reissner membrane,** separates the scala vestibuli and cochlear duct, whereas the basilar membrane separates the scala tympani and cochlear duct.

Two openings or windows are located between the cochlea and the middle ear: the **oval window** into the scala vestibuli and the **round window** into the scala tympani (Fig. 12-1). The footplate of the stapes occupies the oval window; the round window is occupied by a flexible membrane. When the stapes moves inward, the round window moves outward, and vice versa. The in-ward and outward movements of the stapes produce perilymphatic pressure waves between the scala vestibuli and the scala tympani and set the cochlear duct into motion. Because the cochlear duct rests on the basilar membrane, it, too, is set into motion. Movement of the basilar membrane stimulates the auditory receptors located on this membrane.

Tonotopic localization occurs in the basilar membrane, which increases in width from its base, the part nearest the oval window, to its apex at the end of the two and one-half coils (Fig. 12-1). In addition, the structure of the basilar membrane is such that its narrow end is taut but its wide end is more flexible. Consequently, the highest frequencies set the base in motion, whereas the lowest frequencies set the apex in motion.

AUDITORY RECEPTORS

The **spiral organ (of Corti)** consists of neuroepithelial receptor and supporting cells (Fig. 12-4A). The neuroepithelial receptor cells are classified as inner and outer hair cells. The inner hair cells are arranged in a single row, whereas the outer hair cells increase from three rows at the base of the cochlea to four or five rows at the apex (Fig. 12-1B). Of the 16,000 hair cells in each cochlea, about one fourth are inner hair cells and about three-fourths outer hair cells. Projecting from the free surface of

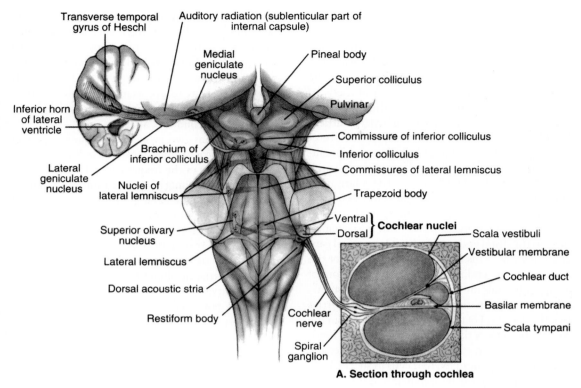

Figure 12-2 Three-dimensional dorsal view of auditory pathways. **A.** Transverse section through cochlea.

the hair cells are stereocilia of varying lengths. The tips of the longest stereocilia are in contact with or actually embedded in the overlying tectorial membrane. Therefore, when the basilar membrane is moved by fluid movement in the scala tympani, the stereocilia bend, resulting in changes in the membrane potentials of their hair cells.

The inner and outer hair cells are innervated by primary auditory neurons in the spiral ganglion. At least 90% of these neurons synapse on the inner hair cells. Each inner hair cell has a 1:1 synaptic relationship with as many as 20 spiral ganglion cells, thereby playing the major role in tonotopic discrimination.

The outer hair cells are innervated by relatively few spiral ganglion cells, each of which synapses with more than 10 outer hair cells. The outer hair cells are also innervated by efferent olivocochlear fibers that arise from the superior olivary nucleus in the pons. Olivocochlear stimulation results in increased heights of the outer hair cells and increased stiffness of their stereocilia. Both of these influence basilar membrane motion and, therefore, spiral organ function.

COCHLEAR RECEPTION AND TRANSDUCTION OF AUDITORY STIMULI

Transduction of auditory stimuli from airborne pressure waves to electrical signals propagated to the brain is a multistep process beginning at the tympanic membrane. The energy from airborne pressure waves is converted to mechanical energy by vibration of the tympanic membrane and the resultant sequential movements of the malleus, incus, and stapes. The movement of the stapes pulls or pushes against the oval window of the inner ear, creating sinusoidal pressure waves in the perilymph in the scala vestibuli and then the scala tympani. These fluid-borne pressure waves cause the basilar membrane to move up or down. Hair cell receptors sense the vibration of the basilar membrane through the tufts of stereocilia on the surface of each hair cell receptor. These tufts of stereocilia are organized by height in a stepped manner with the tallest stereocilia oriented in the direction toward the end of the tectorial membrane. Pressure waves displace the basilar membrane and cause the hair cell stereocilia to bend as the result of their attachment to the overlying tectorial membrane. The stereocilia are directionally sensitive so that when the basilar membrane moves upward toward the scala vestibuli, the stereocilia are bent and the hair cells are depolarized. Movement of the basilar membrane downward toward the scala tympani results in the hair cells being hyperpolarized. Depolarization results from the bending stereocilia opening ionic channels in the apical membrane, leading to the influx of K+ from endolymph in the scala media. The K+-evoked depolarization opens voltage-gated Ca2+ channels in the base of the hair cells that triggers the presynaptic vesicular release of neurotransmitter onto postsynaptic sites on the distal ends of dendrites from spiral ganglion neurons. This leads to the activation of the afferent nerve endings and the propagation of action potentials into the central nervous system.

A change in the biomechanical properties (width, elasticity) of the basilar membrane from the base to the apex of the cochlea underlies the tonotopic organization of auditory inputs. Progressing from the base to the apex, hair cells in successively small segments of the basilar membrane are selectively responsive to high (20 kHz) and to low (20 Hz) frequency sounds (Fig. 12-3). A simple

sound such as that generated by a single piano key activates hair cells in a single very small segment of the basilar membrane and a corresponding limited number of primary auditory afferents. Complex sounds such as those generated by speech or music activate receptors in multiple and different segments of the basilar membrane and different populations of auditory afferents.

Sound has two properties frequency (tone) and intensity or loudness measured in decibels (dB). Neural coding of the frequency and intensity of a sound occurs primarily in the multiple synaptic connections between single inner hair cells and spiral ganglion afferents. A number of spatially contiguous hair cells are responsive to a specific frequency of stimulation. A low-intensity stimulus (10 dB) at this frequency will activate only some postsynaptic afferents. Increasing the stimulus intensity (50 dB) increases the firing frequency of action potentials in these activated afferents until they become saturated, at which time other afferents, which were silent earlier because of their higher thresholds for activation, begin to fire. In this manner several afferents contacting each hair cell receptor are activated by the same stimulus frequency but are differentially activated at disparate stimulus intensities.

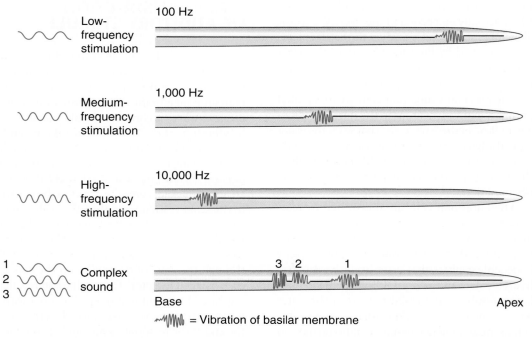

Figure 12-3   Drawing of motion of the basilar membrane to auditory stimulation of different frequencies.

AUDITORY PATHWAY

The primary or first-order auditory neurons are located in the spiral ganglion (Figs. 12-2, 12-4). The dendrites of these bipolar neurons synapse on the hair cells of the spiral organ. Their central processes form the cochlear nerve, which passes toward the cranial cavity in the internal acoustic meatus and enters the brainstem in the cerebellar angle.

CLINICAL CONNECTION

The relation of the cochlear nerve to the vestibular and facial nerves in the internal acoustic meatus is of medical importance, especially in the case of an **acoustic neurinoma,** as illustrated in the clinical case at the beginning of this chapter. This benign Schwann cell tumor almost always arises from part of the vestibular nerve in the internal acoustic meatus. After its initial growth within the meatus, the tumor spreads into the cerebellar angle. This phenomenon results in a sequence of signs and symptoms that are caused by pressure damage to the structures in the internal acoustic meatus: cochlear nerve = progressive deafness, vestibular nerve = dysequilibrium, and facial nerve = facial weakness. Later, in the posterior cranial fossa near the cerebellar angle, there is loss of the corneal reflex and, occasionally, somatosensation in the face and ipsilateral limb ataxia, attributable to the trigeminal nerve and cerebellar pathways, respectively.

The cochlear nerve terminates on second-order neurons in the dorsal and ventral cochlear nuclei, which hang on the inferior cerebellar peduncle like saddlebags (Fig. 12-5). The dorsal cochlear nucleus is posterolateral to the inferior cerebellar peduncle and forms the acoustic tubercle in the floor of the lateral recess of the fourth ventricle. The ventral cochlear nucleus is slightly more rostral and is located anterolateral to the inferior cerebellar peduncle.

As axons from the dorsal and ventral cochlear nuclei pass toward the midline before decussating, they travel rostrally into the pons and form three groups of acoustic striae named for their locations in the caudal pontine tegmentum: dorsal, intermediate, and ventral. Of the three acoustic striae, the ventral is most prominent, and as it decussates it forms the **trapezoid body** (Figs. 12-2, 12-4, 12-5).

After decussating, fibers from all three acoustic striae join the **lateral lemniscus,** which ascends through the pons to the midbrain. On reaching the midbrain, all auditory fibers in the lateral lemniscus enter the inferior colliculus and synapse. Most of the fibers from the inferior colliculus emerge laterally and ascend along the lateral surface of the midbrain as the **brachium of the inferior colliculus (inferior brachium).**

CLINICAL CONNECTION

This bundle of the inferior colliculus forms a conspicuous eminence on the lateral surface of the rostral half of the midbrain and has been used as a landmark for the surgical interruption of pain fibers traveling in the spinothalamic tract, which is located several millimeters medial to the brachium.

The brachium of the inferior colliculus terminates in the medial geniculate nucleus (Figs. 12-2, 12-4, 12-5). This thalamic auditory center then gives rise to the **auditory radiation,** which passes laterally to join the posterior limb of the internal capsule beneath the posterior part of the lentiform nucleus. Hence, the auditory radiation lies in the **sublenticular part** of the posterior limb. From here it travels to the primary auditory cortex, located in the transverse temporal gyri (of Heschl), especially the more anterior gyrus. These gyri are on the dorsal surface of the superior temporal gyrus and are buried in the lateral fissure (Fig. 12-4). Tonotopic localization exists in the primary auditory cortex; high tones are represented posteromedially and low tones anterolaterally.

BILATERALISM IN THE AUDITORY PATHWAYS

The central auditory pathways are unlike other ascending sensory paths owing to (1) the presence of accessory nuclei that are intimately related to the ascending paths and (2) the bilateral representation of auditory impulses on each side.

Three groups of nuclei are found along the auditory pathways between the cochlear nuclei and the inferior colliculus. These are the superior olivary nucleus, the nuclei of the trapezoid body, and the nuclei of the lateral lemniscus.

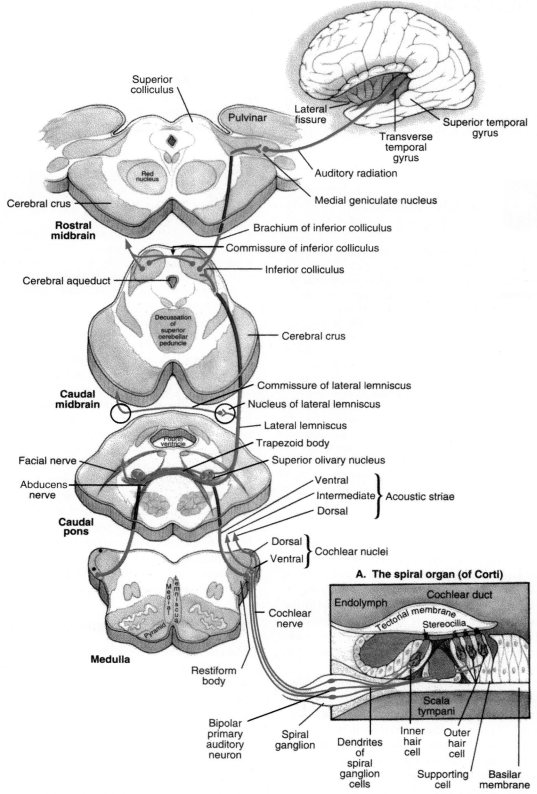

Figure 12-4   Schematic diagram showing auditory paths. **A.** Histologic features of spiral organ.

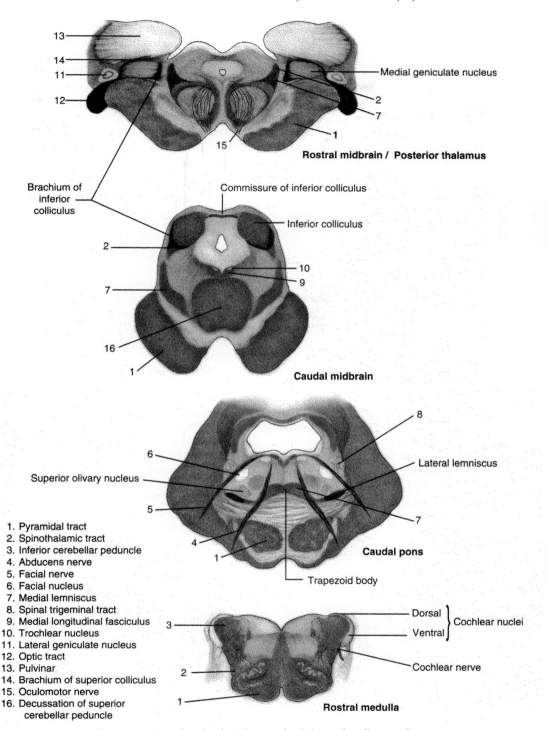

Figure 12-5   Transverse sections showing locations and relations of auditory pathways.

The superior olivary nucleus is located in the caudal pons near the lateral border of the trapezoid body (Figs. 12-2, 12-4, 12-5). It receives input from the ipsilateral and contralateral cochlear nuclei, and it gives rise to fibers that join the ipsilateral and contralateral lateral lemnisci. The superior olivary nucleus plays a key role in the localization of sounds in space. The nuclei of the trapezoid body are scattered among the trapezoid bundles, and its afferent and efferent connections are similar to those of the superior olive.

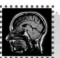

CLINICAL CONNECTION

A unilateral lesion of the auditory cortex or of the ascending paths distal to the cochlear nuclei results in virtually no loss of hearing. The abnormality most often accompanying such a lesion is impairment of the ability to localize the direction and distance of sounds reaching the contralateral ear.

The nuclei of the lateral lemniscus are located in and adjacent to the lateral lemniscus at middle and rostral pontine levels. They receive lemniscal fibers and their collaterals, and these nuclei send axons to both the ipsilateral and the contralateral lateral lemnisci. The nuclei of the inferior colliculi also aid in the bilateralism of the auditory paths by sending axons to the contralateral side via the commissure of the inferior colliculus (Figs. 12-2, 12-4, 12-5).

CLINICAL CONNECTION

U nilateral lesions in the spiral organ, spiral ganglion, cochlear nerve, or cochlear nuclei produce deafness on the ipsilateral side. Because of the bilateralism of auditory impulses as they ascend in the brainstem, unilateral lesions in the pathway beyond the cochlear nuclei result in deficits not nearly as serious as those resulting from unilateral lesions of the other sensory pathways.

AUDITORY MODULATION

Reciprocal connections between the various auditory central nuclei permit descending mod-

ulation of ascending auditory activity. Thus, the auditory cortex sends axons back to the medial geniculate nucleus and inferior colliculus. The inferior colliculus, along with the lateral lemniscus and superior olivary nuclei, sends fibers to the cochlear nuclei. Moreover, the efferent olivocochlear bundle, which arises from neurons in the superior olivary nuclei, terminates on the outer hair cells of the spiral organ and on the afferent terminals innervating them. This auditory feedback system provides a mechanism for regulating selective attention to certain sounds.

CLINICAL CONNECTION

C onduction deafness results from any interference with the passage of sound waves through the external or middle ear (air-ossicular route). Bone conduction (transmission of sound waves through the cranial bones) can still occur. Therefore, conduction deafness is never complete or total.

Nerve deafness (perception deafness) results from damage to the receptor cells of the spiral organ or to the cochlear nerve. The defect or damage is in the portion of the auditory mechanism common to both air and bone conduction and, therefore, hearing failure or loss in both routes occurs. The degree of hearing loss is, of course, related to the amount of damage to the spiral organ or nerve.

Two tuning fork tests may be used to determine types of deafness. The **Weber tuning fork test** is performed by placing the stem of a vibrating tuning fork at the middle of the forehead and asking the patient in which ear the tone is heard. In a patient with normal hearing, the tone is perceived equally in both ears. A patient with unilateral nerve deafness hears the tone in the normal ear because that ear is more sensitive. The patient with unilateral conduction deafness hears the tone louder in the affected ear.

The **Rinne tuning fork test** compares hearing via air conduction and bone conduction. A vibrating tuning fork is held near the patient's auricle (air conduction) until it can no longer be heard. Then the stem of the vibrating tuning fork is placed in contact with the mastoid process (bone conduction). Normally the sound is heard louder and longer by air conduction.

Chapter Review Questions

12-1. Bending of the stereocilia as a result of vibration of the basilar membrane toward the scala vestibuli results in what physiologic response?

12-2. Frequency (tone) and intensity (loudness) of an auditory stimulus is primarily signaled in what receptor cells?

12-3. Account for the bilateral representation of sound in the auditory system.

12-4. Where in the auditory system does a unilateral lesion produce total deafness in the ipsilateral ear?

12-5. As an acoustic neurinoma on the vestibular nerve in the internal acoustic meatus expands, what other nerves become impaired:

   a. in the internal acoustic meatus?
   b. in or near the cerebellar angle?

12-6. Contrast conduction deafness and neural deafness.

13

The Vestibular System: Vertigo and Nystagmus

ON IRRIGATION OF the right external auditory canal with cold water in one comatose patient, the eyes turn toward the right and remain in that position until the irrigation is stopped. Similar irrigation in a second comatose patient results in one eye turning up and out and the other eye turning down and in.

The two chief functions of the vestibular system are to keep the head and body lined up on an even keel and to keep the eyes fixed on a target during brief movements. In other words, the vestibular system is intimately involved in motor mechanisms that maintain equilibrium via vestibulospinal reflexes and maintain visual fixation via vestibulo-ocular reflexes.

All vestibular activity is reflex in nature and normally occurs subconsciously. In cases of excessive vestibular stimulation or when an imbalance exists between input from the right and left sides, **vertigo** occurs. The cortical area associated with vertigo is in the postcentral gyrus at the base of the intraparietal sulcus. This area receives input from the ventral posterior and posterior thalamic nuclei. The vestibular ascending brainstem paths to these nuclei are not known.

The vestibular system has strong connections with the cerebellum and with autonomic centers in the reticular formation as occur in motion sickness. In addition, strong commissural connections between the right and left vestibular nuclei exist and play a key role in the compensatory mechanisms that alleviate the vertigo occurring immediately after unilateral vestibular abnormalities.

VESTIBULOSPINAL SYSTEM AND EQUILIBRIUM

Equilibrium depends on input from three sources: visual, proprioceptive, and vestibular. The proprioceptive input comes from receptors chiefly in the neck, vertebral column, and lower limbs. Equilibrium can be maintained by any two of these inputs, but not by only one. This can be readily demonstrated in a person whose proprioceptive paths in the spinal cord have degenerated, commonly as a result of pernicious anemia. In such a case, when the person closes the eyes or is in a dark room, equilibrium will be lost because, of the three inputs, the vestibular is the only one remaining.

RECEPTORS

The receptors that respond to linear acceleration or position of the head, as well as the receptors that respond to rapid rotation of the head, are located

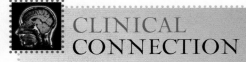

in the bony labyrinth of the internal ear. The vestibular parts of the bony labyrinth consist of the vestibule and semicircular canals. Within the fluid-filled cavity of the bony labyrinth is the membranous labyrinth, which includes the **utricle** and

saccule in the vestibule and the **semicircular ducts** in the semicircular canals. All three contain vestibular receptors. Those in the utricle and saccule are chiefly associated with the vestibulospinal system, and those in the semicircular ducts are chiefly associated with the vestibulo-ocular system.

In the walls of each utricle and saccule is a small, thickened area called the **macula.** The maculae are oriented at right angles to each other, with that of the utricle being almost in the horizontal plane and that of the saccule in almost the sagittal plane. Linear acceleration or changes in position of the head in any direction stimulate a macula on each side. Each macula consists of neuroepithelial hair cells and supporting cells (Fig. 13-1A). Over-

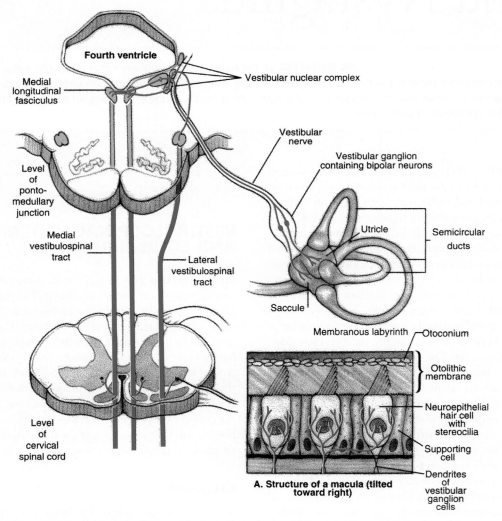

Figure 13-1 Schematic diagram of principal vestibulospinal connections. **A.** Structure of a macula (tilted to right side).

laying the hair cells is the gelatinous **otolithic membrane,** which contains calcium carbonate crystals, the **otoliths** (ear stones) or **otoconia** (ear sand). With linear acceleration or when the position of the head changes, the otolithic membrane shifts, bending the neuroepithelial **stereocilia** embedded in it. As occurs with stimulation of auditory hair cell receptors, bending of the stereocilia on vestibular hair cells is transduced into an electrical receptor potential that then depolarizes and excites the dendrites of the bipolar vestibular ganglion cells, which are in synaptic contact with the hair cells.

VESTIBULAR NERVE

The axons of the vestibular ganglion cells whose dendrites synapse on neuroepithelial cells in the maculae travel centrally in the vestibular part of cranial nerve VIII (Fig. 13-1). The vestibular nerve enters the brainstem with the cochlear nerve at the pontomedullary junction, in the area bounded by the pons, medulla, and cerebellum and called the **cerebellar angle.** Vestibular nerve fibers then pass dorsally to reach the vestibular nuclear complex (Fig. 13-2). Some continue uninterrupted into the cerebellum as the direct vestibulocerebellar fibers, which pass through the **juxtarestiform**

body (Fig. 13-2), the more medial part of the inferior cerebellar peduncle.

VESTIBULAR NUCLEI

The vestibular nuclear complex consists of four nuclei located beneath the vestibular area in the floor and wall of the fourth ventricle (Figs. 13-1, 13-2). The inferior vestibular nucleus is in the rostral medulla. The medial vestibular nucleus is located in the lateral part of the floor of the fourth ventricle in the rostral medulla and caudal pons. The lateral vestibular nucleus is limited to the region of the pontomedullary junction and it contains a population of neurons referred to as Deiters nucleus. The superior vestibular nucleus is limited to the caudal pons where it is located in the wall of the fourth ventricle.

Vestibular nerve fibers carrying input from the maculae synapse in the medial, lateral, and inferior vestibular nuclei. These vestibular nuclei project to the spinal motor nuclei via the lateral and medial vestibulospinal tracts.

VESTIBULOSPINAL TRACTS

The lateral vestibulospinal tract, which arises from the lateral vestibular nucleus, strongly facilitates

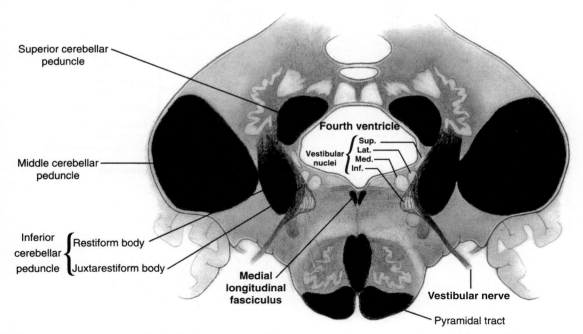

Figure 13-2   Section at the level of the pontomedullary junction showing the relations of the vestibular nerve and nuclei (inf, inferior; lat, lateral; med, medial; sup, superior).

the extensor muscles in the ipsilateral limbs. The medial vestibulospinal fibers arise from the medial and inferior vestibular nuclei, descend bilaterally via the medial longitudinal fasciculus, and influence muscles of the head, neck, trunk, and proximal parts of the limbs. Thus, the vestibulospinal reflexes, key mechanisms for equilibrium, include three main groups of neurons (Fig. 13-1):

1. Afferent neurons in the vestibular ganglion;
2. Interneurons in the vestibular nuclei;
3. Efferent or lower motor neurons in the spinal cord.

VESTIBULO-OCULAR REFLEX

The other main function of the vestibular system is to keep the eyes fixed on a target when the head is rotated quickly. Thus, the eyes always reflexly turn opposite to the direction of rotation of the head. The anatomic basis for this phenomenon is the very strong **vestibulo-ocular reflex,** which includes three groups of neurons (Fig. 13-3):

1. Afferent neurons in the vestibular ganglion;
2. Interneurons in the vestibular nuclei;
3. Efferent or lower motor neurons in the oculomotor, trochlear, and abducens nuclei.

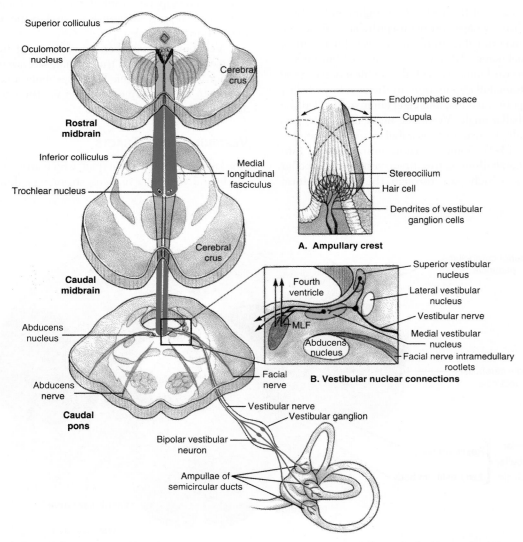

Figure 13-3   Schematic diagram of principal connections of vestibulo-ocular reflex. **A.** Histology of ampullary crest. **B.** Connections of vestibular nuclei (MLF, medial longitudinal fasciculus).

RECEPTORS

The receptors for the vestibulo-ocular reflex are located in the ampullae of the three semicircular ducts of the internal ear (Fig. 13-3). The anterior and posterior ducts are oriented vertically but at right angles to each other, whereas the lateral duct is oriented horizontally. Thus, rotation of the head in any direction stimulates the receptors in functional pairs of semicircular ducts. At one end of each duct is an enlargement, the ampulla. In each ampulla, a part of the wall is thickened and projects into the cavity of the duct as the **ampullary crest.** The ampullary crest is a vestibular receptor organ composed of sensory neuroepithelial hair cells and supporting cells (Fig. 13-3A). Overlaying each ampullary crest is a gelatinous substance, the **cupula,** in which are embedded the free ends of the stereocilia of the hair cells of the crests. One of the hairs in each hair cell is longer and is called the **kinocilium.**

When the head begins to rotate, the endolymph in the semicircular duct lags behind and prevents the cupula from moving. As a result, the stereocilia embedded in the cupula are bent in the direction opposite that of the rotation. When the rotation is stopped suddenly, the endolymph continues to move, causing the cupula to bend in the direction of the rotation. The hair cells are polarized so that when the stereocilia are bent toward the kinocilium they are depolarized, whereas when they are bent away from the kinocilium they are hyperpolarized. In this way, the receptors in the right and left semicircular ducts work in pairs: when one side is excited, the other is inhibited. The hair cells are in synaptic contact with the dendrites of bipolar vestibular ganglion cells (Fig. 13-3).

NUCLEI AND PATHS

The axons of the vestibular ganglion cells whose dendrites synapse on neuroepithelial cells of the cristae pass centrally in the vestibular nerve and, on entering the brainstem, proceed dorsally to terminate in the superior and medial vestibular nuclei (Figs. 13-3B, 13-4). Vestibulo-ocular fibers then pass to the ocular motor nuclei chiefly via the medial longitudinal fasciculus (MLF). The vestibulo-ocular reflex connections for horizontal rotation to the right are shown in Figure 13-5.

CLINICAL CONNECTION

Superimposed on a background of tonic unitary activity in vestibular afferents is complex phasic activity reflecting the collective stimulation of hair cells in the five vestibular receptor organs. Generally vestibular input is balanced, resulting in normal vestibulospinal and vestibulo-ocular reflex activity. When vestibular afferent activity is abnormally increased or decreased, there may be very debilitating effects on the patient. **Ménière disease** is a relatively common disorder affecting hair cell receptors. Altered activity in vestibular hair cells results in intermittent and relapsing vertigo, postural instability, and nausea occurring coincident with abnormal activity in auditory hair cells resulting in tinnitus. The pathophysiologic basis for Ménière's disease is thought to be attributable to abnormal endolymphatic fluid hemodynamics. Diuretics in most instances or, in severe cases, pharmacologic ablation of hair cells with streptomycin or surgical labyrinthectomy are used as therapy for Ménière's disease.

VESTIBULO-OCULAR NYSTAGMUS

Nystagmus refers to involuntary rhythmic movements of the eyes that include two components: a slow drifting away from the target and a fast return to the target. Nystagmus can be induced by stimulating the vestibular apparatus either by rotating the head (vestibular nystagmus) or by irrigating the external auditory canal with cold or warm water (caloric nystagmus). Both methods induce currents in the endolymphatic fluid in the semicircular ducts, the rotation because of the fluid inertia and the irrigation because of convection currents. The fluid inertia or the convection currents bend stereocilia and stimulate the hair cells of the cristae, thereby initiating the powerful vestibulo-ocular reflex. The slow phases of vestibular and caloric nystagmus are caused by this vestibulo-ocular reflex, whereas the fast phases are triggered by the cerebral cortex. In all cases, nystagmus is described according to the fast phase because it is more obvious than the slow phase.

In the case of caloric nystagmus, the fast phase will be toward the side opposite irrigation with cold water and toward the same side irrigated with warm water. Thus, **"COWS"** (cold opposite, warm same) represents the fast phases of caloric nystagmus. In the case of rotary nystagmus occurring immediately after the cessation of rotation, the fast phase will be toward the direction of the rotation.

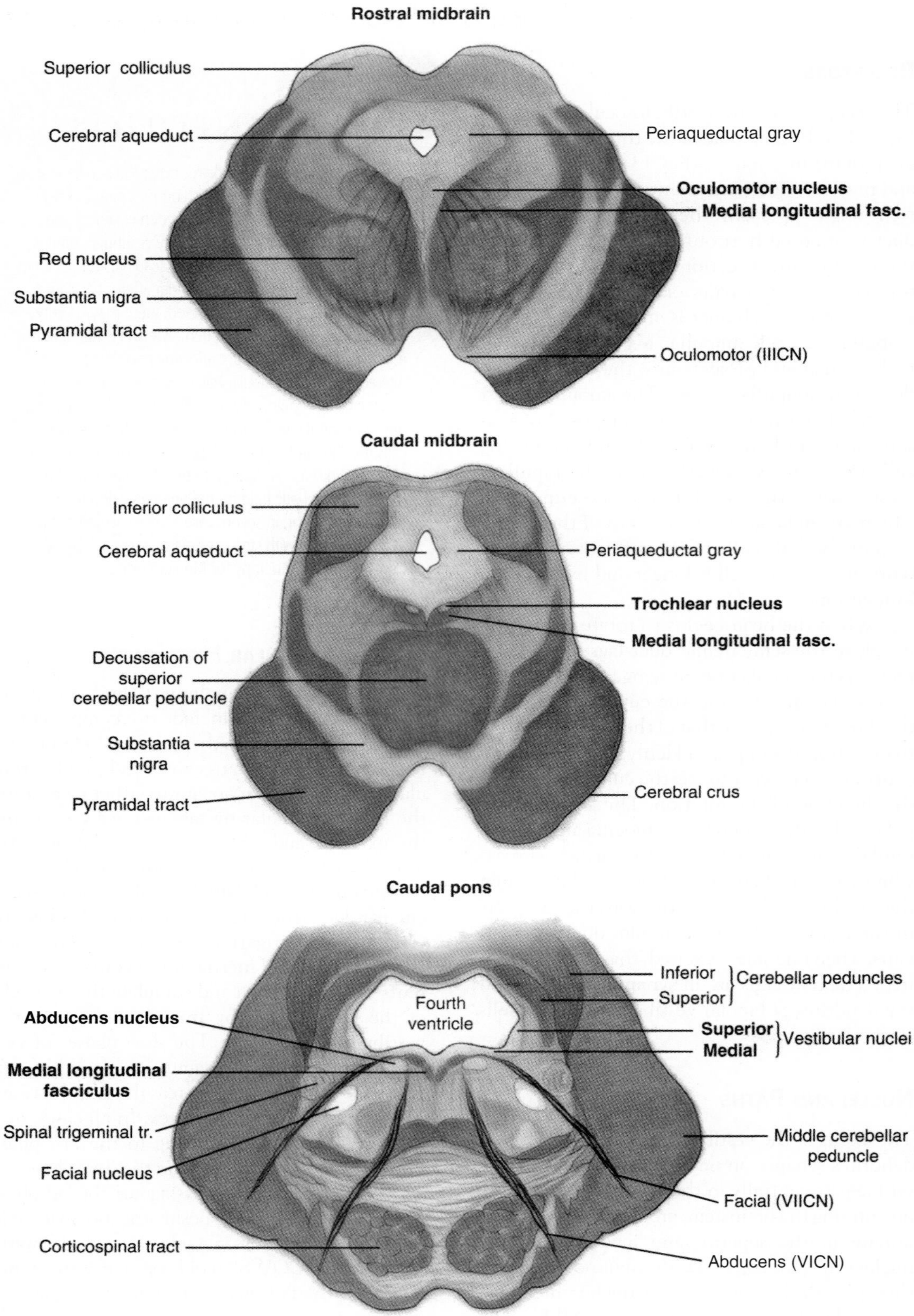

Figure 13-4 Relations of vestibulo-ocular paths in transverse section (bolded terms relate to ocular motor paths) (CN, cranial nerve; fasc, fasciculus; tr, tract).

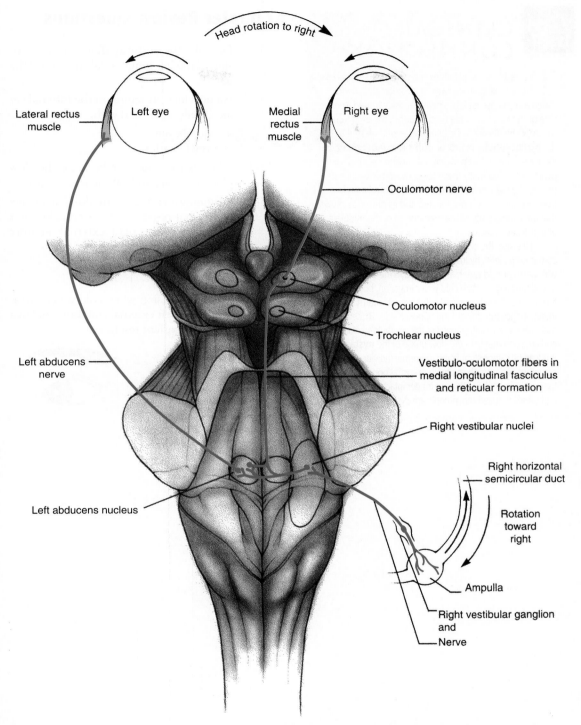

Figure 13-5   Schematic drawing of dorsal aspect of brainstem showing the vestibulo-ocular reflex on rotation to the right.

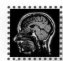

CLINICAL CONNECTION

The vestibulo-ocular reflex can be used to assess levels of brainstem damage in a comatose patient. When a comatose patient's head is briskly turned to one side or the other, or is tilted up or down, the eyes turn in the opposite direction. This phenomenon, referred to as the **oculocephalic reflex** or **doll's eye movement,** is indicative of an intact pathway subserving the vestibulo-ocular reflex. Normally these reflex movements are suppressed by the cerebral cortex. In the comatose patient, however, the reflex is disinhibited and its presence shows that the central parts of the tegmentum of the midbrain and pons are intact.

Likewise, the oculocephalic reflex can be induced in comatose patients by irrigating the external auditory canal with warm or cold water, as described in the case that introduced the chapter. With cold water irrigation, both eyes turn toward the side irrigated, whereas with warm water irrigation they turn toward the opposite side. These movements are also manifestations of the vestibulo-ocular reflex and are comparable to the slow phase of the **nystagmus** induced by caloric stimulation in normal individuals. In a comatose patient with midbrain or rostral pons impairment the vestibulo-ocular path is no longer intact and doll's eye and caloric induced movements are dysfunctional.

Chapter Review Questions

13-1. Describe the pathway that causes extension of the left limbs on falling toward the left.

13-2. Name which structures in the internal ear are chiefly associated with:

a. equilibrium
b. visual fixation

13-3. What is the anatomic basis for the slow phase of rotary and caloric nystagmus?

13-4. Assuming an intact vestibulo-ocular reflex path, what response occurs on cold water irrigation of the right external auditory meatus in a patient who is:

a. conscious
b. comatose

13-5. Locate the lesion when cold water irrigation of the left external auditory canal in a comatose patient results in:

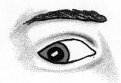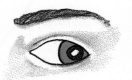

14

The Visual System: Anopsia

A HYPERTENSIVE PATIENT, admitted because of stroke, is found to have paralysis of the left upper and lower limbs, left hemianesthesia, and blindness of the left half of the field of vision in both eyes.

We receive most of the information about our surroundings through the visual system. The medical importance of this system includes the fact that blindness is the most devastating of all sensory deficits and that clinical examination of the visual system provides precise localization of lesions.

We "see" when light rays are focused on the retina; these rays are transduced by photoreceptor cells into retinal potentials, and nerve impulses are transmitted to the thalamus and thence to the cerebral cortex. Three anatomic features of the visual pathways are of medical significance:

1. These pathways extend from the front to the back of the head.
2. They are entirely supratentorial.
3. Visual information travels in both crossed and uncrossed paths.

THE EYE

The eye is composed of (1) a wall made up of three coats, and (2) internal refractive media that bend the light rays as they pass toward the photoreceptors (Fig. 14-1). The three coats or layers of the eye are the outer or fibrous layer, the middle or vascular layer, and the inner or retinal layer. The fibrous layer consists of the **sclera** and **cornea.** The sclera is posterior and forms the "white of the eye." Its

strength helps to maintain the shape of the eyeball and it gives attachment to the external ocular muscles. The cornea is the avascular, translucent anterior part of the fibrous layer. Its translucency is attributable to a number of anatomic factors: nonkeratinizing epithelium; absence of blood vessels and pigment; cellular components with a uniform regular arrangement and the same index of refraction; and the arrangement of its collagen fibrils.

CLINICAL CONNECTION

The outer layers of the cornea are easily replaced if damaged. Damage to the deeper layers, however, results in scar formation. Because the cornea is avascular, it can be transplanted into allogeneic recipients without immunologic rejection.

The **middle** or **vascular layer,** also referred to as the **choroid** or **uvea,** is responsible for focusing and regulating the intensity of light. It consists of three parts: the **choroid proper,** the **ciliary body,** and the **iris.** The choroid is a highly vascular and pigmented membrane lining the posterior five sixths of the eye deep to the sclera. Anteriorly it

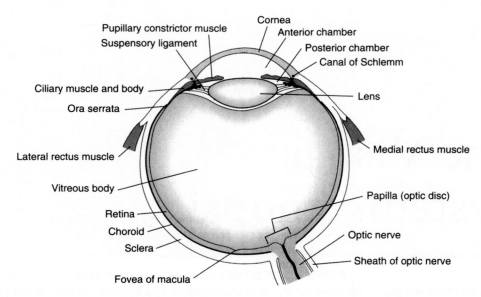

Cornea
Anterior chamber
Posterior chamber
Canal of Schlemm
Pupillary constrictor muscle
Suspensory ligament
Ciliary muscle and body
Ora serrata
Lens
Lateral rectus muscle
Medial rectus muscle
Vitreous body
Papilla (optic disc)
Retina
Choroid
Optic nerve
Sclera
Sheath of optic nerve
Fovea of macula

Figure 14-1 A cross section of the human eye illustrating the major anatomic features. (Modified with permission from Kingsley, Concise Text of Neuroscience, 1996: Williams & Wilkins.)

becomes the ciliary body (Fig. 14-2). The **ciliary body** is involved in the production of **aqueous humor** and some constituents of the **vitreous humor,** and in **accommodation of the lens.** It is attached to the lens by the suspensory ligament and contains smooth muscles, which are under the influence of **parasympathetic** impulses. Contraction of the ciliary muscles results in decreased tension on the suspensory ligament and, in turn, on the lens. This allows the lens to increase its thickness, thereby focusing the light rays from a near object onto the retina.

The iris projects inwardly from the anterior part of the ciliary body, and its free margin forms the rim of the **pupil.** The size of the pupil is regulated by **constrictor** and **dilator smooth muscles** in the iris. The **constrictor** muscle is under the influence of **parasympathetic** impulses, whereas the **dilator** is under **sympathetic** control.

The **inner** or **retinal layer** is located between the choroid and the vitreous body and may be divided into two strata, **pigmented** and **cerebral.** The pigmented or external stratum, not nervous in nature, is composed of a single layer of pigmented cells. The cerebral or internal stratum is transparent and consists of nine layers. Altogether the retina comprises 10 layers, which will be described subsequently.

Light entering the eye passes through a number of structures before it reaches the retina. These structures form the **refractive apparatus** or media and consist of the cornea, aqueous humor, lens, and vitreous body.

The cornea has a marked curvature and a different refractive index than air. Thus, the light rays are bent by the cornea. In fact, the cornea is the main refractive structure of the eye.

The **aqueous humor** has about the same index of refraction as the cornea. It is thought to be secreted by the epithelium lining the ciliary body and is similar in composition to protein-free plasma. On its formation it enters the posterior chamber of the eye, flows through the pupil into the anterior chamber, and drains into a trabecular meshwork (the spaces of Fontana) located at the junction of the iris, cornea, and sclera. These trabeculae then empty into the sinus venosus sclerae (canal of Schlemm), a large, branching circumferential vessel that drains into the episcleral veins.

After passing through the cornea, the anterior chamber, and the pupil, light rays strike the lens. Although the lens is not as refractive as the cornea, it is essential for focusing because its refractile power can be altered. The lens is suspended from the ciliary body by the suspensory ligament. This

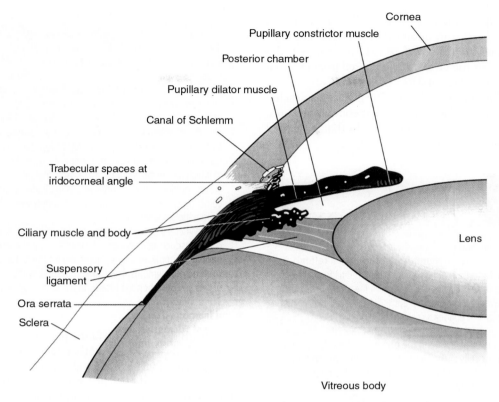

Figure 14-2 Anatomic features of anterior part of eye. (Modified with permission from Kingsley, Concise Text of Neuroscience, 1996: Williams & Wilkins.)

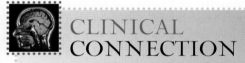
CLINICAL
CONNECTION

Besides its role as a refractive medium the aqueous humor is also important in the maintenance of intraocular pressure. In fact, intraocular pressure is intimately related to aqueous humor dynamics. Decreased drainage of aqueous humor or, occasionally, increased production, may result in an increased intraocular pressure and **glaucoma,** which causes progressive degeneration of retinal ganglion cells, optic nerve damage, and impaired vision. Glaucoma is the leading cause of blindness worldwide, affecting more than 67 million people.

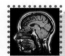
CLINICAL
CONNECTION

When the eye is at rest the suspensory ligament is taut and exerts a pull on the lens capsule, thereby keeping it relatively flat. When vision is shifted from a far to a near object, reflex contraction of the ciliary muscle causes the ciliary body to move forward and decreases the tension on the suspensory ligament. This allows the inherently elastic lens to bulge and increase its anteroposterior diameter, thereby shortening the focal distance between the lens and retina. With age the lens becomes harder and its power of accommodation is decreased, a condition termed **presbyopia.** Opacification of the lens is called a **cataract.**

consists of delicate but strong fibrils that attach to the lens capsule near the equator.

The vitreous body is a clear, gelatinous substance that fills the posterior four-fifths of the eyeball. It not only supports the structures within the eye but also provides a transparent medium.

THE RETINA

The retina contains seven types of cells: the receptors for vision, the first two neurons in the visual pathway, two types of interneurons, supporting cells, and pigment epithelial cells. The cells and their processes are arranged in 10 layers. The light rays pass from internal to external through the retina, but the layers are numbered from external to internal (Fig. 14-3).

The outermost layer is the pigment epithelial layer, a single layer of cells that contain melanin. The pigment cells absorb the light that has passed through the retina.

CLINICAL CONNECTION

Two clinical conditions related to the pigment epithelial layer are **retinitis pigmentosa** and **retinal detachment.** In retinitis pigmentosa, debris from photoreceptor cells accumulates between the photoreceptor cell layer and the pigment epithelial cell layer. Normally the pigment epithelial cells phagocytose this debris.

Retinal detachment occurs between the pigment epithelial cell layer and the photoreceptors. The photoreceptor cells at the site of detachment cease to function, resulting in blurred vision in the affected part of the visual field.

Layer two contains the photoreceptors, the rods and cones. The human retina contains 110 to 125 million rods and 6 to 7 million cones. The cones are responsible for visual acuity and color vision (**photopic vision**); the rods are responsible for vision in light of low intensity (**scotopic vision**). The rods are uniformly slender, whereas the cones have wide bases and tapered, narrow ends. Each rod and cone cell consists of four parts: outer segment, inner segment, cell body, and synaptic terminal (Fig. 14-3). Actually, the photoreceptor layer contains only the outer and inner segments of the photoreceptors.

CLINICAL CONNECTION

The outer segments contain the visual photopigments, **rhodopsin** in the rods and **iodopsin** in the cones. On absorbing light, rhodopsin is broken down into retinal, the light-absorbing molecule, and opsin. After absorbing light, rhodopsin is then restored by a series of chemical reactions, some of which depend on **vitamin A.**

The rods, which are much more sensitive to light than the cones, are chiefly used in dim or nocturnal vision. Because of its vital role in the restoration of rhodopsin, vitamin A deficiency reduces nocturnal vision, a condition called **night blindness.** Although only one type of rod exists in the human eye, there are three types of cones: red-, green-, and blue-sensitive cones. The light-absorbing molecule in each cone type appears to be similar to the retinal found in rods. Different wavelength sensitivities are determined by the specific type of opsin to which the retinal is bound. The absence of the red-, green-, or blue-sensitive cones results in blindness to that color. Thus, cones respond to colors, but only when the illumination is great enough.

Whereas the outer segments of the photoreceptor cells transduce light rays into electrical energy, the inner segments supply the energy necessary for the restoration of the visual pigments. This is accomplished by the numerous mitochondria located in the inner segments.

With the exception of the pigment epithelial cells in layer one, all the other cell bodies are in retinal layers four, six, and eight (Fig. 14-3). Layer four, the external nuclear layer, contains the cell bodies and nuclei of the rods and cones. Layer six, the internal nuclear layer, contains chiefly the cell bodies of the bipolar neurons, the first neurons in the visual pathway.

Local circuit neurons, the **horizontal cells** and **amacrine cells,** are interspersed among the bipolar neurons. The horizontal cells, located in the outer part of layer six, modulate the synaptic activity between the photoreceptors and bipolar cells, whereas the amacrine cells, located in the inner part of layer six, modulate such activity between the bipolar and the second neurons in the visual path, ganglion cells. Most of the cell bodies of the supporting cells of the retina, the **Müller cells,** are located in the internal nuclear layer also.

Layer eight is the ganglion cell layer, formed by the cell bodies of the second neurons in the visual pathway. The axons of these second-order neurons form layer nine, the optic nerve fiber layer. Until they emerge from the eye, these axons are unmyelinated, an optical advantage because myelin is highly refractile.

The remaining layers of the retina are the external and internal plexiform layers, layers five and seven, respectively, and the external and internal limiting membrane layers, layers three and ten, respectively. The plexiform layers are the synaptic layers and consist of the axons and dendrites of

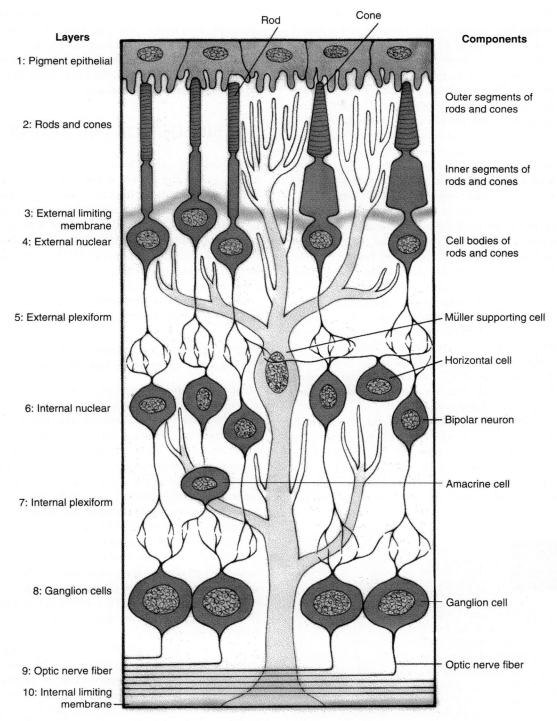

Figure 14-3   The retina: layers, cells, and their connections.

the cells in the adjacent layers. The limiting membranes are formed by the external and internal ends of the Müller supporting cells, the modified glial cells of the retina.

Two parts of the retina that are structurally and functionally different from the rest of the retina are the central area and the **optic disc.** The central area contains the **macula lutea** and the **fovea centralis.** At the fovea, the inner layers of the retina are displaced, forming a pit or **foveola.** Only cones are present in the floor of the foveola. The fovea is the area for acute vision and, therefore, the line connecting it with the viewed object is the visual axis.

Acuity occurs at the fovea not only because of displacement of the inner retinal layers, which allows the light rays to reach the cones without having to traverse the other layers, but also because cones are densest in the fovea, where they number about 200,000 per square millimeter.

The rest of the retina participates in nonacute paramacular and peripheral vision. Most of the photoreceptors in the paramacular and peripheral parts of the retina are the rods. Because of their longer outer segments, the rods can detect very small amounts of light, and because the impulses from many rods converge on the same bipolar neuron, the rods have low acuity.

The optic disc or papilla is the area at which the unmyelinated optic nerve fibers exit from the retina. At this point the outer eight layers of the retina are interrupted; hence, because of the absence of photoreceptors, it is the **blind spot.** As the fibers emerge to form the optic nerve, they become myelinated.

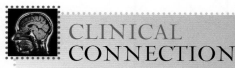

CLINICAL CONNECTION

At the point of attachment of the optic nerve to the back of the eye, the external layer of the eye, the sclera, becomes continuous with the dura mater that completely encloses the nerve. The optic nerve, therefore, is surrounded by the dura as well as the arachnoid and pia mater (Fig. 14-1). Hence, increased intracranial pressure can exert pressure via the cerebrospinal fluid-filled subarachnoid space onto the optic nerve, especially at its emergence from the eyeball. When this occurs, the axoplasmic flow in the individual optic nerve axons is obstructed, and they become swollen at the optic disc. This condition is known as **disc edema, papilledema,** or **choked disc** and can be observed with an ophthalmoscope.

Embryologically, the retina develops from the diencephalon; hence, it is a central nervous system (CNS) derivative. As a result, the optic nerve, unlike all other cranial nerves, is a CNS structure. Like other CNS structures, the optic nerve fibers do not regenerate when damaged.

PHYSIOLOGY OF THE RETINA

The physiology of the visual system is the most complex of all the sensory systems. As noted earlier, visual stimuli are received directly in the CNS by neurons in the retina where significant processing of the photic stimuli begins and continues progressively through the lateral geniculate nucleus, the primary visual cortex (V1), and finally in multiple association areas of the temporal and parietal cortices. In each step of the pathway the stimulus properties that activate a neuron become progressively more specific.

PHOTOTRANSDUCTION AND INITIAL PROCESSING OCCURS IN THE RETINA

Light in a limited range (approximately 400 to 700 nm) of the electromagnetic spectrum activates the human retina. Phototransduction occurs as the result of a photon of light triggering the dissociation of the visual pigments rhodopsin or iodopsin, thereby initiating a biochemical cascade in the outer part of the receptor segments. This leads to graded membrane changes in the inner segment of the receptors that synaptically depolarize or hyperpolarize bipolar cells. The time course for this photic-biochemical transduction process can be appreciated by the time it takes to visually accommodate when moving from a dark to a brightly lit area or vice versa. Potential changes in bipolar cells are electronically conducted to tonically active ganglion cells, resulting in an increased or decreased firing of action potentials.

The most elementary photic stimulus is a small spot of light on contiguous receptors. On-center bipolar and connected ganglion cells are excited when the light spot is centered in a circular receptive field and inhibited by light applied to a ring area surrounding the center (center surround inhibition). Off-center bipolar and ganglion cells respond just the opposite (Fig. 14-4). On- and off-center bipolar and ganglion neurons enable the retina to optimally detect subtle differences in contrast and rapid changes in light intensity.

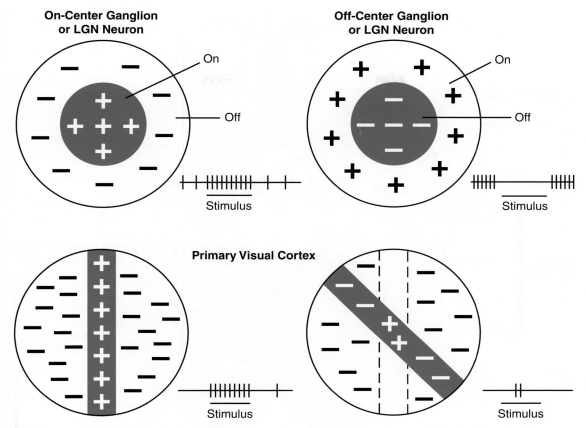

Figure 14-4 Ganglion cells in the retina and neurons in the lateral geniculate nuclei (LGN) have circular receptive fields and respond to focal light stimuli in an on-center or off-center manner. Neurons in the primary visual cortex respond to line stimuli with a specific orientation.

VISUAL PATHWAY

Light rays striking the retina travel from the internal layers to the external layers where the rods and cones are stimulated. The visual impulses then pass from the external to the internal layers. Thus, within the retina the light rays and visual impulses travel in opposite directions.

The visual impulses from the rods and cones are transmitted to the bipolar cells, the primary or first-order neurons in the visual system. Axons from the bipolar neurons synapse with the dendrites of the retinal ganglion cells, the second neurons in the pathway. The optic nerve axons coming from the ganglion cells radiate toward the optic disc, where they become myelinated and emerge to form the optic nerve. The optic nerves from each eye proceed posteriorly and medially, enter the cranial cavity through the optic foramina, and unite to form the optic chiasm (Fig. 14-5).

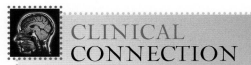

CLINICAL CONNECTION

The optic chiasm rests on the diaphragma sellae in close relation to the stalk of the pituitary gland. Laterally, it is related to the internal carotid arteries. A pituitary tumor may damage the median portion of the chiasm, whereas an **aneurysm** on one of the internal carotid arteries may damage the lateral part of the chiasm.

Leaving the optic chiasm is the optic tract, which passes posterolaterally along the surfaces of the hypothalamus and cerebral crus and enters the ventral surface of the lateral geniculate nucleus. Here, axons from the retinal ganglion cells finally reach the tertiary visual path neurons.

The lateral geniculate nucleus has a triangular shape, somewhat similar to a Napoleonic hat.

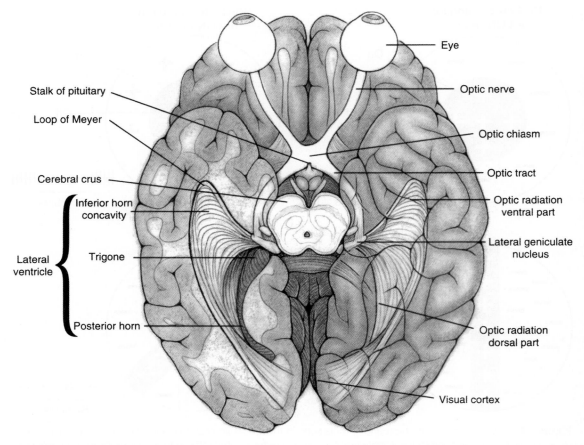

Stalk of pituitary

Loop of Meyer

Cerebral crus

Inferior horn concavity

Lateral ventricle

Trigone

Posterior horn

Eye

Optic nerve

Optic chiasm

Optic tract

Optic radiation ventral part

Lateral geniculate nucleus

Optic radiation dorsal part

Visual cortex

Figure 14-5 Three-dimensional ventral view of the visual path with right temporal lobe dissected.

It consists of six layers. The two ventral layers are composed of large neurons, whereas the four dorsal layers consist of small neurons. Both types are the tertiary neurons that send axons to the cerebral cortex. The magnocellular layers are the part of the visual pathway concerned with the location and movement of an object in the visual field, whereas the parvicellular layers are concerned with the color and form of the object. Hence, the magnocellular is part of the "where" pathway and the parvicellular is part of the "what" pathway.

The tertiary lateral geniculate neurons give rise to the geniculocalcarine tract or optic radiation, which initially enters the retrolenticular part of the posterior limb of the internal capsule. As it enters the internal capsule, the optic radiation forms a conspicuous triangular area referred to as **Wernicke zone** (Fig. 14-6).

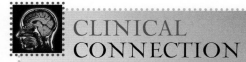

CLINICAL CONNECTION

The location of the optic radiation in the triangular zone of Wernicke is of clinical importance. Because of its close anatomic relation to the pyramidal tract and somatosensory thalamocortical radiations that are immediately adjacent in the posterior limb of the internal capsule, a small lesion (approximately 1.5 cm) in this area gives rise to a contralateral paralysis and hemianesthesia and blindness in the opposite half of the field of vision in each eye (as given in the case introducing this chapter). These abnormalities usually result from anterior choroidal artery disease.

From the internal capsule, the fibers of the optic radiation sweep to the lateral surface of the lateral ventricle (Fig. 14-5). The more dorsal fibers proceed directly posteriorly, initially within the

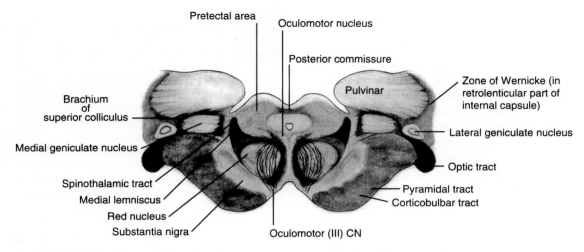

Figure 14-6   Transverse section at rostral midbrain and overlapping thalamus (CN, cranial nerve).

parietal lobe and then the occipital lobe. The more ventral fibers pass anteriorly and loop over the inferior horn of the lateral ventricle. Those fibers that proceed most anteriorly form the **loop of Meyer.** Therefore, after emerging from the internal capsule, the ventral part of the optic radiation is located initially in the temporal lobe and then in the occipital lobe.

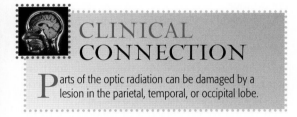

CLINICAL CONNECTION

Parts of the optic radiation can be damaged by a lesion in the parietal, temporal, or occipital lobe.

The optic radiation sweeps posteriorly near the lateral wall of the posterior horn of the lateral ventricle and terminates in the primary visual cortex located in the walls of the calcarine sulcus (Fig. 14-7). The more dorsal fibers terminate in the cuneus; the more ventral fibers pass to the lingual gyrus. The visual cortex is also referred to as the striate cortex because, unlike other parts of the cerebral cortex, it contains a very conspicuous horizontal stripe, called the line of Gennari. Within the visual cortex, the macula of the retina is represented in the posterior half and the paramacular and peripheral parts of the retina are represented successively more anteriorly (Fig. 14-7A).

PROCESSING OF VISUAL INFORMATION

Neurons with on-center and off-center receptive fields are also present in the lateral geniculate nucleus. Circular on- and off-center receptor field properties are maintained in geniculocortical input to layer four of V1, but columns of neurons above and below layer four transform this input to linearly shaped receptor fields characterized as lines or bars with discrete boundaries. Most neurons in each column are responsive to line stimuli of the same spatial orientation. These individual columns are called orientation columns through which many circular fields are converted to a rectilinear receptive field with a specific axis of orientation. Immediately adjacent V1 orientation columns contain neurons activated by visual stimuli to the same area of the retina but with different orientations. Thus, the convergence of parallel on- and off-center inputs from the lateral geniculate nucleus and the resultant processing in the orientation columns enable objects to be perceived by their shapes. Fewer and more complex neurons in each orientation column respond to movement of the linear shape across the receptive field in the retina.

Binocular inputs remain segregated in the different layers of the lateral geniculate nucleus and in ocular dominance columns in layer four in V1. These alternating inputs from the right or left eye in adjacent ocular dominance columns are important for binocular interactions and depth perception. Finally, there are also regularly spaced columns of neurons in the upper layers of V1 that are responsive to colors. Functionally related columns are richly interconnected by horizontally oriented axonal connections that integrate activity from across wide areas of the retina.

Visual perception involves four major attributes: form or shape, depth, motion, and color. Although each of these attributes is processed in the striate cortex, the conscious interpretation of the input occurs in extrastriate areas of cortex. The parvocellular (P) and magnocellular (M) parallel pathways transmit functionally different information from the retina through the lateral geniculate nucleus to V1. The anatomic and functional divergence of the two paths continues in their termination in different parts of layer four. From V1 ventral and dorsal cortical pathways emerge to the extrastriate cortex. The ventral pathway is the continuation of the P pathway and is directed to the inferior temporal lobe, whereas the dorsal path transmits the flow of information from the M pathway to posterior areas of the parietal lobe. Motion is analyzed primarily through the dorsal pathway to the parietal lobe (the where), whereas perception of shape and color necessary for object identification (the what) occurs through the ventral pathway to the inferior temporal cortex.

COLOR VISION

Normal color vision in humans depends on cone receptors being activated preferentially to one of three particular wavelengths of reflected light. The mixing of the signals from the different cone receptors allows for the perception of a wide spectrum of color. Color stimuli are transmitted mainly by neurons forming the P pathway from the retina and lateral geniculate nucleus. In V1 color perception is limited to the regularly arranged columns in layers two and three. As visual stimuli flow from V1 to extrastriate areas the transformation of color information occurs in concert with that regarding the shape of an object, thereby collectively allowing for the identification of an object. For example, a shiny red object with a shape of a well-recognized piece of fruit would be interpreted as an apple.

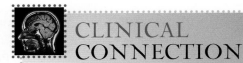

CLINICAL CONNECTION

True color blindness is rare, but many individuals have impaired color vision as a result of congenital abnormalities. Instead of normal trichromatic vision, some people have only a dichromatic vision, typically seen in males, suggesting the X chromosome encodes the synthesis of visual pigments in cones. The loss of one type of cone receptor pigment results in dichromatic vision making it difficult to distinguish colors, especially on surfaces with multiple colors. This can be demonstrated using the Ishihara test where within a pattern of different colored dots an embedded number can be recognized by an individual with normal trichromatic vision but not by individuals with dichromatic vision. Acquired diseases of the eye such as retinitis pigmentosa and glaucoma can also selectively damage one type of cone receptor resulting in dichromatic vision.

VISUAL FIELDS AND VISUAL PATHS

Lesions in various parts of the visual path are described according to the visual field deficits that result. Knowledge of the representation of the fields of vision in the visual paths is of medical importance.

The field of vision is divided into four quadrants: upper right, upper left, lower right, and lower left. The quadrants are demarcated by imaginary horizontal and vertical lines through the **fixation point,** that is, the point on which vision is focused.

These visual field quadrants are projected onto each retina in a reversed and inverted pattern through the action of the lens (Fig. 14-7). Within the optic chiasm, the optic nerve fibers from the nasal or medial halves of the retinae cross, but those from the temporal or lateral halves of the retinae do not cross. This partial decussation serves to bring all of the optic nerve fibers transmitting impulses from either the right or the left half of the field of vision into the contralateral optic tract. Thus, the right and left visual pathways distal to the chiasm are carrying all of the impulses from the contralateral halves of the visual field.

Moreover, because of the point-to-point relations that exist between the retina, lateral geniculate nucleus, and primary visual cortex, impulses

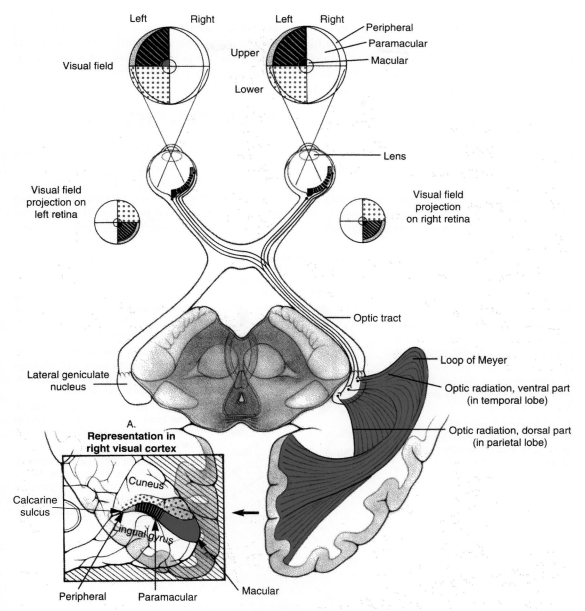

Figure 14-7 Visual field representation in visual paths. **A.** Visual field and retinal representation in primary visual cortex.

from the upper and lower halves of the visual field are located in different parts of the optic radiation. Impulses from the contralateral upper quadrant take a ventral course and sweep into the white matter of the temporal lobe before proceeding posteriorly into the occipital lobe where they end in the lower wall of the calcarine sulcus, the lingual gyrus (Fig. 14-7A). Impulses from the contralateral lower

quadrant, however, take a dorsal course and sweep posteriorly through the white matter of the parietal lobe to the occipital lobe, where they end in the upper wall of the calcarine sulcus, the cuneus.

Damage to the visual pathways results in the loss of vision, anopsia, which is described according to the field of vision that is lost. Visual defects are **homonymous** when confined to the same part of the visual field in each eye. They are **heterony-mous** when the part of the visual field lost in each eye is different. A homonymous defect results from lesions in the visual pathway distal to the optic chiasm. Thus, total destruction of the optic tract, lateral geniculate nucleus, geniculocalcarine tract, or visual cortex results in loss of the entire opposite field of vision in each eye, a phenomenon referred to as contralateral homonymous hemianopsia.

Lesions of the optic chiasm cause several types of heteronymous defects. Most commonly, the crossing fibers are involved and this results in an interruption of the nasal retinal fibers, which are carrying impulses from the temporal fields of

vision. The defect in this case is referred to as **bitemporal hemianopsia.** Examples of lesions in various parts of the visual pathway, the visual field defects, and the principal causes of the lesions that result are given in Figure 14-8.

VISUAL REFLEXES

The size of the pupil and the curvature of the lens are governed by three groups of visual reflexes whose afferent components include parts of the visual system and whose efferent components involve, with only one exception, the autonomic system. These reflexes are the light or pupillary con-

Visual field defects

A. **Right optic nerve:** Blindness of right eye (trauma, optic neuritis).

B. **Optic chiasm:** Complete midline transection causes bitemporal hemianopsia (pituitary tumors, craniopharyngiomas).

C. **Right angle of chiasm:** Right nasal hemianopsia (pressure by aneurysm of internal carotid artery).

D. **Right optic tract:** Left homonymous hemianopsia (abscess or tumor of temporal lobe that compresses optic tract against the crus cerebri).

E. **Complete capsular destruction of right optic radiation:** Left homonymous hemianopsia (anterior choroidal artery dysfunctions, tumors).

F. **Right Meyer loop or lower part of geniculocalcarine tract:** Left homonymous superior quadrantic anopsia (temporal or occipital lobe tumor).

G. **Upper part of right geniculocalcarine tract:** Left homonymous inferior quadrantic anopsia (parietal or occipital lobe tumor).

H. **Right striate area (visual cortex):** Left homonymous hemianopsia. Macular vision may be preserved if posterior part of the visual cortex is not involved (posterior cerebral artery dysfunctions, tumors, trauma).

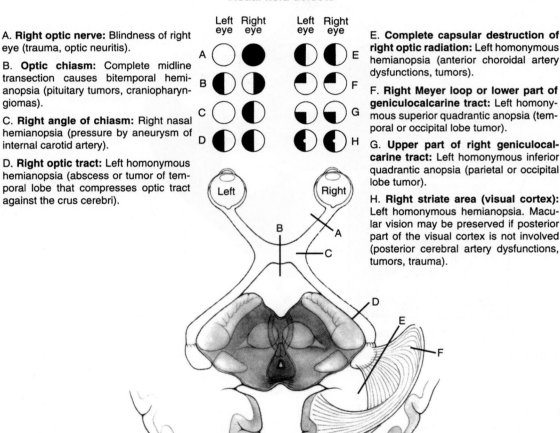

Figure 14-8 Visual field defects resulting from lesions in various parts of the visual pathway, and chief causes of the lesions.

striction reflex, the pupillary dilation reflex, and the accommodation reflexes.

THE LIGHT REFLEX

When light entering the eye becomes brighter, the pupil constricts. The reflex pupillary constriction of this eye is referred to as the **direct light reflex.** In addition to the pupillary constriction of the stimulated eye, constriction in the opposite eye also occurs; this reflex is referred to as the **consensual light reflex.**

The afferent components of the light reflex involve the receptor and neuronal elements of the retina, the optic nerve, the optic chiasm, and the optic tracts (Fig. 14-9). From each optic tract, the impulses enter the brachium of the superior colliculus (superior brachium; Fig. 14-6), which carries them to the light reflex center in the pretectal region.

CLINICAL CONNECTION

The light reflex may be used to distinguish an optic tract lesion from lesions more distal in the visual pathway, all of which result in hemianopsia. With lesions distal to the optic tract, that is, in the lateral geniculate nucleus, optic radiation, or visual cortex, a small beam of light directed into only the blind halves of each retina results in pupillary constriction because the visual pathway is interrupted beyond the optic tract and superior brachium. In other words, the afferent components of the light reflexes in the optic tract are intact. Conversely, when either the optic tract or the superior brachium is damaged, shining light into the blind halves of each retina does not elicit the light reflexes because the afferent limb from the blind hemifield is interrupted.

Neurons in the pretectal region have axons that terminate on visceromotor parasympathetic neurons of the oculomotor nuclear complex, commonly referred to as the Edinger-Westphal nucleus. For the consensual phenomenon, crossing occurs in the optic chiasm or in the posterior commissure, thus involving the contralateral Edinger-Westphal nucleus.

The efferent limb of the light reflex involves preganglionic parasympathetic axons from the Edinger-Westphal nucleus that travel in the oculomotor nerve and its branches to the ciliary gan-

glion. Postganglionic fibers from this ganglion course to the eye through the short ciliary nerves and terminate on the constrictor muscle of the iris.

The preganglionic pupilloconstrictor fibers in the oculomotor nerve are usually the first components affected when the nerve is compressed. Thus, an early sign of oculomotor nerve compression, such as occurs in herniation of the brain into the tentorial notch, is ipsilateral pupillary dilation.

CLINICAL CONNECTION

Total destruction of the retina or optic nerve interrupts the afferent limb of the light reflex and abolishes both the direct and the consensual responses from the blind eye. However, both pupils react when the good eye is stimulated by increased light. An oculomotor nerve lesion interrupts the efferent limb of the reflex, resulting in pupillary dilation (mydriasis) and a loss of both the direct and consensual responses in the ipsilateral eye.

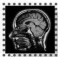

CLINICAL CONNECTION

In the afferent pupillary defect (APD) or Marcus Gunn pupil, which occurs after unilateral partial retinal or optic nerve lesion, both pupils have reduced constriction when light is shined in the affected eye but normal constriction when light is shined in the normal eye.

THE PUPILLARY DILATION REFLEX

Pupillary dilation occurs passively when the parasympathetic tone is decreased, and actively when sympathetic tone is increased. The latter is usually a result of emotional expressions (fear, rage, and so forth) or pain. Impulses from sympathetic centers in the posterior hypothalamus travel via the brainstem reticular formation to the **ciliospinal center,** which is composed of preganglionic sympathetic neurons located at the C8 and T1 spinal cord segments (Fig. 14-10). These preganglionic sympathetic neurons have axons that emerge with the ventral roots of spinal nerves T1 and T2, traverse the white communicating rami to enter and ascend in the sympathetic trunk, and terminate in the superior

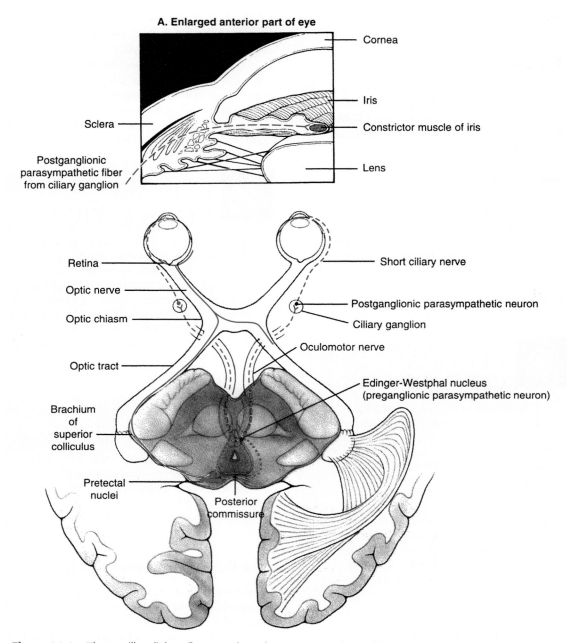

A. Enlarged anterior part of eye

Cornea

Iris

Constrictor muscle of iris

Sclera

Lens

Postganglionic
parasympathetic fiber
from ciliary ganglion

Retina

Short ciliary nerve

Optic nerve

Postganglionic parasympathetic neuron

Optic chiasm

Ciliary ganglion

Oculomotor nerve

Optic tract

Edinger-Westphal nucleus
(preganglionic parasympathetic neuron)

Brachium
of
superior
colliculus

Pretectal
nuclei

Posterior
commissure

Figure 14-9   The pupillary light reflex. **A.** Enlarged anterior part of eye showing innervation of constrictor muscle of iris.

cervical ganglion. Postganglionic sympathetic fibers then travel in the **carotid plexuses** and via the nasociliary and long ciliary nerves to the dilator muscle of the iris. Interruption of this pathway, centrally as it descends from the hypothalamus to the ciliospinal center in the spinal cord, in the spinal cord at C8 to T1, or in the periphery, leads to constriction of the pupil (miosis) as a result of the unopposed action of the parasympathetically innervated pupillary constrictor. In spite of the miosis the pupil still reacts to light and accommodation.

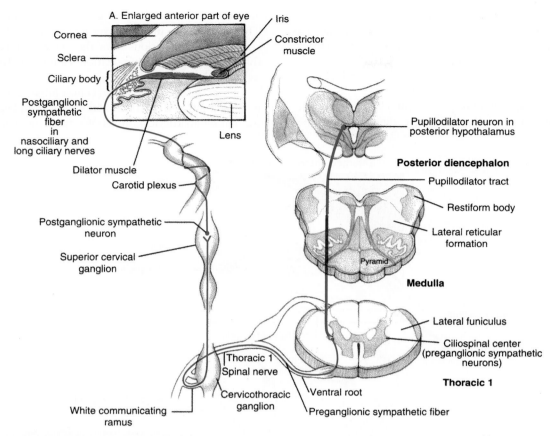

Figure 14-10   The pupillodilator reflex. **A.** Enlarged anterior part of eye showing innervation of dilator muscle iris.

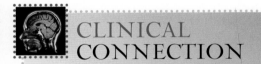

CLINICAL CONNECTION

The miosis resulting from interruption of the pupillary dilation path is included in a triad of symptoms referred to as **Horner syndrome.** In addition to the miosis, the syndrome includes a mild ptosis (drooping of the eyelid) and an **anhidrosis** (loss of sweating). The mild ptosis occurs because of the denervation of smooth muscle in the upper eyelid (Müller muscle). The anhidrosis occurs because of the sympathetic denervation of facial sweat glands.

Horner syndrome commonly results from tumors or vascular lesions involving the lateral medulla; cervical spinal cord injuries, tumors, or syringomyelia; trauma to T1 and T2 ventral roots; cervical sympathetic trunk involvement by pulmonary carcinoma; and diseases of the internal carotid artery.

THE ACCOMMODATION REFLEXES

Accommodation is the process in which a clear visual image is maintained as gaze is shifted from a distant to a near point. There are three components of the accommodation reaction commonly referred to as the **near triad:** convergence of the eyes, pupillary constriction, and thickening of the lens.

When vision is changed from a distant object to a near one the light rays become more divergent on passing through the lens. For the image to remain focused on the retina, the curvature of the lens increases. The mechanism for this accommodation of the lens is based on an inherently elastic lens that is suspended by ligaments from the ciliary body. On contraction of its muscles the ciliary body moves closer to the lens, thereby decreasing the tension on the suspensory ligaments. This allows the lens to increase its anteroposterior diameter by bulging. To facilitate visual acuity further, convergence of the eyes and constriction of the pupils are combined with the accommodation of the lens. The accompanying constriction of the pupil enhances visual acuity by keeping light rays from the more peripheral part of the lens where chromatic and spherical aberrations are more likely to result.

The stimulus for accommodation is the perception of an object. The accommodation reflexes

are initiated by the occipital cortex (Fig. 14-11). The afferent limbs in the reflexes are represented by corticotectal projections from the occipital lobe that pass to the **accommodation center** in the region of the oculomotor nuclei.

From the accommodation center impulses go to appropriate nuclei of the oculomotor complex: the parasympathetic Edinger-Westphal nucleus

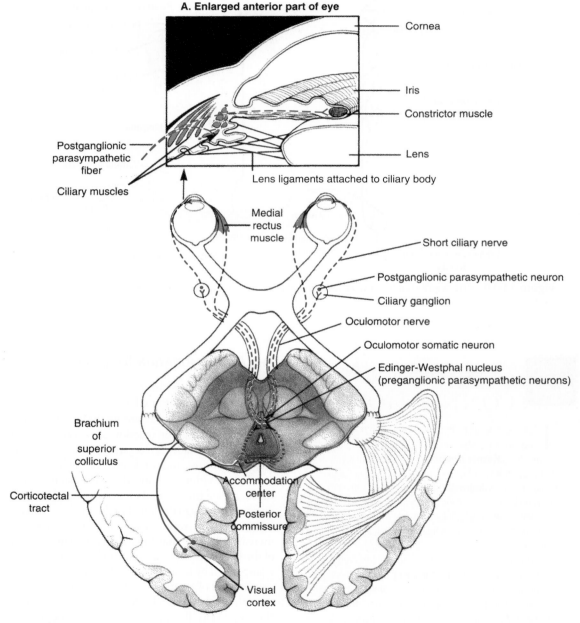

Figure 14-11   The accommodation reflexes. **A.** Enlarged anterior part of eye showing innervation of ciliary muscles and constrictor muscle of iris.

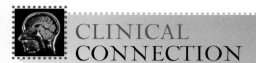

CLINICAL CONNECTION

In certain pathologic conditions, such as tabes dorsalis resulting from neurosyphilis or tumors near the posterior part of the third ventricle, an Argyll Robertson pupil sign occurs. This sign is characterized by a small pupil that does not react to increased light, but does react well on accommodation. The underlying mechanism is not understood, but probably involves bilateral lesions in the pretectal light reflex centers or their connections with the Edinger-Westphal nuclei.

for changes in the lens and pupil and the somatic nuclei for convergence of the eyes. The efferent limb is the oculomotor nerve with a synapse in the ciliary ganglion for the parasympathetic impulses responsible for the involuntary accommodation and constriction. Short ciliary nerves carry the postganglionic parasympathetic fibers to the eye. The somatic impulses for convergence pass un-interruptedly from lower motor neurons of the oculomotor complex to the medial rectus muscles.

Chapter Review Questions

14-1. How does glaucoma differ from cataract?

14-2. Between what layers does detachment of the retina occur?

14-3. What morphologic features are common to retinal layers four, six, and eight?

14-4. Night blindness is associated with functional deficits in what structures? What vitamin may be involved?

14-5. Color blindness is associated with functional deficits in what structures?

14-6. Compare the fovea centralis and optic disc as to morphology and function.

14-7. What is the medical significance of the morphologic features unique to the optic nerve?

14-8. How is transduction of a sensory stimulus in the retina different from transduction in most other sensory systems?

14-9. What visual field deficits result from destructive lesions of the following?
  a. left optic nerve
  b. median part of optic chiasm
  c. retrolenticular part of right internal capsule
  d. left loop of Meyer
  e. right striate cortex

14-10. How is processing of visual stimuli different in the retina and lateral geniculate nucleus compared with the primary visual cortex?

14-11. The conscious interpretation of shape, motion, and color occurs in what area(s) of the cerebral cortex?

14-12. What cranial nerves and which parts of the brain are essential for the integrity of the direct and consensual light reflexes?

14-13. Name three CNS and three peripheral nervous system structures that when damaged interrupt the pupillodilator path unilaterally.

14-14. Describe the phenomenon associated with accommodation and give its neural substrate.

The Gustatory and Olfactory Systems: Ageusia and Anosmia

A 50-YEAR-OLD PATIENT has right facial paralysis, right hyperacusis, and the loss of taste on the anterior two-thirds of the right side of the tongue.

Taste and smell are chemical senses that provide information about a wide range of stimuli, from the pleasant taste of certain foods and drinks to the unpleasant or noxious odors of decay and danger. Both senses arise from specific chemical receptors, which when activated transmit neural impulses to the cerebral cortex, where perception occurs.

GUSTATORY SYSTEM

Taste arises chiefly from receptors embedded in the mucosa of the tongue. A few receptors may also exist on the epiglottis and adjacent part of the pharynx. The gustatory pathway consists of three neurons: the first neuron is in the ganglia of cranial nerves (CN) VII, IX, and X; the second neuron is in the medulla; and the third neuron is in the thalamus.

GUSTATORY RECEPTORS

Taste receptors, or gustatory receptors, are activated by sweetness, saltiness, bitterness, and sourness. Perhaps there is an additional taste quality, umami, which has been described as being associated with monosodium glutamate by some investigators or "meaty" by others. All qualities of taste are elicited from all regions of the tongue containing taste buds.

The taste buds are composed of 50 to 100 gustatory receptor cells, supporting cells, and basal stem cells (Fig. 15-1). At the apex of each gustatory cell, microvilli form the gustatory hairs, which project into a small cavity beneath the gustatory pore. The base of each taste bud is penetrated by nerve fibers that branch and spiral around the receptor cells. Individual receptor cells have a life span of approximately 2 weeks and are replaced from the basal stem cells.

Transduction begins in the microvilli with tastants interacting directly with ion channels or receptors. Directly or indirectly this leads to a depolarization of the base of the taste cells that form synaptic contacts with the gustatory afferents, resulting in the propagation of action potentials centrally.

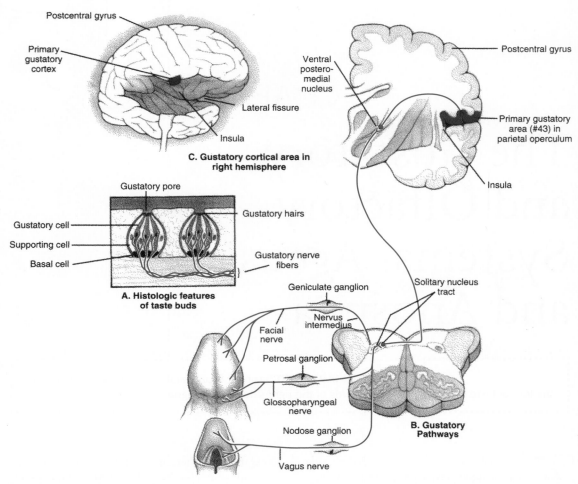

Figure 15-1 Schematic diagram of gustatory pathways. **A.** Histology features of taste buds. **B.** Gustatory pathways. **C.** Gustatory cortical area in right hemisphere.

GUSTATORY PATHWAY

Taste buds in different parts of the tongue are innervated by different cranial nerves (Fig. 15-1). Taste buds in the anterior two-thirds of the tongue are innervated by the facial nerve as illustrated in the case history at the beginning of this chapter; taste buds in the posterior third of the tongue are innervated by the glossopharyngeal nerve; and taste buds in the epiglottic and palatal portions of the oral cavity are innervated by the vagus nerve. The primary or first-order neurons in the gustatory pathway are unipolar cells in the geniculate ganglion of the facial nerve (VII CN), inferior or petrosal ganglion of the glossopharyngeal nerve (IX CN), and inferior or nodose ganglion of the vagus nerve (X CN).

The axons of these ganglia cells enter the brainstem, pass to the solitary tract, and synapse in the rostral part of the solitary nucleus, commonly referred to as the gustatory nucleus (Figs. 15-1–15-3). Secondary connections of the gustatory nucleus ascend near either the medial lemniscus or central tegmental tract to reach the ventral posteromedial (VPM) nucleus of the thalamus. The most medial part of the VPM nucleus, the small cell parvicellular part, receives projections from the gustatory nucleus. From this parvicellular part, fibers travel in the gustatory radiation through the posterior limb of the internal capsule to the cortical gustatory area. The primary gustatory cortex is located in the parietal operculum and the adjacent part of the insula.

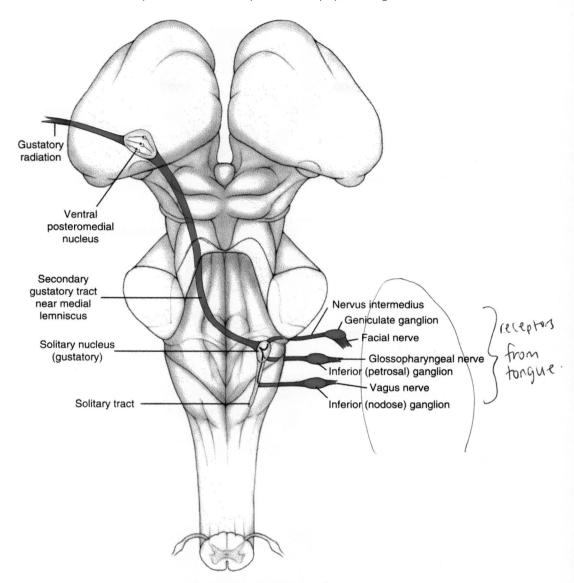

Gustatory radiation

Ventral posteromedial nucleus

Secondary gustatory tract near medial lemniscus

Solitary nucleus (gustatory)

Solitary tract

Nervus intermedius

Geniculate ganglion

Facial nerve

Glossopharyngeal nerve

Inferior (petrosal) ganglion

Vagus nerve

Inferior (nodose) ganglion

} receptors from tongue.

Figure 15-2 Three-dimensional dorsal view of gustatory pathways.

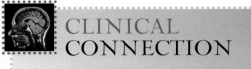

CLINICAL CONNECTION

According to clinical reports, damage to the VPM nucleus or to the gustatory cortex results in a loss of taste on the contralateral side of the tongue.

OLFACTORY SYSTEM

Humans are microsmatic, i.e., their sense of smell is poorly developed; hence, the sense of smell and its pathways are considerably less important clinically than the visual, auditory, and somatosensory senses and their pathways. The central nervous system (CNS) structures associated with olfaction form the rhinencephalon "nose-brain," which chiefly includes the olfactory structures on the base of the brain and the medial parts of the temporal lobe in the vicinity of the uncus.

OLFACTORY RECEPTORS

The primary olfactory neurons are located in the yellowish olfactory mucosa, which consists of about 1 square inch of epithelium on the superior nasal

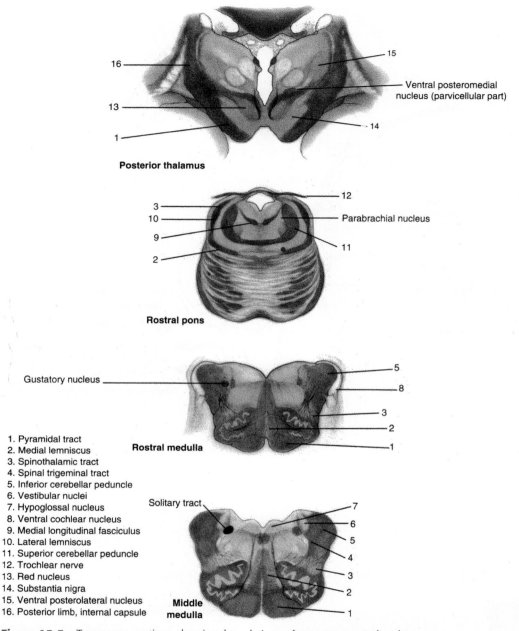

Posterior thalamus

15 — Ventral posteromedial nucleus (parvicellular part)

Rostral pons

Parabrachial nucleus

Gustatory nucleus

Rostral medulla

1. Pyramidal tract
2. Medial lemniscus
3. Spinothalamic tract
4. Spinal trigeminal tract
5. Inferior cerebellar peduncle
6. Vestibular nuclei
7. Hypoglossal nucleus
8. Ventral cochlear nucleus
9. Medial longitudinal fasciculus
10. Lateral lemniscus
11. Superior cerebellar peduncle
12. Trochlear nerve
13. Red nucleus
14. Substantia nigra
15. Ventral posterolateral nucleus
16. Posterior limb, internal capsule

Solitary tract

Middle medulla

Figure 15-3 Transverse sections showing the relations of gustatory central pathways.

concha and the upper part of the nasal septum. The olfactory neurons are bipolar and number several million on each side. Each neuron possesses a dendrite that extends to the surface, where it expands to form a bulbous olfactory vesicle. Each of these vesicles, in turn, gives rise to a number of olfactory cilia (Fig. 15-4). These cilia spread over the surface of the olfactory mucosa and are bathed in mucus secreted mainly by specialized glands and by cells in the olfactory epithelium and the neighboring nasal mucosa. For odors to be smelled, odorants must dissolve in the mucus to stimulate receptors in the cilia. There may be as many as 1,000 receptors responsive to different odorant stimuli. Odorant receptor binding is transduced to a depolarization of the primary olfactory neuron by acti-

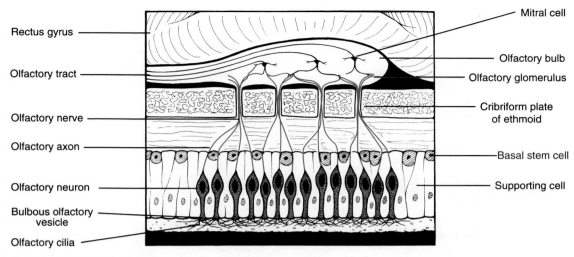

Figure 15-4   Histologic features of olfactory receptors, nerves, and bulb.

vation of an intermediary second messenger cyclic nucleotide pathway that controls ionic channels that lead to the generation of an action potential.

A unique feature of the primary olfactory neurons is that they are constantly replaced throughout a person's lifetime. It is estimated that the life span of these neurons is only 4 to 6 weeks and, on degenerating, new neurons are formed from undifferentiated basal stem cells in the deeper part of the olfactory epithelium.

OLFACTORY PATHWAY

The central branches of the bipolar olfactory neurons form the axons of the olfactory nerves (Fig. 15-4). These nonmyelinated fibers are collected into about 20 bundles, which traverse the foramina in the cribriform plate of the ethmoid

bone. Collectively these bundles form the olfactory nerve and they terminate in the olfactory bulb located on the floor of the anterior cranial fossa above the cribriform plate. How the axons of olfactory neurons newly formed throughout life reach synaptic sites on the secondary neurons in the olfactory bulb is not known.

The olfactory bulb is the flattened oval structure on the orbital surface of the frontal lobe near the anterior end of the olfactory sulcus (Fig. 15-5). It is composed of several types of cells, the most prominent of which are the mitral cells (Fig. 15-4). The synaptic contacts between the olfactory nerve fibers and the mitral cells are made via dense arborizations that form the olfactory glomeruli. In these structures, thousands of olfactory nerve fibers may synapse on the dendrites of one mitral cell. The axons of the mitral cells enter the olfactory tract.

The olfactory tract is the narrow band that continues posteriorly from the olfactory bulb along the olfactory sulcus. It is mainly composed of the efferent fibers of the bulb, although it does contain clumps of neurons that form the anterior olfactory nucleus as well as centrifugal fibers from the contralateral anterior olfactory nucleus and from neurons in the basal forebrain whose axons modulate the olfactory bulb neurons.

At the posterior end of the olfactory tract is the olfactory trigone (Fig. 15-5), where the fibers of the tract diverge to form two bundles, the lateral and medial olfactory striae, which border the anterior perforated substance. The fibers of the medial olfactory stria arise chiefly in the anterior

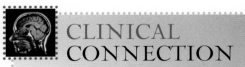

CLINICAL CONNECTION

The sudden loss of smell (anosmia) is not uncommon after sudden blows to the head. Anosmia occurs most frequently as the result of head injuries that injure the olfactory nerves or nasal infections that damage the olfactory receptors. However, the gradual loss of smell may be related to the growth of a tumor at the base of the anterior cranial fossa; hence, this type of loss should be investigated.

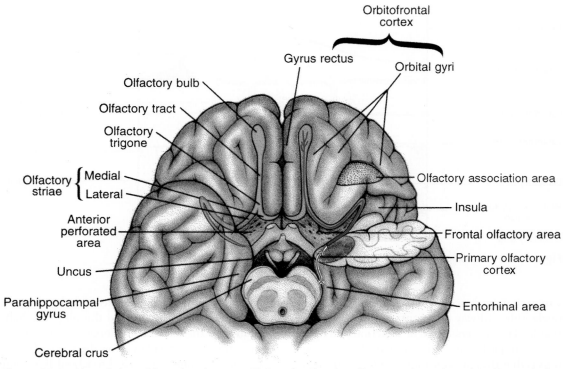

Figure 15-5   Ventral view of frontal and temporal lobes showing the olfactory pathway from the olfactory bulb to the primary olfactory cortex. Left temporal lobe removed from temporal pole to uncus to expose pathway.

olfactory nucleus and project via the anterior or olfactory part of the anterior commissure to the contralateral olfactory bulb. The medial olfactory stria becomes buried in the anterior perforated substance shortly after emerging from the olfactory trigone.

The lateral olfactory stria carries the efferent projections of the olfactory bulb toward the insula, where they bend medially to enter the temporal lobe. On entering the temporal lobe, the fibers of the lateral olfactory stria terminate in the primary olfactory cortex in the uncus. The uncus is the enlargement in the anterior part of the parahippocampal gyrus and is located on the medial surface of the temporal lobe (Fig. 15-5). The uncus is actually the medial part of the amygdaloid nucleus, which sends axons to the medial dorsal nucleus of the thalamus. The medial dorsal nucleus, in turn, sends axons to the posterolateral part of the orbitofrontal cortex, the neocortical olfactory association area important for discrimination and identification of odors.

Olfactory sensations may also reach the orbitofrontal cortex without passing through the thalamus. This nonthalamic pathway passes from the uncus to more posterior parts of the parahippo-

campal gyrus, which, in turn, sends axons via the uncinate fasciculus directly to the orbitofrontal cortex. In addition to the olfactory connections destined for the orbitofrontal cortex, olfactory sensations transmitted from the uncus to the hypothalamus mediate the behavioral and autonomic responses to odors.

Projections from olfactory and gustatory cortical areas converge in the medial orbitofrontal cortex, where there appears to be a center that integrates smell and taste, thereby producing flavor.

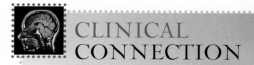

CLINICAL CONNECTION

Lesions in the olfactory area of the orbitofrontal cortex result in the loss of ability to discriminate different odors. Irritative lesions in the region of the uncus result in olfactory hallucinations, usually disagreeable in character. These olfactory hallucinations commonly occur in temporal lobe epilepsy and frequently constitute the aura that precedes the phenomenon referred to as "uncinate fits."

Chapter Review Questions

15-1. Which cranial nerves contain taste fibers and what are their peripheral distributions and central connections?

15-2. Locate the primary gustatory area in the cerebral cortex.

15-3. Give the location and morphologic features of the olfactory membrane.

15-4. Locate the primary olfactory area.

The Cerebral Cortex: Aphasia, Agnosia, and Apraxia

A 62-YEAR-OLD PATIENT experiences sudden loss of speech, accompanied by weakness of the right lower facial muscles and the right hand.

*T*he cerebral cortex is the "highest center" in the brain and, as such, it perceives sensations, commands skilled movements, provides awareness of emotions, and is necessary for memory, thinking, language abilities, and all other higher mental functions.

SUBDIVISIONS OF THE CEREBRAL CORTEX

There are three types of cortex in the human brain: neocortex, paleocortex, and archicortex. The neocortex appeared last in evolution and constitutes about 90% of the total cerebral cortex. The paleocortex is restricted to the base of the cerebral hemispheres and is associated with the olfactory system, whereas the archicortex, the phylogenetically oldest cortex, makes up the **hippocampus.** Both the paleocortex and archicortex are parts of the limbic system, which is described in Chapter 17.

The cerebral cortex reaches its greatest development in the human. It contributes about half the total brain weight and consists of a sheet of neurons 2.5 square feet in area that is folded or convoluted with only about one-third of the neocortex found on the surface and the remainder buried in the grooves between the convolutions. A fold or convolution is called a gyrus (pl. gyri), and the groove between adjacent gyri is called a sulcus (pl. sulci).

HISTOLOGIC FEATURES

The young adult cortex contains billions of neurons. The two main neuronal cell types are the **pyramidal** and **granule cells** (Fig. 16-1). The pyramidal cells have a pyramid-shaped cell body with a large apical dendrite directed toward the surface of the cortex and several large basal dendrites that pass horizontally from the base of the cell. The axon proceeds from the base of the cell and in most cases leaves the cortex to reach other cortical areas or subcortical nuclei. The pyramidal cells are the chief cortical efferent or output neurons.

The granule or stellate cells are the main interneurons of the cortex and greatly outnumber the

Layers   Cells

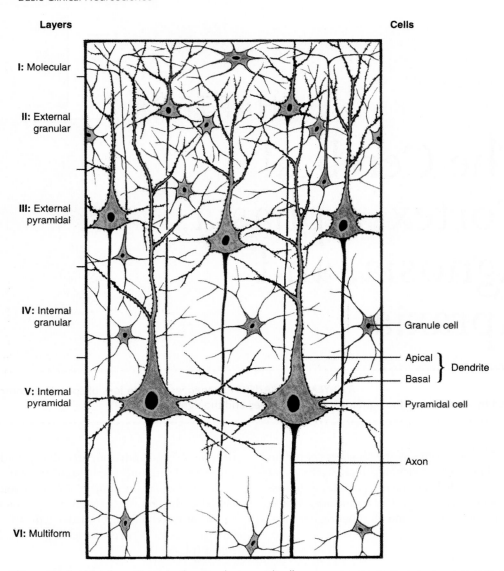

I: Molecular

II: External
granular

III: External
pyramidal

IV: Internal
granular   Granule cell

                                                                            Apical ⎫
                                                                                   ⎬ Dendrite
                                                                            Basal ⎭

V: Internal
pyramidal   Pyramidal cell

                                                                            Axon

VI: Multiform

Figure 16-1   Histology of cerebral cortex: layers and cells.

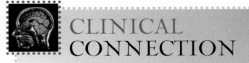

CLINICAL CONNECTION

The surfaces of the dendrites of mature pyramidal cells contain numerous synaptic sites, called spines (Fig. 16-1). During postnatal maturation of the cortex, the pyramidal cell dendritic trees expand and the number of spines increases. The finding that the faulty development of these dendritic trees and their spines is seen in cases of mental retardation such as **Down syndrome** suggests that these phenomena may be related to learning.

pyramidal cells. These small cells have numerous short dendrites that extend in all directions and a short axon that arborizes on other neurons in the vicinity. Granule cells occur in large numbers in all cortical areas and are especially numerous in the sensory and association areas.

FUNCTIONAL HISTOLOGY

The neurons of the neocortex are arranged in six horizontal layers. The most superficial is the cell-poor molecular layer (I), and the deepest is the multiform layer (VI). In between these layers are alternating external and internal granular layers (II and IV) and pyramidal layers (III and V), each of which is named according to its predominant cell type (Fig. 16-1).

Although the neurons of the cortex are arranged in six layers oriented parallel to the surface, the functional units of cortical activity are organized in groups of neurons oriented perpendicular to the surface. These vertically oriented functional units are called **cortical columns,** each of which is a few millimeters in diameter and contains thousands of neurons that are interconnected in the vertical direction.

Within each cortical column the internal granular layer (IV) is the chief input layer (Fig. 16-2) and receives afferent fibers from the thalamic nuclei. The infragranular layers (V and VI) are for output, layer V giving rise to fibers destined for the corpus striatum, brainstem, and spinal cord. Layer VI projects fibers to the thalamus. The supragranular layers (I, II, and III) are associative and connect with other parts of the cerebral cortex.

CORTICAL CONNECTIONS

The connections of each cortical column are of four types: intracortical, association, commissural, and subcortical (Fig. 16-2).

INTRACORTICAL FIBERS

Intracortical connections are quite short and occur chiefly through horizontally oriented neurons in layer I and the horizontally coursing branches of pyramidal cell axons.

ASSOCIATION FIBERS

Association connections occur from gyrus to gyrus and from lobe to lobe in the same hemisphere. The short association fibers, called arcuate fibers or loops, connect adjacent gyri, and the long association fibers form bundles connecting more distant gyri (Fig. 16-3). The long association bundles give fibers to and receive fibers from the overlying gyri along their routes. The main long association bundles are the **superior longitudinal fasciculus** and

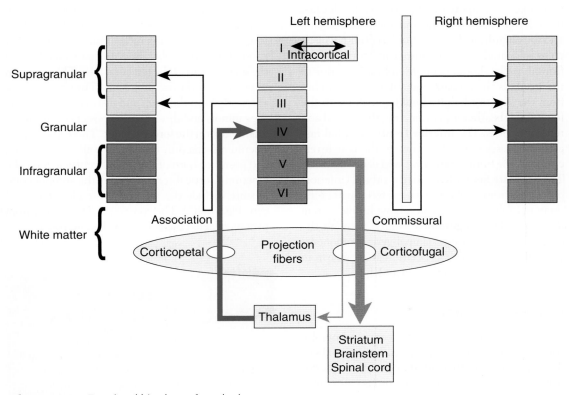

Figure 16-2   Functional histology of cerebral cortex.

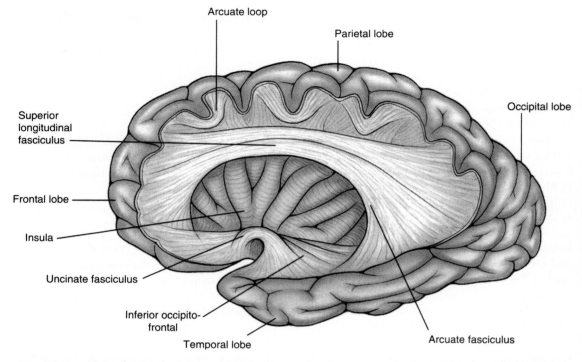

Arcuate loop

Parietal lobe

Occipital lobe

Superior longitudinal fasciculus

Frontal lobe

Insula

Uncinate fasciculus

Inferior occipito-frontal

Temporal lobe

Arcuate fasciculus

Figure 16-3   Three-dimensional drawing of the major association bundles dissected from the lateral aspect.

its temporal component, the **arcuate fasciculus,** the inferior occipitofrontal and uncinate fasciculi, and the **cingulum.** The superior longitudinal fasciculus is located above the insula and connects the frontal, parietal, and occipital lobes. Posterior to the insula is the arcuate fasciculus, which arches from the superior longitudinal fasciculus into the temporal lobe, thereby connecting the frontal and temporal lobes. The **inferior fronto-occipital fasciculus** passes ventral to the insula as it interconnects the frontal, temporal, and occipital lobes. The **uncinate fasciculus** joins the orbital (inferior) part of the frontal lobe with the anterior part of the temporal lobe, both of which have limbic system functions. The **cingulum** is located beneath the cingulate and parahippocampal gyri, components of the limbic lobe. The association fibers arise from pyramidal neurons chiefly in layer III.

COMMISSURAL FIBERS

Commissural connections occur between homologous areas of the two hemispheres. Two major bundles exist: the corpus callosum and the anterior commissure (Fig. 16-4A). The corpus callosum is divided, from anterior to posterior, into **rostrum,** **genu, trunk,** and **splenium.** The rostrum and genu interconnect the anterior part of the frontal lobe (Fig. 16-4B). The trunk interconnects the posterior part of the frontal lobe, the entire parietal lobe, and the superior part of the temporal lobe. The splenium interconnects the occipital lobes. The fibers arching anteriorly from the genu and rostrum form the **forceps minor,** and those arching posteriorly from the splenium form the **forceps major.** Those fibers of the splenium located in the lateral wall of the atrium and posterior horn of the lateral ventricle form the **tapetum.** Cortical connections of the anterior commissure include the inferior and middle temporal gyri (Fig. 16-4C). The commissural fibers arise from pyramidal cells chiefly in layer III (Fig. 16-2).

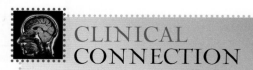

CLINICAL CONNECTION

Surgical transection of the corpus callosum is sometimes performed for the relief of epilepsy. Such **split brain** patients have served to elucidate the importance of the corpus callosum, especially for language functions.

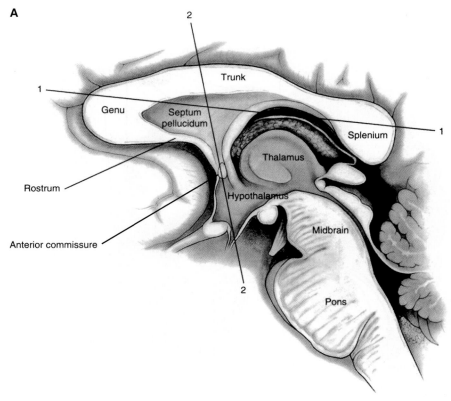

A

2

Trunk

1

Genu

Septum
pellucidum

Splenium

1

Thalamus

Rostrum

Hypothalamus

Anterior commissure

Midbrain

2

Pons

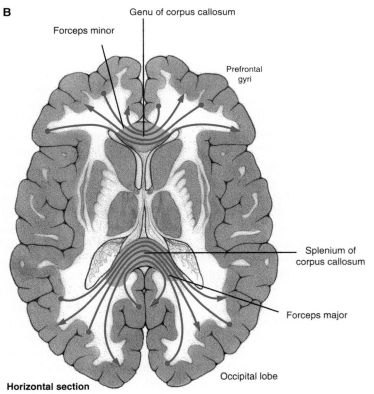

B

Genu of corpus callosum

Forceps minor

Prefrontal
gyri

Splenium of
corpus callosum

Forceps major

Occipital lobe

Horizontal section

Figure 16-4   A. Median brainstem showing locations of hemispheric commissural
fibers: the corpus callosum and anterior commissure. **B.** Plane of horizontal section
through genu and splenium of corpus callosum (line 1-1). Connections of genu and
splenium of corpus callosum: forceps minor and major. (*continued*)

C

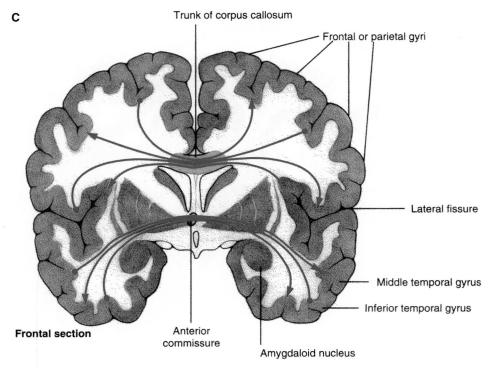

Trunk of corpus callosum

Frontal or parietal gyri

Lateral fissure

Middle temporal gyrus

Inferior temporal gyrus

Frontal section

Anterior commissure

Amygdaloid nucleus

Figure 16-4 (*Continued*) **C.** Plane of coronal section through corpus callosum and anterior commissure (line 2-2). Connections of anterior commissure and trunk of corpus callosum.

PROJECTION FIBERS

Projection fibers connect the cerebral cortex with subcortical nuclei and are classified as **corticofugal** or efferent if they carry impulses away from the cortex, or **corticopetal** or afferent if they carry them toward the cortex (Fig. 16-2). The corticofugal projection fibers are distributed to the corpus striatum and nuclei at all levels of the brainstem and spinal cord. The major corticofugal projections are described with the motor system (Chapters 6–9). Corticopetal projection fibers arise predominantly in the thalamus and are called thalamic radiations. These radiations can be distributed to specific or to widespread cortical areas. In most cases the connections between the thalamic nuclei and the cerebral cortex are reciprocal.

As projection fibers course between the thalamus and the corpus striatum, they are gathered together in a conspicuous band called the internal capsule. In the horizontal plane, the internal capsule is V-shaped (Fig. 16-5) and is divided into an anterior limb located between the head of the caudate and lentiform nuclei, a posterior limb located between the thalamus and lentiform nucleus, and a genu where the two limbs meet. The anterior limb of the internal capsule is for prefrontal connections exclusively, e.g., corticofugal projections to the striatum and pontine nuclei and corticopetal projection fibers from the anterior and medial thalamic nuclei. The genu and adjacent part of the posterior limb contain corticopetal projection fibers from the motor thalamus (i.e., the ventral anterior and ventral lateral nuclei), which project to the premotor and motor areas, respectively. Posteriorly, the posterior limb contains the corticonuclear (corticobulbar) and corticospinal (pyramidal) tracts as well as the somatosensory thalamic radiations from the ventral posterior nucleus. The precise location of the corticonuclear and corticospinal tracts in the posterior limb varies according to the superior-inferior level of the capsule. Superiorly, the pyramidal tract is in the anterior half of the posterior limb, whereas inferiorly it is in the posterior half (Fig. 16-5). The corticobulbar tract

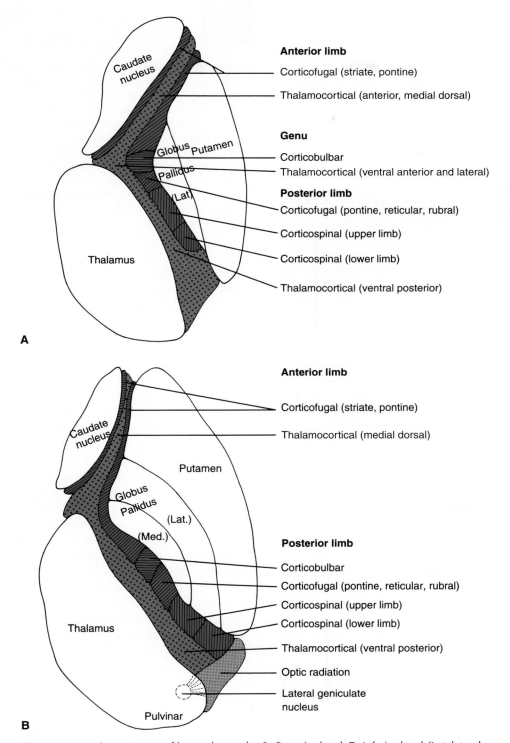

Figure 16-5 Components of internal capsule. **A.** Superior level. **B.** Inferior level (Lat, lateral; Med, medial).

is slightly anterior to the pyramidal tract. The part of the internal capsule lateral to the thalamus and posterior to the lentiform nucleus is the retrolenticular limb and contains the optic radiations as they emerge from the lateral geniculate nucleus (Fig. 16-5B). The auditory radiations from the medial geniculate nucleus are located in that part of the internal capsule lateral to the thalamus and ventral to the lentiform nucleus, the sublenticular limb of the internal capsule.

CLINICAL CONNECTION

The posterior limb of the internal capsule is of great clinical importance because it is the most frequent site of cerebral hemorrhage or "stroke." Moreover, when this area is damaged the signs and symptoms are more widespread than those associated with a lesion of comparable size anywhere in the nervous system. After a capsular stroke, the patient has contralateral spastic hemiplegia, resulting from damage to the corticospinal tract, and contralateral hemianesthesia, resulting from damage to the somatosensory thalamic radiation. In addition, contralateral lower facial paralysis results from damage to the corticobulbar tract. If the damaged capsular area includes the retrolenticular limb, contralateral homonymous hemianopsia results from interruption of the optic radiation.

FUNCTIONAL AREAS

Anatomically, the cerebral cortex is described according to lobes (frontal, parietal, temporal, occipital, limbic, and insular) that are subdivided into gyri (Figs. 16-6A, 16-7A). Functionally, the cortex is described according to the numbered areas (Figs. 16-6B, 16-7B) that were originally demarcated by Brodmann. Interestingly, Brodmann designated these areas not on the basis of function but of cytoarchitecture. A summary of the cortical areas, the localization of cortical functions, and the effects of destructive lesions is given in Table 16-1.

FRONTAL LOBE

The frontal cortex constitutes about one-third of the entire cerebral cortex, and its size and connections are far more differentiated in humans

CLINICAL CONNECTION

Because the density of the pyramidal and granule cells and the thickness of the various cortical layers are not uniform, the various parts of the cortex have different patterns or cytoarchitecture. On the basis of its different cytoarchitecture, the cerebral cortex was divided into numbered areas by Brodmann in 1909. With the advent of functional studies by electrical stimulation of the human cortex, it became apparent that the Brodmann numbered map corresponded well with functions of the various cortical areas. Hence, **Brodmann numbered areas** have become functional areas in addition to cytoarchitectonic areas.

than in any other animal, including the highest subhuman primates. It contains the following six main functional areas: (1) primary motor, (2) premotor, (3) supplementary motor, (4) frontal eye field, (5) prefrontal, and (6) Broca speech.

The primary motor area (MI) corresponds to Brodmann area 4 and occupies the posterior part of the precentral gyrus and the adjoining part of the paracentral lobule (Figs. 16-6B, 16-7B). Within the motor cortex somatotopic localization of contralateral movements is represented in an upside-down fashion with the lower limb in the paracentral lobule, the upper limb in the dorsal part of the precentral gyrus, and the face most ventral (Figs. 16-6C, 16-7C). The size of the area representing various movements is directly proportional to the degree of skill or finesse associated with the particular movement. Lesions of the primary motor area result in a weakness in the body part contralateral to the specific area damaged (Figs. 16-6D, 16-7D).

The premotor cortex, area 6, is located in the precentral gyrus anterior to the MI cortex on the lateral surface of the hemisphere. Electrical stimulation of this area also produces contralateral movements, but they are slower in nature and include larger groups of muscles as compared with MI stimulation. The premotor area is involved in the programming or organizing of the postural adjustments necessary to perform a skilled movement. The supplementary motor area consists of the extension of area 6 into the medial aspect of the frontal lobe (Fig. 16-7B). Thus, it lies in superior frontal gyrus anterior to the MI cortex at the convexity of the hemisphere and the paracentral lobule on the medial surface. Stimulation of this area results in posturing responses such as turning the head and eyes toward the elevated contralateral arm. This area is involved in motor planning, that is organizing complex movements. Functional magnetic resonance imaging studies show that when performing a complex movement both the MI cortex and the supplementary motor cortex are active; however, when only thinking about the movement the supplementary motor cortex alone is active.

CLINICAL CONNECTION

Focal lesions in the supplementary motor area often result in **motor apraxia,** the inability to perform purposive movement even though no paralysis exists. For example, an apraxic patient who is unable to protrude the tongue when asked spontaneously does so a few minutes later to lick the lips. Apraxia may also occur after lesions in premotor or parietal association areas.

The frontal eye field, area 8, is located immediately in front of area 6, chiefly in the middle frontal gyrus, although it may extend into the superior frontal and precentral gyri as well (Fig. 16-6B). Stimulation of this area produces conjugate deviation of the eyes to the contralateral side; a unilateral destructive lesion here results in a transient deviation of the eyes to the same side and paralysis of contralateral gaze (Fig. 16-6D).

The prefrontal cortex includes almost one fourth of the entire cerebral cortex and is located on the lateral, medial, and inferior surfaces of the frontal lobe in front of areas 6, 8, and 45 (Figs. 16-6B, 16-7B). It is referred to as the frontal association cortex and is divided into two main regions: orbital and lateral. The orbital region, sometimes called the orbitofrontal region, is located on the inferior surface of the frontal lobe and includes the orbital gyri, as well as on the medial surface anterior to the corpus callosum. The lateral area, frequently called the dorsolateral prefrontal region, includes the superior and middle frontal gyri on the convexity of the frontal lobe in front of the motor areas. The orbitofrontal area has strong limbic system connections and is associated with social behavior, whereas the dorsolateral area is concerned with such intellectual abilities as concentration, conceptualizing, planning, judgment, and problem solving. Bilateral lesions of the prefrontal cortex result in loss of initiative or ambition and responsibility, as well as judgment and foresight. The patient becomes easily distracted and careless of appearance and dress, and loses the sense of acceptable social behavior. Prefrontal leucotomy, isolation of the prefrontal cortex by cutting its connections with the rest of the brain, or prefrontal lobotomy, removal of the prefrontal cortex, were once fairly common surgical procedures used to treat patients with severe behavioral disorders.

CLINICAL CONNECTION

Insight into the functions of the prefrontal cortex was first reported in the middle of the 19th century when a railroad construction foreman, Phineas Gage, suffered prefrontal lobotomy when a dynamite tamping rod was accidentally blown through the front of his head. Before the accident, Gage was a model employee—punctual, hardworking, gentlemanly, and highly respectable. After recovery from the accident, Gage lost all sense of responsibility, became impulsive, irascible, and profane, and drifted aimlessly the rest of his life.

Even though many functions are attributed to the prefrontal cortex, massive bilateral lesions often result in changes so subtle they are difficult to detect. As a result, it has been suggested that instead of having specific functions, the prefrontal cortex may be the orchestrator for other cortical areas and may elicit the behavior appropriate to the situation at hand.

The **Broca area,** located in the triangular and opercular parts of the inferior frontal gyrus, is associated with speech and is described later.

PARIETAL LOBE

The parietal cortex constitutes slightly more than one-fifth of the entire cerebral cortex and contains the following four functional areas: (1) primary somatosensory, (2) secondary somatosensory, (3) gustatory, and (4) association.

The primary somatosensory area (SI) occupies the postcentral gyrus and the adjoining part of the paracentral lobule (Figs. 16-6A, 16-7A). It consists of three longitudinal zones: area 3 that includes the cortical tissue in the floor and posterior wall of the central sulcus, area 1 in the anterior two-thirds of

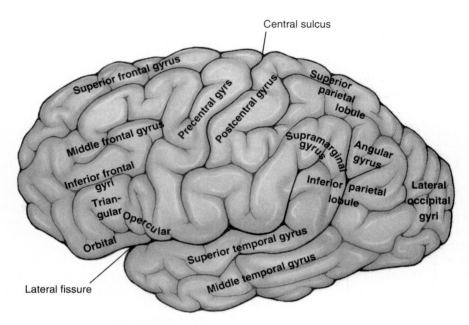

A. Principal gyri and sulci

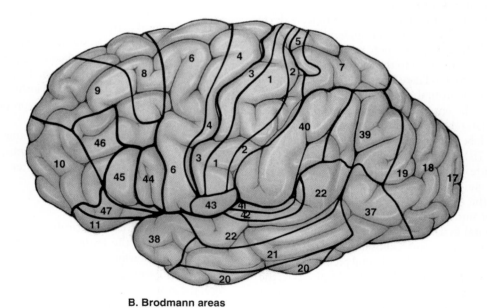

B. Brodmann areas

Figure 16-6   Lateral views of left hemisphere. **A.** Gyri and sulci. **B.** Brodmann areas.

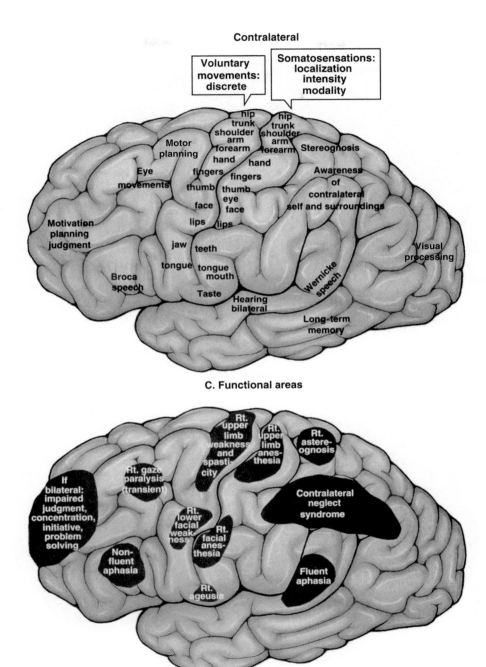

C. Functional areas

D. Results of lesions

Figure 16-6 (*Continued*)   **C.** Functional areas. **D.** Results of lesion (Rt, right).

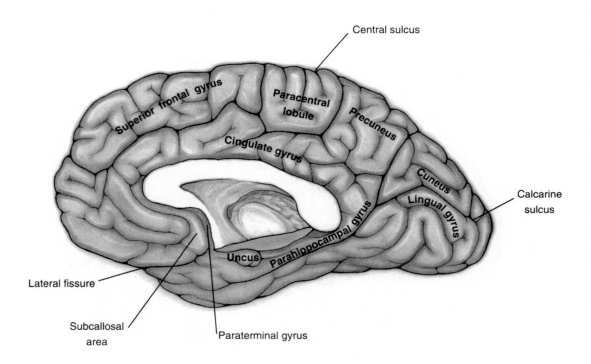

Central sulcus

Superior frontal gyrus

Paracentral lobule

Precuneus

Cingulate gyrus

Cuneus

Calcarine sulcus

Lingual gyrus

Parahippocampal gyrus

Uncus

Lateral fissure

Subcallosal area

Paraterminal gyrus

A. Principal gyri and sulci

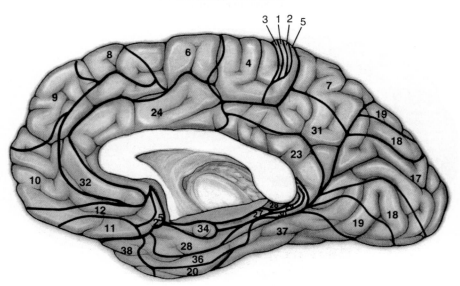

B. Brodmann areas

Figure 16-7   Medial views of right hemisphere. **A.** Gyri and sulci. **B.** Brodmann areas.

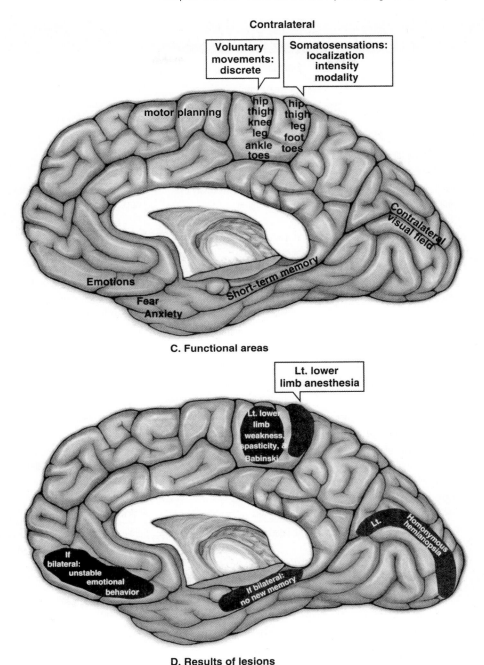

C. Functional areas

D. Results of lesions

Figure 16-7 (*Continued*)   **C.** Functional areas. **D.** Results of lesions (Lt, left).

the convex surface of the postcentral gyrus, and area 2 in the remaining one-third of the convex surface and the adjoining anterior wall of the postcentral sulcus. The somatotopic representation is contralateral with parts of the head located ventrally and the upper limb located dorsally in the

postcentral gyrus (Fig. 16-6C), and the lower limb medially, in the posterior part of the paracentral lobule (Fig. 16-7C). The total area associated with a particular region of the body is directly related to the sensitivity of the particular region and not to its size. Stimulation of the pri-

TABLE 16-1 Cortical Functions and Lesion Abnormalities

Lobe	Structure	Function	Destructive Lesion
Frontal	Precentral g. (in ant. wall of central sulcus) and paracentral lobule (ant. part)	MI area: commands movements—head and upper limb and lower limb	Contralateral paralysis or paresis: lower face and upper limb and lower limb; Babinski response also
	Precentral g. (surface)	Premotor area: programs MI area	Motor apraxia
	Superior frontal g. (post. and med. parts)	Supplementary motor area: motor planning	Motor apraxia
	Middle frontal g. (post. part and adjacent sup. frontal and precentral)	Frontal eye field: voluntary eye movements	Transitory paralysis of conjugate gaze to opposite side
	Inferior frontal g. (opercular and triangular parts in dominant hemisphere)	Broca speech: word production	Nonfluent aphasia
	Sup., med., inf., frontal g. (ant. parts)	Dorsolateral prefrontal: executive cortex (problem solving, judgment, planning, etc.)	Bilateral lesions: impaired ability to concentrate, easily distracted, loss of initiative, apathy, cannot make decisions
	(med. parts)	Orbitofrontal prefrontal: social behavior and emotions	Unstable emotions; unpredictable and frequent unacceptable behavior
	Orbital g.: (posterolat. part)	Olfactory association	Inability to discriminate odors
Parietal	Postcentral g. and paracentral lobule (post. part)	SI area: general sensory head and upper limb and lower limb	Contralateral anesthesia: head and upper limb and lower limb
	Opercular postcentral g. (and adjacent insula)	Taste	Impairment of taste in contralateral side of tongue
	Sup. parietal lobule Inf. parietal lobule (supramarginal and angular g.)	Processing of somatic and visual information	Tactile and visual agnosia, visual disorientation, neglect of contralateral self and surroundings
	Angular g. (dominant hemisphere)	Names of objects Mathematics	Anomic aphasia Acalculia
Temporal	Transverse temporal g. (of Heschl)	AI: hearing (bilateral)	Subtle decrease in hearing and ability to localize sounds, both contralaterally
	Sup. temp. g.–(post. part in dominant hemisphere)	Wernicke speech: language understanding and formulation	Fluent aphasia
	Middle and inferior temporal g.	Long-term memory	Bilateral lesions: memory impairment of past events
	Occipitotemporal g. (post. part)	Recognition of faces	Prosopagnosia
	Parahippocampal g. (entorhinal part)	Recent memory	Bilateral lesions: anterograde amnesia
	Uncal region	Olfaction	Bilateral lesions: anosmia
Occipital	Cuneus and lingual g. (walls of calcarine fissure)	Vision	Contralateral homonymous hemianopsia
	Parastriate and peristriate areas	Visual association	Bilateral lesions: color agnosia and loss of spatial relationships (cannot draw floor plan of home, map of route to work or church, etc.)

AI, primary auditory; ant, anterior; g, gyrus; inf, inferior; med, medial; MI, primary motor; post, posterior; posterolat, posterolateral; SI, primary sensory; sup, superior.

mary sensory cortex in humans produces sharply localized contralateral sensations described as tingling or numbness. Lesions of this area result in the loss of tactile discrimination and proprioception on the contralateral side (Figs. 16-6D, 16-7D). In addition, the precise localization, sharpness, and intensity of pinprick, as well as temperature sensations, are impaired. Pain cannot be elicited from this area nor is it abolished or relieved after its ablation.

The secondary somatosensory area (SII) is composed of a strip of cortex that extends from the parietal operculum into the posterior part of the insula. The parietal operculum (operculum means lid) is the cortical tissue continuous with the postcentral gyrus that forms the upper wall of the lateral fissure. Hence, it overlies and covers the insula. Somatotopic localization in the SII area is poorly defined and bilateral.

The primary gustatory cortex appears to be in area 43 of the parietal operculum (Fig. 16-6B). It extends along the wall of the lateral fissure toward the insula and is adjacent to the tongue regions of the primary sensory and motor areas. A lesion in this area results in contralateral ageusia, i.e., loss of taste (Fig. 16-6D).

The parietal association area consists of the superior and inferior parietal lobules. The superior parietal lobule contains areas 5 anteriorly and 7 posteriorly (Figs. 16-6B, 16-7B). Area 5 receives input primarily from the SI cortex, whereas area 7 has widespread connections with the visual and motor areas of the cortex and is involved in the control of eye movements (Chapter 10). The inferior parietal lobule includes two gyri: the supramarginal (area 40) and the angular (area 39) gyri. These receive input from the other parts of the parietal lobe as well as from association areas in the frontal, occipital, temporal, and limbic lobes. The parietal association areas process tactile and visual information and are intimately concerned with the cognition of the body itself and the objects surrounding it. These areas are also important in the orderly or sequential performance of tasks, especially those involving the hands. Lesions in the parietal association areas are associated with **astereognosis** and the **neglect syndrome,** a perceptual disorder related to recognition of the opposite side of the body and its surroundings (Fig. 16-6D).

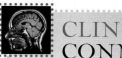

CLINICAL CONNECTION

In the neglect syndrome, the patient fails to recognize the opposite side of the body and its surroundings. For example, when the damage is in the right hemisphere, the patient does not bathe the left side of the body and may actually deny that the left limbs belong to him. Moreover, objects located in the left side of the visual field, e.g., a cup of coffee on the left side of a food tray, do not exist in the mind of the patient.

Lesions in the inferior parietal lobule, especially the angular gyrus and perhaps adjacent parts of the occipital or temporal lobes, usually in the left or dominant hemisphere, result in **Gerstmann syndrome,** which includes (1) finger agnosia (the inability to distinguish the various fingers of each hand), (2) acalculia (the inability to do simple arithmetic), (3) right-left confusion (the inability to distinguish right from left), (4) agraphia (the inability to write), and (5) sometimes alexia (the inability to read).

TEMPORAL LOBE

The temporal cortex forms almost one-fourth of the entire cortex and contains the primary auditory area as well as areas associated with emotions and higher mental functions such as memory and speech. The AI or primary auditory cortex (area 41) is situated in the transverse temporal gyri of Heschl, which are buried in the floor of the lateral fissure (Figs. 12-3, 16-6). The AI cortex is mostly in the anterior gyrus but extends slightly into the adjacent part of the posterior gyrus. Immediately adjacent to area 41 is area 42, the secondary auditory area, and adjacent to this area is the auditory association part of area 22, located in the superior temporal gyrus. Electrical stimulation of the primary auditory area results in noises described as humming, buzzing, clicking, or ringing, whereas stimulation of the auditory association part of area 22 produces sounds perceived as a whistle, a bell, and so forth. A unilateral lesion in the primary auditory area results in no significant hearing loss because of the bilateralism of the central auditory pathways. Such a lesion does, however, cause difficulty in recognizing the distance and direction from which sounds are coming, especially in the ear contralateral to the lesion.

The anterior and ventromedial parts of the temporal lobe (temporal pole and parahippocampal gyrus) are strongly connected with the limbic system and are concerned with mechanisms related to visceral activity, emotions, behavior, and some forms of memory. The inferolateral and ventral parts of the temporal lobe (middle temporal, inferior temporal, and occipitotemporal gyri) appear to record and store experiences. Electrical stimulation here produces illusions of past events that include not only the scenes and sounds but also the emotions associated with them. Lesions of the left posterior temporal cortex may impair the learning or remembering of verbally based information, whereas lesions of the right posterior temporal cortex may impair the learning and remembering of visually based information. Bilateral lesions of the posterior parts of the occipitotemporal gyri result in prosopagnosia, the inability to recognize the faces of others and themselves.

OCCIPITAL LOBE

The occipital cortex makes up only about one eighth of the entire cortex and contains the primary visual (VI) and visual association areas. The primary visual cortex (area 17), also called the striate area, receives the optic radiation and is located in the gyri forming the walls of the calcarine fissure (Fig. 16-7A, B). The cuneus forms the upper wall of the calcarine fissure and herein is represented the lower half of the contralateral hemifield of vision. The upper half of the contralateral visual hemifield is represented in the lingual gyrus that forms the lower wall of the calcarine fissure. Macular vision is represented in the entire posterior half of area 17 (Fig. 14-4A). Unilateral lesions of the VI cortex result in contralateral homonymous hemianopsia (Fig. 16-7D). However, in the case of a vascular lesion involving the calcarine artery, which is a branch of the posterior cerebral artery, macular sparing may occur because of an intact vascular supply to the occipital pole from the middle cerebral artery.

The rest of the occipital lobe consists of area 18, which borders area 17 and is called the parastriate cortex, and area 19, the peristriate cortex, which is larger and forms most of the lateral surface of the occipital lobe. These areas receive visual information from the striate areas bilaterally and are important in the complex visual perceptions related to color, movement, direction of objects, and so forth. Lesions in the visual association areas and the adjoining parts of the temporal lobe result in visual agnosia, the inability to recognize objects and their colors.

HEMISPHERIC LATERALIZATION OF FUNCTION

In terms of motor and sensory functions (other than olfaction), each cerebral hemisphere contains contralateral representation of the body and its surroundings. Thus, lesions in the primary motor, primary somatosensory, or primary visual areas in one hemisphere result in contralateral hemiparesis, contralateral hemianesthesia, or contralateral hemianopsia. Higher functions such as analytical thinking, language comprehension and production of emotional and intuitive thinking, spatial orientation, and artistic and music abilities—to cite only a few—are functions centered more in one than the other hemisphere. The hemisphere that contains the centers for language comprehension and production is called the **dominant hemisphere.**

As the result of numerous tests to determine the language-dominant hemisphere in patients in need of neurosurgical removal of cerebral cortical tissue, it has been found that language is represented in the left hemisphere in a high percentage of people: almost all right-handed persons and more than 50% of left-handed persons.

Handedness and language dominance develop before a child has learned to speak. A unilateral lesion in the left hemisphere of a child does not hinder the development of speech because the right hemisphere assumes dominance. Furthermore, lesions occurring in children even toward the end of the first decade of life usually result in language difficulties only until the other hemisphere assumes the language function.

In addition to language dominance, the left hemisphere excels in intellectual processes such as analytical thinking or rationalizing, calculating, and verbalization (Fig. 16-8). In contrast, the nondominant hemisphere, usually the right, excels in sensory discrimination, in emotional, nonverbal thinking, and in artistic skills such as drawing and composing music spatial perception, and, perhaps, recognition of faces.

LANGUAGE AREAS AND APHASIA

Language is represented chiefly in cortical areas bordering the lateral fissure of the dominant hemisphere. Two main areas exist: **Broca** and **Wernicke** (Fig. 16-9). Broca area, the motor or expressive speech center, is located in the left inferior frontal

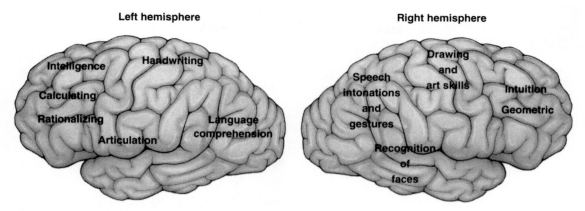

Figure 16-8 Higher mental functions of right and left hemispheres.

gyrus, especially the opercular and triangular parts, areas 44 and 45, respectively (Fig. 16-6A). Broca area contains the motor programs for the production of words, and it projects fibers to the parts of the motor cortex that control the muscles used in articulation, i.e., the muscles in the vocal cords, tongue, and lips. A lesion in the Broca area is associated with an **expressive** or **motor aphasia,** characterized as **nonfluent** (Fig. 16-6D) because of the slow and prolonged output of words, poor articulation, and short sentences containing only the necessary verbs, nouns, and pronouns. If a lesion is actually limited to the Broca area in the inferior frontal gyrus, the aphasia is mild and transient. A severe and persisting Broca aphasia occurs when the lesion is larger and includes the adjacent parts of the frontal lobe and the underlying white matter as illustrated in the case history at the beginning of this chapter. The Broca aphasia in this case may result in **mutism,** the inability to speak, and frequently **agraphia,** the inability to write.

The Wernicke area, the sensory or receptive speech area, is in the posterior part of area 22 in the superior temporal gyrus. This area contains the mechanisms for the comprehension and formulation of language. A lesion in the Wernicke area, associated with **receptive** or **sensory aphasia,** is characterized as **fluent** (Fig. 16-6D) because production of words is normal but the use of words is defective. The patient substitutes one word for another, inserts meaningless words, or strings together words or phrases of great length but no meaning. The patient with Wernicke aphasia is fluent but cannot comprehend language in any form—heard, read, or spoken—and cannot write (agraphia). A more severe and persisting Wernicke aphasia occurs when the lesion is larger and includes the middle temporal gyrus and underlying white matter.

The Wernicke area projects into the Broca area via association fibers in the arcuate and superior longitudinal fasciculi (Figs. 16-3, 16-9). A lesion interrupting these fibers has been thought to produce a **conduction aphasia** in which speech deficiency is similar to a receptive aphasia. But, because comprehension remains intact, the patient makes repeated attempts to say the right words. In addition, conduction aphasia includes impairment in attempting to name objects and pictures. More severe and persistent conduction aphasia is now thought to result from larger lesions including not only left superior temporal gyrus but also the angular and supramarginal gyri.

Other forms of aphasia also exist and may result from lesions not only in the cortical tissue bordering the lateral fissure (the perisylvian language areas) but also in cortical areas some distance from these and even in some subcortical structures, such as the thalamus or caudate nucleus. **Transcortical motor aphasia,** in which fluency is impaired but repetition, naming, and reading are normal, occurs with lesions in the left supplementary motor area or the left prefrontal cortex anterior and dorsal to the Broca area. **Transcortical sensory aphasia,** in which fluency is excessive and repetition normal but naming, reading, and comprehension are impaired, occurs with lesions at the junction of the left temporal, parietal, and occipital lobes. Anomic aphasia, impairment in naming objects, occurs with lesions usually at the junction of the angular gyrus and adjacent occipital lobe. **Global aphasia,** the most severe aphasia, combines the deficits seen in the Broca, Wernicke, and conduction aphasias so

CLINICAL CONNECTION

The simplified pathway for a spoken description of an object or a scene is as follows:

1. Visual input to area 17 bilaterally with further processing in areas 18 and 19 (Fig. 16-9);
2. Input from the visual association areas to the left angular gyrus where the objects are recognized and named;
3. Input to the Wernicke area, where words are assembled into sentences and the appropriate impulses are sent via the arcuate and superior longitudinal fasciculi to the Broca area;
4. Motor programs in the Broca area are projected to the motor cortex, which then elicits speech via the appropriate brainstem centers and the muscles under their control.

that the loss of language is almost complete. It is accompanied by paralysis of the right lower facial muscles and the right upper limb and results from a massive lesion caused by occlusion of the middle cerebral artery. Anterior Broca-like and posterior Wernicke-like language areas exist in the nondominant hemisphere. These areas produce or interpret prosody, the rhythm melody and intonation associated with the emotional aspects of speech.

CLINICAL CONNECTION

Lesions in the right inferior frontal gyrus result in impairment of the production of speech intonation, whereas lesions in the right posterior superior temporal gyri result in impairment in interpreting the speech intonations of others.

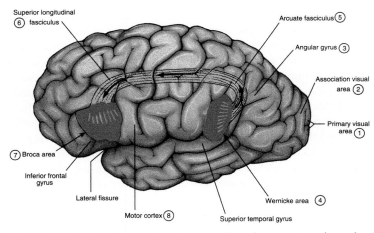

Figure 16-9 Speech areas. Structures numbered represent pathway for spoken description of an object or scene.

Chapter Review Questions

16-1. How many layers are present in the neocortex and what are the connections of each?

16-2. The planning of complex movements occurs in what area of the cerebral cortex?

16-3. Locate the cortical area whose damage results in the following:

a. left lower limb anesthesia, weakness, and a Babinski response
b. paralysis of gaze to the right
c. left homonymous hemianopsia
d. weakness of right upper limb
e. fluent aphasia
f. left neglect syndrome

16-4. Locate the smallest lesion in a 63-year-old patient who experiences sudden loss of speech, accompanied by weakness of the right lower facial muscles and the right hand.

16-5. Locate the smallest lesion in a 55-year-old patient who has left spastic hemiplegia, lower facial weakness, hemianesthesia, and homonymous hemianopsia.

The Limbic System: Anterograde Amnesia and Inappropriate Social Behavior

AT 12 MONTHS OF AGE a male infant appears emotionally flat: no smiling or warm, happy expressions. Also, the mimicking of sounds, facial expressions, and spontaneous babbling are absent. At 16 months the child does not say single words and at 24 months does not link two or three words into meaningful statements such as "want drink." Continued development is marked by the lack of socialization with other toddlers, the lack of attentiveness to his parents when talking to him, diminished "normal" play, obsessive attention directed to objects, and the lack of spontaneous expressions of normal emotions coupled with abnormal tantrums.

The term limbic system is the arbitrary name of a functional system of cortical and subcortical neurons. The interconnections between these neurons form complex circuits that play an important role in memory and behavior.

LIMBIC LOBE

The term limbic means border. Limbic was first used by Broca in 1878 to describe a lobe on the medial surface of the cerebral hemisphere bordering the corpus callosum and rostral brainstem. The limbic lobe (Fig. 17-1) comprises the cingulate gyrus and its anterior extension and **septal area,** both of which border the corpus callosum, and the parahippocampal gyrus of the temporal lobe bordering the rostral brainstem.

The limbic lobe is anatomically and functionally connected with other structures. The entire complex is called the limbic system. The two centers most closely related to the limbic lobe are the hippocampus, deep to the posterior part of the parahippocampal gyrus, and the **amygdala**

219

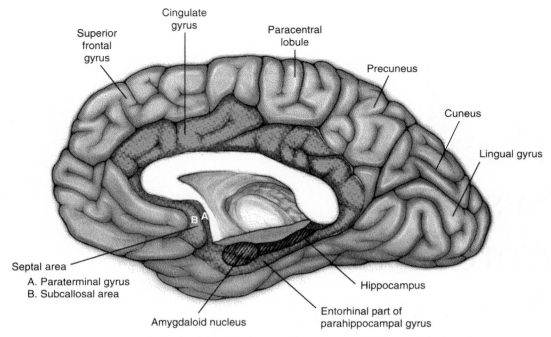

Figure 17-1   Location of the limbic lobe (shaded), the hippocampus, and amygdaloid nucleus.

or amygdaloid nucleus, deep to the anterior part of the parahippocampal gyrus (Fig. 17-1). These two structures are the key functional centers of the limbic system. Also closely associated with the limbic system is the hypothalamus, which has abundant connections with the hippocampus and amygdaloid nucleus.

HIPPOCAMPUS

The hippocampus plays a key role in memory and learning. It is composed of three parts: dentate gyrus, hippocampus proper, and subiculum (Fig. 17-2). The dentate gyrus and hippocampus proper are the archicortex, the phylogenetically oldest part of the cerebral cortex. The subiculum is a transitional zone of cortex between the hippocampus proper and **entorhinal area,** part of the parahippocampal gyrus. The parahippocampal gyrus is neocortex, the phylogenetically newest part of the cortex.

CONNECTIONS

The hippocampus resembles a sea horse about 2 inches long in the floor of the temporal horn of the lateral ventricle (Fig. 17-3). The major input to the hippocampus comes from the entorhinal part of the parahippocampal gyrus. The entorhinal area receives input from widespread cortical association areas dealing with multiple sensory perceptions via the cingulum. The hippocampi in the right and left hemispheres are connected via the hippocampal commissure.

The hippocampus is the initial center in a reverberating pathway called the **Papez circuit** (Fig. 17-4). A major part of the Papez circuit is the fornix, which connects the hippocampus to the hypothalamus. The fornix originates from the alveus of the hippocampus as the **fimbria of the fornix** (Figs. 17-2–17-4). Beneath the splenium of the corpus callosum, the fibers of the fimbria leave the hippocampus and become the **crus of the fornix.** As the two crura converge toward the midline they exchange fibers, forming the **hippocampal commissure.** Each crus then continues forward as the **body of the fornix.** The body passes forward beneath the corpus callosum suspended in the free margin of the septum pellucidum and arches downward toward the anterior commissure as the **column of the fornix.** At the anterior commissure, the fornix separates into two parts: a precommissural part, located in front of the anterior

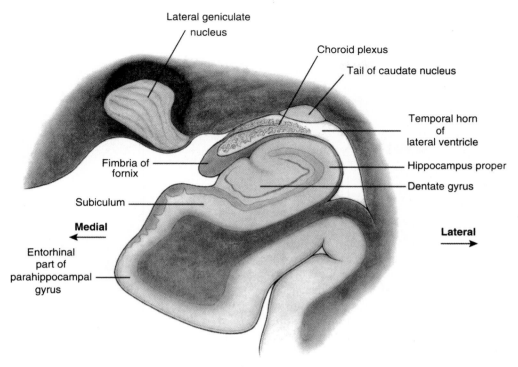

Figure 17-2   Coronal section of the hippocampus showing its relations.

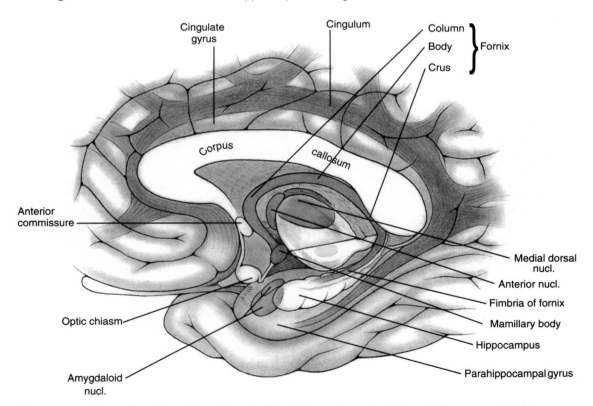

Figure 17-3   Three-dimensional view of cerebral hemisphere showing relations of hippocampus, fornix, and cingulum (nucl, nucleus).

A

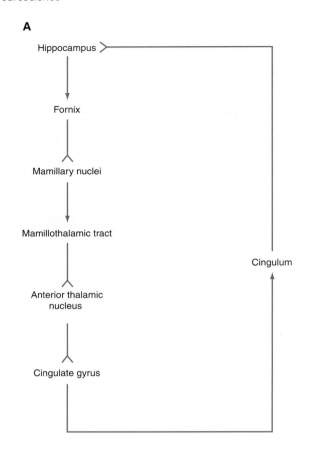

B

1. Hippocampus
2. Fimbria of fornix
3. Body of fornix
4. Column of fornix
5. Mamillary body
6. Mamillothalamic tract
7. Anterior nucl.
8. Thalamocingulate radiation
9. Cingulate gyrus
10. Cingulum
11. Entorhinal area
12. Medial dorsal nucl.

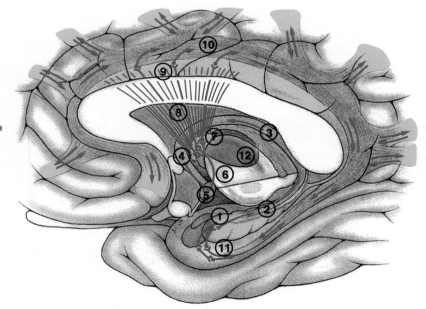

Figure 17-4   Papez circuit (**A**) and other connections of the hippocampus (**B;** nucl, nucleus).

commissure, and a postcommissural part, located behind it. The precommissural fibers arise from the hippocampus proper and terminate in the septal region and basal forebrain structures. The postcommissural fibers arise from the subiculum and are distributed primarily to nuclei in the mamillary body.

The mamillary body gives rise to the mamillothalamic tract, which passes dorsally between the medial and lateral thalamic nuclei and terminates in the anterior thalamic nucleus (Fig. 17-4). This nucleus then projects axons via the thalamocingulate radiation to the cingulate gyrus, which projects to the cingulum, an association bundle deep to the gyrus. From the cingulum, impulses reach the entorhinal area of the parahippocampal gyrus and then pass to the hippocampus, thus completing the Papez circuit.

Besides the fornix, another important output of the hippocampus is from both the hippocampus proper and the subiculum directly to the entorhinal area, from which impulses reach the association areas in all lobes of the cerebral hemisphere.

FUNCTION

The hippocampus is essential for the consolidation of memory and learning. Bilateral damage of the hippocampi such as occurs with severe hypoxia results in a profound loss of recent or short-term memory and the ability to learn. Persons who have survived such an event cannot remember anything that has occurred longer than a few minutes beforehand (anterograde amnesia). Memories of the distant past and intelligence remain intact.

The hippocampus receives all types of information from the sensory association areas. When particular items of information are important to remember or one desires to remember them, or even when there is no desire, the hippocampus emits the signals that reverberate over and over in the Papez circuit until they are stored permanently in the areas of the cerebral cortex for long-term memory.

AMYGDALA

The amygdala or amygdaloid nucleus plays an important role in behavior and emotions. It resem-

CLINICAL CONNECTION

Alzheimer disease is characterized by progressive dementia in patients younger than 65 years of age. In patients older than 65 years of age, progressive dementia is referred to as senile dementia. In both cases, the individuals become increasingly forgetful and develop progressive abnormalities of memory, cognition, orientation, and behavior. These types of dementia are associated with (1) a loss of neurons in the hippocampus and adjacent parahippocampal cortex (Fig. 17-5) and (2) a reduction in the cholinergic innervation of the cerebral cortex. The neurons lost in the parahippocampal cortex are those providing input to the hippocampus from the association and limbic cortices. The neurons lost in the hippocampus are those providing output from the hippocampus to the association cortices and diencephalon. Thus, the loss of these hippocampal connections with the neocortex undoubtedly accounts for the characteristic loss of recent memory in persons with these dementias. The reduction in the cholinergic innervation of the cerebral cortex is the result of the degeneration of the large cholinergic neurons in the **basal nucleus of Meynert** located in the anterior perforated substance, more commonly referred to as the **substantia innominata.** The anterior perforated substance extends from the olfactory striae anteriorly to the optic tracts posteriorly. Normally, the axons of these cholinergic neurons in the basal nucleus provide acetylcholine to the neocortex. The absence of neocortical acetylcholine may account for the cognitive deficits that occur in more advanced stages of dementia.

CLINICAL CONNECTION

Korsakoff syndrome or psychosis is characterized by the loss of recent memory and often a tendency to fabricate accounts of recent events. This syndrome most often results from chronic alcoholism and associated nutritional deficiency. Although morphologic changes have been described in the hippocampus and the mamillary bodies, the most frequent alterations occur in the medial parts of the medial dorsal thalamic nuclei (Fig. 17-5).

bles an almond and is located beneath the uncus near the dorsomedial tip of the temporal lobe. It consists of a number of subnuclei that are divided into a large basolateral group and small corticomedial and central groups.

Limbic system syndromes

‡‡‡‡ Alzheimer: loss of
‡‡‡‡   recent memory

vvvv Klüver-Bucy: behavioral
vvvv   changes

▨ Korsakoff: loss of recent
     memory and confabulation

Structures

1. Hippocampus
2. Amygdala
3. Medial dorsal nucleus
4. Parahippocampal gyrus
5. Uncus
6. Mamillary body
7. Mamillothalamic tract

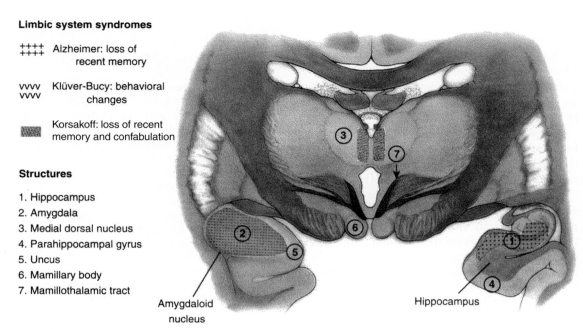

Amygdaloid
nucleus

Hippocampus

Figure 17-5   Coronal section at mamillary bodies showing sites associated with limbic system syndromes.

CONNECTIONS

The basolateral nuclear group is especially well developed in humans and receives strong connections from temporal, prefrontal, and parietal association areas as well as the cingulate gyrus. The corticomedial nucleus is poorly developed in humans and receives olfactory input directly from the olfactory bulb via the lateral olfactory stria. The central nucleus receives input from brainstem visceral paths and from the basolateral nucleus.

The major output of the amygdala (Fig. 17-6) is the ventral amygdaloid path. This output courses within the anterior perforated substance (Fig. 17-7) and provides input to the hypothalamus, septal nuclei, and medial dorsal thalamic nucleus. The medial dorsal nucleus has strong reciprocal connections with the prefrontal cortex. A minor output of the amygdala is the stria terminalis, which passes forward in the angle between the caudate nucleus and thalamus and terminates in the hypothalamus, accumbens nucleus, and septal nuclei.

FUNCTIONS

The amygdala associates experiences with consequences and then programs the appropriate behavioral response to an experience. In animals that largely depend on the sense of smell to seek food, search for a mate to reproduce, and sense danger,

olfactory sensations are the primary input to the amygdala. On receiving the aforementioned types of information, the amygdala programs the appropriate behavioral responses by emitting signals to the various centers that control appropriate activities. In these types of animals the amygdala is comparable to the human corticomedial amygdala, which enhances digestive processes and the craving for food in response to pleasant aromas or induces the loss of appetite and even nausea and vomiting in response to foul or putrid odors. Human behavior, however, is based chiefly on nonolfactory experiences that are projected from the cerebral cortex to the large basolateral amygdala. After assessing the nature of the input, i.e., friendly, unfriendly, frightening, dangerous, and so on, the basolateral amygdala sends signals to centers in the hypothalamus that elicit the appropriate autonomic and motor responses. Signals are also sent from the basolateral amygdala via the medial dorsal thalamic nucleus to the orbitofrontal cortex. The orbitofrontal cortex provides the perception of emotions, whereas the hypothalamus provides the expression of emotions.

Bilateral lesions of the amygdalae result in behavioral alterations, especially a profound loss of fear. Surgical lesions of the amygdalae in patients with socially unacceptable aggressive behavior result in placid behavior and decreased emotional excitability.

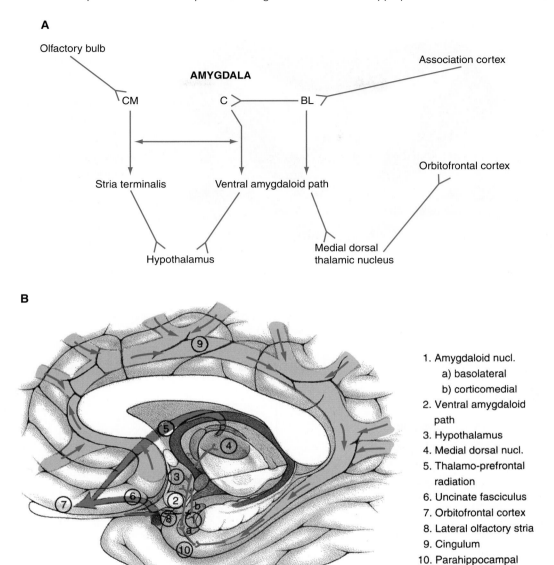

A.

Olfactory bulb

AMYGDALA

Association cortex

CM   C   BL

Stria terminalis   Ventral amygdaloid path

Orbitofrontal cortex

Hypothalamus

Medial dorsal
thalamic nucleus

B.

1. Amygdaloid nucl.
   a) basolateral
   b) corticomedial
2. Ventral amygdaloid
   path
3. Hypothalamus
4. Medial dorsal nucl.
5. Thalamo-prefrontal
   radiation
6. Uncinate fasciculus
7. Orbitofrontal cortex
8. Lateral olfactory stria
9. Cingulum
10. Parahippocampal
    gyrus

Figure 17-6   **A.** Principal connections of amygdala (C, central; CM, corticomedial; BL, basolateral).
B. Three-dimensional medial view of the connections of the amygdaloid nucleus (nucl, nucleus).

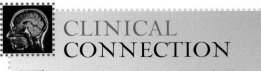

CLINICAL CONNECTION

The **Klüver-Bucy syndrome** is characterized by:

1. An absence of emotional responses so that fear, rage, and aggression cease to exist;
2. A compulsion to be overly attentive to all sensory stimuli, to examine all objects visually, tactilely, and orally;
3. Hypersexuality;
4. Psychic blindness or visual agnosia, in which objects are not recognized visually.

These disturbances are seen experimentally and clinically after bilateral removal of the temporal lobes as far posteriorly as the auditory areas. The docility, compulsive attentiveness, oral tendencies, and hypersexuality result from the bilateral destruction of the amygdaloid nuclei (Fig. 17-5); the visual agnosia results from damage to the neocortical parts of the temporal lobe.

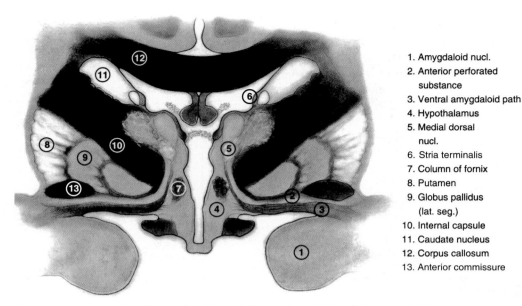

1. Amygdaloid nucl.
2. Anterior perforated
   substance
3. Ventral amygdaloid path
4. Hypothalamus
5. Medial dorsal
   nucl.
6. Stria terminalis
7. Column of fornix
8. Putamen
9. Globus pallidus
   (lat. seg.)
10. Internal capsule
11. Caudate nucleus
12. Corpus callosum
13. Anterior commissure

Figure 17-7 Coronal section at tuberal hypothalamus showing hypothalamic and thalamic connections of the amygdala (lat, lateral; nucl, nucleus; seg, segment).

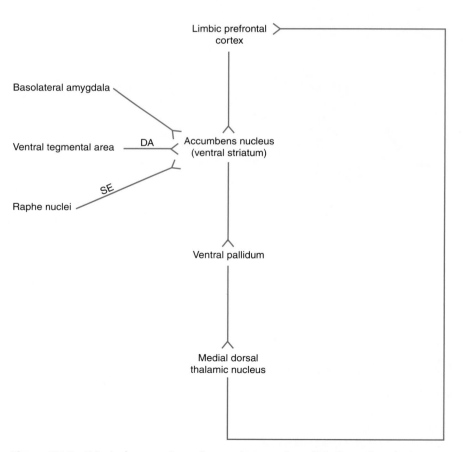

Figure 17-8 Principal connections of accumbens nucleus (DA, dopaminergic; SE, serotonergic).

ACCUMBENS AND SEPTAL NUCLEI

The accumbens nucleus, or ventral striatum, is located between the head of the caudate nucleus and the putamen in the vicinity of the anterior commissure. It is closely related to the septal nuclei located in the septum pellucidum. The septal nuclei are the subcortical components of the septal region, which also includes a cortical component, the septal area, composed of the pararterminal gyrus and subcallosal area (Fig. 17-1).

CONNECTIONS

The accumbens nucleus is the striatal component of the limbic loop. It receives input chiefly from the basolateral amygdala, prefrontal cortex, and brainstem monoaminergic nuclei (Fig. 17-8) and projects to the ventral pallidum located deep to the lateral part of the anterior commissure. The

ventral pallidum projects to the medial dorsal thalamic nucleus, which completes the loop by projecting to the prefrontal cortex.

The septal nuclei receive input chiefly from the amygdala, hippocampus, and brainstem reticular formation (Fig. 17-9). Outputs of the septal nuclei travel via the **medial forebrain bundle** to the hypothalamus and brainstem reticular formation and via the **stria medullaris of the thalamus** to the habenular nuclei and thence via the **fasciculus retroflexus** to the midbrain reticular formation.

FUNCTIONS

The accumbens and septal nuclei are associated with reward mechanisms and pleasure. Electrical stimulation of the septal region or the medial forebrain, which contains dopaminergic fibers, is associated with pleasure phenomena. On stimulation of electrodes placed in the septal region, patients have described sexual feelings.

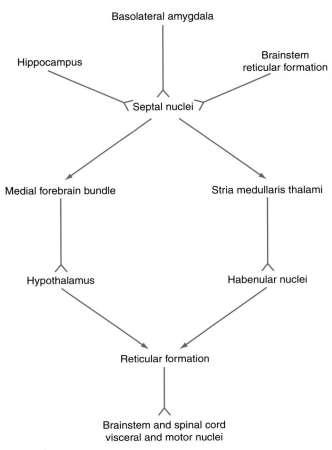

Figure 17-9 Principal connections of septal nuclei.

The accumbens nucleus is related to the euphoria associated with the use of psychostimulants such as amphetamine and cocaine. Dopaminergic projections from the ventral tegmental area in the midbrain and serotonergic projections from the raphe nuclei appear to play important roles in these phenomena.

LIMBIC CORTICAL AREAS

Several areas in the cerebral cortex are strongly associated with limbic system phenomena. The temporal poles and most anterior parts of the parahippocampal gyrus, which are anatomically related to the amygdala, are associated with fear and anxiety. These areas have strong connections with the orbitofrontal cortex via the uncinate fasciculus (Fig. 17-6B).

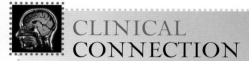

CLINICAL CONNECTION

Abnormal activity in the anterior parts of the parahippocampal gyri have been reported in cases of panic attack syndrome.

The orbitofrontal cortex both ventrally and medially is associated with social behavior such as described in the case of Phineas Gage in Chapter 16. Prefrontal lobotomy, commonly performed in the 1930s on patients with severe psychoses, depression, and even neuroses, in many cases resulted in "cures" worse than the original abnormality, so that the lobotomized patients developed inappropriate behavior and the lowering of moral standards as seen in Phineas Gage. Recent evidence also suggests that the medial orbitofrontal cortex is strongly associated with depression.

The anterior part of the cingulate gyrus appears to contain an inhibitory control center. This center may elicit second thoughts or caution before undertaking an action. Reports suggest that the inhibitory control area may become abnormal in drug addicts who cannot control their addiction even though they are aware of consequences.

CLINICAL CONNECTION

Autism is a behavioral disorder diagnosed in approximately 0.5% of children between 2 and 4 years of age. Autism is characterized clinically by a triad of behavioral deficits including social, communication, and attentional impairments with repetitive behaviors and obsessive interests, as illustrated in the case at the beginning of this chapter. The cause of autism is clearly attributable to a developmental disorder affecting prenatal and postnatal brain development. Neuropathologic findings are observed most often in the limbic system, frontal cortex, and cerebellum. Microscopically, neurons in the entorhinal area, hippocampus, and amygdala are abnormally small and relatively more densely packed. Conversely, in the frontal cortex, pyramidal neurons are larger than normal. In the cerebellum, Purkinje cells in the vermis and posterior-inferior hemispheres degenerate. Macrencephaly secondary to increased brain size is a common observation in autistic children up to about 5 years of age. During this time magnetic resonance imaging studies have reported increased gray and white matter volumes in the frontal and temporal lobes and reduced gray and white matter volumes in the cerebellum. The increase in frontal lobe volume and decreased cerebellar volume appear linked, possibly reflecting developmentally early overexcitation of the frontal cortex related to diminished inhibition of cerebellar nuclear neurons as a result of the Purkinje cell degeneration. After 5 years of age, brain maturation in autistic children appears to be slower compared with that in unaffected children.

Chapter Review Questions

17-1. What are the parts of the limbic lobe and the limbic system?

17-2. What are the two key functional centers of the limbic system and where are they located?

17-3. Describe the Papez circuit.

17-4. Based on clinical evidence, what are the functions of the hippocampus and amygdaloid nuclei?

17-5. Bilateral alterations in what limbic system structures are most commonly associated with Alzheimer disease, the Klüver-Bucy syndrome, and Korsakoff psychosis?

17-6. What is the limbic loop of the basal ganglia and its functional significance?

18

The Hypothalamus: Vegetative and Endocrine Imbalance

DURING THE PAST YEAR, a 15-year-old girl became obese and listless, had episodes of high fever without apparent cause, ceased menstruating, drank copious amounts of water owing to severe thirst, passed excessive amounts of urine, frequently fell asleep during the day, often had reversed sleep–wake cycles, and on occasion erupted into a violent state of rage without provocation.

The hypothalamus controls visceral activity and, as the chief effector of the limbic system, elicits the phenomena associated with emotions. Because it has both neural and endocrine components, the hypothalamus exerts its influence through the nervous system and the circulatory system. It plays an important role in self-preservation and in preservation of the species. Through its neural and vascular connections it influences water balance, food intake, the endocrine system, reproduction, sleep, behavior, and the entire autonomic nervous system.

HYPOTHALAMIC SUBDIVISIONS AND NUCLEI

Despite its enormous number of connections and functions, the hypothalamus is extremely small,

weighing approximately 4 g and making up less than 1% of the total human brain mass. In the median plane, the hypothalamus extends from the lamina terminalis anteriorly through the mamillary bodies posteriorly. The hypothalamus is divided into anterior or chiasmatic, intermediate or tuberal, and posterior or mamillary regions (Fig. 18-1). Lateral to the lamina terminalis, the chiasmatic region consists of the preoptic area, which extends anteriorly to the septal nuclei and basal forebrain and is considered by some as an additional subdivision.

The **hypothalamus** is also divided into three sagittal zones: lateral and medial, which are on either side of the fornix, and periventricular, which is deep to the ependyma of the third ventricle (Fig. 18-2). Although numerous hypothalamic nuclei are described, it is difficult to define the precise boundaries of most of them.

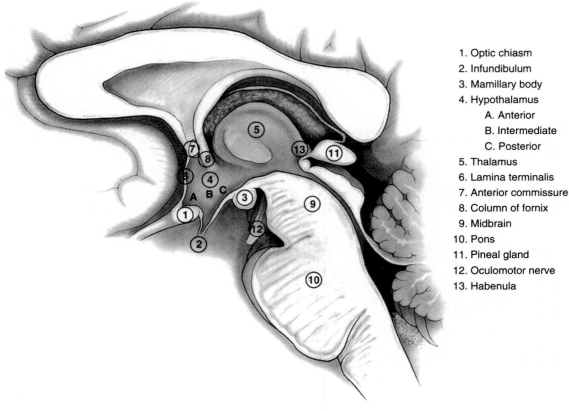

1. Optic chiasm
2. Infundibulum
3. Mamillary body
4. Hypothalamus
    A. Anterior
    B. Intermediate
    C. Posterior
5. Thalamus
6. Lamina terminalis
7. Anterior commissure
8. Column of fornix
9. Midbrain
10. Pons
11. Pineal gland
12. Oculomotor nerve
13. Habenula

Figure 18-1   Median view of brainstem and diencephalon.

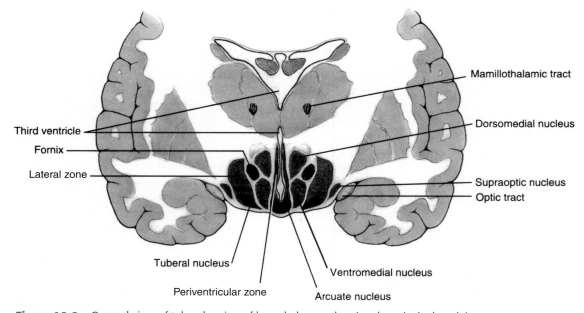

Figure 18-2   Coronal view of tuberal region of hypothalamus showing the principal nuclei.

The lateral zone, interspersed with longitudinally arranged fibers, contains diffuse neurons and influences widespread areas of the cerebral cortex. The longitudinal fibers in the lateral zone belong to the medial forebrain bundle, a diffuse system of axons interconnecting the orbitofrontal cortex, accumbens nucleus, septal region, hypothalamus, and brainstem reticular formation. It also projects to the medial zone.

The medial and periventricular zones consist of many nuclei (Fig. 18-3). The anterior region contains the preoptic, supraoptic, paraventricular, anterior, and suprachiasmatic nuclei; the intermediate region has the dorsomedial, ventromedial, and arcuate nuclei (Fig. 18-2); and the posterior region contains the mamillary and posterior nuclei. The periventricular zone also contains the periventricular system of fibers that extends into the periaqueductal gray of the midbrain as the dorsal longitudinal fasciculus.

CONNECTIONS

INPUT

Input to the hypothalamus is both neural and humoral. The neural input is primarily from the limbic system. As previously described, afferent projections to the hypothalamus from the hippocampus travel via the fornix to the mamillary nuclei (Figs. 17-4, 18-3) and from the amygdala via (1) the ventral amygdaloid path to the lateral hypothalamus and preoptic nuclei (Figs. 17-6, 17-7) and (2) the stria terminalis to the medial hypothalamus

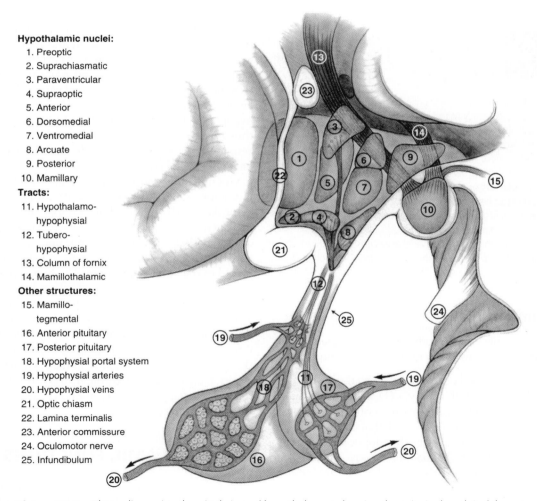

Hypothalamic nuclei:
1. Preoptic
2. Suprachiasmatic
3. Paraventricular
4. Supraoptic
5. Anterior
6. Dorsomedial
7. Ventromedial
8. Arcuate
9. Posterior
10. Mamillary

Tracts:
11. Hypothalamo-
    hypophysial
12. Tubero-
    hypophysial
13. Column of fornix
14. Mamillothalamic

Other structures:
15. Mamillo-
    tegmental
16. Anterior pituitary
17. Posterior pituitary
18. Hypophysial portal system
19. Hypophysial arteries
20. Hypophysial veins
21. Optic chiasm
22. Lamina terminalis
23. Anterior commissure
24. Oculomotor nerve
25. Infundibulum

Figure 18-3 Three-dimensional sagittal view of hypothalamus showing the principal nuclei of the medial zone and their connections with the pituitary gland, thalamus, and midbrain tegmentum.

and preoptic nuclei. Projections also reach the hypothalamus from the orbitofrontal cortex, the medial dorsal thalamic nucleus, the retina, and the mamillary peduncle, which carries fibers from the midbrain reticular formation. The medial forebrain bundle interconnects the basal forebrain and septal region with the lateral hypothalamic area and midbrain reticular formation.

The humoral input is vascular, and through it various hypothalamic neurons are stimulated chemically by substances such as glucose and hormones, and physically by factors such as temperature changes and osmolality. In addition to chemically sensitive or physically sensitive hypothalamic neurons, **circumventricular organs** located in the wall of the third ventricle also detect chemical changes in the cerebrospinal fluid and blood and relay this information to the nearby hypothalamus.

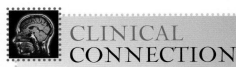

OUTPUT

The output of the hypothalamus is also neural and humoral. The two major targets of neural output are:

1. The cerebral cortex directly from the hypothalamus and indirectly via (1) the anterior thalamic nucleus, a component of Papez circuit, which receives the mamillothalamic tract that relays impulses from the hippocampus after a synapse in the mamillary body (Figs. 17-4, 18-3), and (2) the medial dorsal thalamic nucleus, which relays impulses from hypothalamic nuclei that are targets of the amygdala and septal nuclei.

2. Brainstem and spinal cord motor and autonomic centers, which receive direct and indirect input from the lateral and posterior hypothalamus and the paraventricular nucleus via the dorsal longitudinal fasciculus and mamillotegmental tract (Fig. 18-3).

Pathways from hypothalamic nuclei to autonomic centers in the brainstem and spinal cord are not clearly demarcated. In the midbrain and rostral pons, the dorsal longitudinal fasciculus is located dorsomedially, i.e., near the periaqueductal gray and floor of the fourth ventricle, respectively. From here the path sweeps laterally and descends through the caudal pons and the medulla in the lateral part of the reticular formation. The medial forebrain bundle also connects the lateral hypothalamus to the midbrain reticular formation.

The hypothalamic humoral output influences the endocrine system and occurs directly by secretion into the general circulation and indirectly by secretion into the **hypophysial portal system** (Fig. 18-3). The direct humoral route involves large neurons in the supraoptic and paraventricular nuclei whose axons pass via the hypothalamo-hypophysial tract to the posterior pituitary, where they release **vasopressin** and **oxytocin** into the general circulation. Vasopressin, or **antidiuretic hormone (ADH),** controls water balance, and oxytocin causes constriction of smooth muscle in the uterus and myoepithelial cells in the mammary glands. The indirect humoral route involves small neurons chiefly in the tuberal region that produce **hypothalamic regulatory hormones,** which enter the hypophysial portal system and are transported to the anterior pituitary. The hypophysial portal system is a vascular connection between the hypothalamus and anterior pituitary. Capillaries, derived from the superior hypophysial artery and located in the **median eminence** and infundibulum, form portal vessels that pass down the pituitary stalk to a second capillary bed in the anterior pituitary. It is through this route that the hypothalamic regulatory hormones reach the anterior pituitary.

HYPOTHALAMIC FUNCTIONS

The functions of the tiny hypothalamus are Herculean (Table 18-1). Perhaps they can best be described by considering the manifestations of

TABLE 18-1   Hypothalamic Functions and Nuclei

Anterior	Intermediate	Posterior
Heat loss (preoptic)	Endocrine activity (tuberal and arcuate)	Heat conservation (posterolateral)
Thirst (preoptic)	Satiety (ventromedial)	Arousal (posterolateral)
Water balance, milk ejection, and uterine contraction (supraoptic and paraventricular)	Feeding (lateral) Emotions (dorsomedial)	Aggressive behavior (posterolateral) Analgesia (periventricular)
Circadian rhythm (suprachiasmatic)		Consolidation of memory (mamillary)
Sleep (anterior and preoptic)		
Parasympathomimetic		Sympathomimetic

a hypothalamic lesion as given in the clinical illustration at the beginning of this chapter. The **hypothalamic syndrome** is manifested chiefly by (1) **diabetes insipidus,** (2) endocrine imbalance, (3) impairment of temperature regulation, (4) abnormalities of sleep patterns, and (5) behavioral changes.

Diabetes insipidus occurs as a result of the absence of vasopressin, the ADH that is produced in the large neurons of the supraoptic and paraventricular nuclei and released into the bloodstream in the posterior pituitary or neurohypophysis. ADH increases the permeability of the distal convoluted tubules and collecting ducts of the kidney. In the absence of ADH, the kidney does not reabsorb water, and urine production is extremely high.

Endocrine imbalance is the result of the absence of hypothalamic regulatory hormones that influence the anterior pituitary or adenohypophysis. These hormones are produced by small neurons, particularly in the arcuate nucleus, but also in the paraventricular nucleus. The regulatory hormones are transported via the axons of the tuberoinfundibular tract to capillaries in the infundibulum, where these hormones are released and carried to the anterior pituitary via the hypophysial portal system (Fig. 18-3). Within the pituitary gland these hormones regulate the production and release of the adrenocorticotropic, growth, thyrotropic, follicle-stimulating, and luteinizing hormones. Damage to the hypothalamus or to the hypophysial portal system results in decreased secretion of all the anterior pituitary hormones except prolactin. As a result, the patient exhibits hypoadrenalism, hypothyroidism, and abnormalities in the reproductive system cycles.

Body temperature is regulated in the hypothalamus by a **heat loss center** located anteriorly and a **heat gain center** located posteriorly. Temperature-sensitive neurons located near capillary beds in the hypothalamus respond to very small changes in temperature. Neurons in the preoptic and anterior hypothalamic nuclei are sensitive to a small increase in blood temperature, and these neurons initiate heat loss responses. Neurons in the posterior hypothalamic nucleus are sensitive to decreased blood temperature and initiate heat gain mechanisms. Lesions in the anterior hypothalamus result in **hyperthermia** because the neurons that initiate sweating and cutaneous vasodilation when the body temperature increases are not functional. Lesions in the posterior hypothalamus may result in a decrease in body temperature because of the absence of shivering and vasoconstriction mechanisms. But, most frequently, posterior hypothalamic lesions result in **poikilothermy,** the condition in which body temperature varies with the environment. Poikilothermy occurs because the posterior hypothalamic heat gain center that normally elicits cutaneous vasoconstriction, piloerection, and shivering is no longer functional, and the impulses from the anterior hypothalamic heat loss center, which normally elicit sweating and vasodilation, are interrupted en route to the brainstem reticular formation.

Food intake is influenced by several hypothalamic areas, such as the ventromedial nuclei and the lateral hypothalamic zone. Glucose- or fat-sensitive neurons in these areas influence the endocrine glands associated with metabolism. Bilateral lesions of the "satiety center" in the ventromedial nuclei result in increased appetite and, eventually, obesity. Bilateral lesions of the "feeding center" in the lateral hypothalamus at the tuberal level result in decreased food and drink intake.

Reproduction and sexual functions are influenced by the preoptic, anterior, and ventromedial nuclei. Estrogen-sensitive and androgen-sensitive neurons in these areas elicit the production of appropriate hormones that regulate the production and release of the anterior pituitary gonadotropins. Hypothalamic lesions may result in menstrual cycle disturbances or precocious puberty.

Sleep and the sleep-wake cycle are influenced by several areas of the hypothalamus. The suprachiasmatic nucleus, which receives input from the retina, is the biologic clock that plays a role in the **circadian rhythm** of approximately 24 hours. The anterior and preoptic nuclei can induce sleep, and the posterolateral hypothalamic area is involved in cortical arousal.

It is well known that hypothalamic lesions result in abnormalities of sleep patterns. Lesions in the anterior hypothalamus, particularly the preoptic nuclei, result in insomnia. The most frequent sleep alteration is an impairment of wakefulness that varies from drowsiness to permanent coma. The posterior hypothalamus appears to be associated with this abnormality; lesions here often result in hypersomnia.

The expression of emotions such as anger, fear, embarrassment, and so forth occurs through hypothalamic connections with appropriate brainstem and spinal cord centers. The hypothalamus has reciprocal connections with nuclei associated with behavior such as the amygdala and the medial dorsal thalamic nucleus. Bilateral hypothalamic lesions, especially in or near the ventromedial nuclei, result in extreme viciousness. Animals with such lesions fly into a rage and attack repeatedly without provocation. A similar phenomenon occurs in humans with such hypothalamic lesions. Patients with these lesions exhibit violent, aggressive behavior toward anyone present, including loved ones. It seems probable, therefore, that the ventromedial area of the hypothalamus normally exerts a regulatory effect on more posterolateral parts of the hypothalamus, where the mechanisms associated with aggressive behavior are centered. Such mechanisms include increased heart rate, elevated blood pressure, increased respiration, pupillary dilation, piloerection, and so forth—phenomena that are associated with activity of the sympathetic nervous system. It is generally accepted that the posterior hypothalamus controls sympathetic activity. In contrast, the anterior hypothalamus controls parasympathetic events (Table 18-1).

Chapter Review Questions

18-1. What are the anteroposterior subdivisions of the hypothalamus?

18-2. What is the chief neural output of the hypothalamus?

18-3. What is the hypophysial portal system?

18-4. Which parts of the hypothalamus are associated with the following?

a. temperature regulation
b. parasympathomimetic activity
c. sympathomimetic activity
d. hypothalamic regulatory hormones
e. water balance
f. sleep–wake cycle
g. emotions

The Autonomic Nervous System: Visceral Abnormalities

A 28-YEAR-OLD MAN involved in an automobile accident several months ago, in which he suffered whiplash, has recovered from all the abnormalities resulting from brainstem damage except for a right-sided mild ptosis, miosis, and facial anhidrosis.

The autonomic or involuntary system regulates visceral activity throughout the body. The autonomic system is divided into efferent and afferent parts, both of which innervate the involuntary musculature (as smooth and cardiac) and glandular tissue. The autonomic efferent system is composed of two divisions: sympathetic and parasympathetic. The autonomic afferent system consists of visceral afferent fibers that travel in the nerves making up the sympathetic and parasympathetic divisions. Because all viscera are supplied by both sympathetic and parasympathetic nerves, all visceral organs are innervated by four types of fibers: sympathetic efferents and afferents and parasympathetic efferents and afferents.

AUTONOMIC EFFERENTS

BASIC PRINCIPLES

The anatomic features of the autonomic and somatic efferent systems differ considerably: two efferent neurons exist in the autonomic path, whereas only a single neuron exists in the somatic path (Fig. 19-1).

The autonomic efferent system is divided into two parts: sympathetic and parasympathetic. The basic anatomic features of the two parts significantly differ. First, sympathetic activity enters the peripheral nervous system only via the thoracolumbar spinal nerves, whereas parasympathetic activity enters the peripheral nervous system only via cranial nerves and sacral spinal nerves (Table 19-1). Second, because of its short postganglionic fibers and the small ratio of preganglionic fibers to postganglionic neurons (1:2; Fig. 19-2), the parasympathetic division has a localized influence. The parasympathetic division, with its very localized influence, is associated with the protection, rest, and recuperation of individual organs and bodily functions, i.e., pupillary constriction, decreased heart rate, salivation; and digestion, elimination of waste products from bowel and bladder, and so forth.

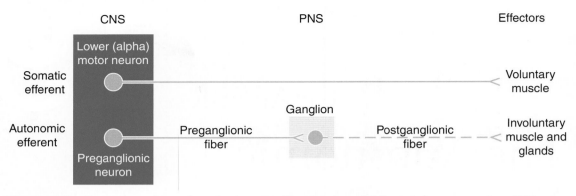

Figure 19-1 Comparison of somatic and automatic efferent systems (CNS, central nervous system; PNS, peripheral nervous system).

Conversely, the sympathetic division, with its long postganglionic fibers and large ratio of postganglionic neurons to preganglionic fibers, has a widespread influence. Because of these anatomic features, sympathetic system activity results in diffuse phenomena associated with emergency situations such as "fight or flight," i.e., increased heart rate and respiration, dilated pupils, increased blood supply to voluntary muscles, and so forth.

PARASYMPATHETIC DIVISION

All activity in parasympathetic nerve fibers originates in the brainstem or spinal cord (Fig. 19-3). The brainstem preganglionic parasympathetic neurons are found in four locations:

1. the Edinger-Westphal nucleus, the visceromotor component of the oculomotor nuclear complex;

2. the superior salivatory nucleus, the viscerosecretory component of the facial nuclear complex;

3. the inferior salivatory nucleus, found near the rostral part of the nucleus ambiguus and contributing viscerosecretory fibers to the glossopharyngeal nerve; and

4. the dorsal nucleus of the vagus as well as neurons scattered near the caudal part of the nucleus ambiguus. The visceromotor and viscerosecretory axons of these neurons emerge in the vagus nerve.

The cranial ganglia that give rise to the postganglionic parasympathetic fibers are the ciliary ganglion, which receives preganglionic fibers from the oculomotor nerve; the pterygopalatine and submandibular ganglia, which receive preganglionic fibers from the facial nerve; and the otic ganglion, which receives preganglionic fibers from

TABLE 19-1	**Principal Features of Autonomic Efferent Divisions**	
	Sympathetic	**Parasympathetic**
Preganglionic location	Thoracolumbar	Craniosacral
Postganglionic location	Paravertebral and prevertebral ganglia	Terminal ganglia
Postganglionic fibers	Relatively long, thus a more diffuse action	Relatively short, thus a more discrete action
Preganglionic to postganglionic ratio	Larger (e.g., 1:17)	Smaller (e.g., 1:2)
Function	Prepares organism for emergencies: "fight or flight"	Prepares organism for "rest and recuperation"

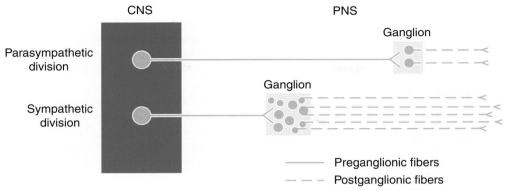

Figure 19-2 Comparison of parasympathetic and sympathetic divisions of automatic efferent system. Preganglionic fibers (solid line); postganglionic fibers (broken line; CNS, central nervous system; PNS, peripheral nervous system).

the glossopharyngeal nerve. The preganglionic fibers in the vagus nerve synapse in terminal ganglia both extrinsic and intrinsic to the thoracic, abdominal, and pelvic viscera that are vagally innervated (Fig. 19-3).

The sacral preganglionic parasympathetic neurons are in and near the intermediolateral nucleus in spinal cord segments S2, S3, and S4. The preganglionic fibers emerge from the spinal cord and pass to the terminal ganglia of the colon and

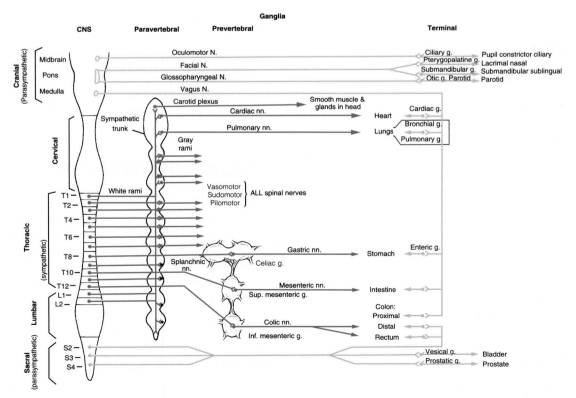

Figure 19-3 Schematic diagram showing basic plan of automatic efferent system (CNS, central nervous system; g, ganglion; inf, inferior; N, nerve; nn, nerves; sup, superior). Sympathetic-dark blue; parasempathetic-light blue.

rectum, urinary bladder, prostate and vaginal glands, and erectile tissues of the penis and clitoris. The sacral parasympathetic nerves control defecation, urination, and erection.

SYMPATHETIC DIVISION

All activity in sympathetic nerve fibers originates in the spinal cord (Fig. 19-3). The preganglionic sympathetic neurons are found in several columns extending from about C8 to L2 or L3. These sympathetic columns are an intermediolateral nucleus in the lateral horn, an intermediomedial nucleus in the medial part of the intermediate zone (lamina VII), and an intercalated nucleus bridging the previous two. Some sympathetic preganglionic neurons are also scattered in the lateral funiculus near the lateral horn.

The sympathetic neurons that give rise to postganglionic fibers are in the paravertebral (sympathetic trunk) ganglia and in the prevertebral (collateral or autonomic plexus) ganglia. The sympathetic trunk ganglia comprise 20 to 25 pair along the vertebral column, whereas the autonomic plexus ganglia are found along the abdominal aorta, especially around the origins of the celiac, superior mesenteric, and inferior mesenteric arteries.

The basic circuitry of the sympathetic system (Fig. 19-4) is as follows:

1. All preganglionic sympathetic fibers emerge from the spinal cord in spinal nerves T1 through L2.
2. The preganglionic sympathetic fibers reach the sympathetic trunk by passing through the ventral roots, the spinal nerves, and the white communicating rami.
3. Within the sympathetic trunk, the preganglionic sympathetic fibers may:
   a. synapse at the same level;
   b. ascend and synapse in a higher or more cranial sympathetic trunk ganglion;
   c. descend and synapse in a lower or more caudal sympathetic trunk ganglion; or
   d. emerge via thoracic splanchnic nerves and lumbar splanchnic nerves without synapsing.
4. The sympathetic trunk neurons give rise to three types of postganglionic fibers:
   a. perivascular, which travel along the walls of blood vessels, e.g., carotid plexus, to their destinations;
   b. spinal, which pass via the gray communicating rami to each spinal nerve, through which they are distributed to blood vessels, sweat glands, and piloerector muscles; and
   c. visceral, which pass directly to the viscera, e.g., cardiac nerves.
5. The autonomic plexus ganglia receive their preganglionic fibers from the splanchnic nerves and send their postganglionic fibers to the viscera via perivascular plexuses around the arteries supplying the abdominal and pelvic viscera, e.g., gastric, mesenteric, colic, and so forth.

GENERAL FUNCTIONS OF AUTONOMIC EFFERENTS

The autonomic efferent system plays an indispensable role in the maintenance of the internal environment. At times the sympathetic and parasympathetic divisions exert antagonistic effects. However, in most instances, the two divisions collaborate, both of them regulating and adjusting visceral functions. Most visceral organs are innervated by both divisions. One division usually produces effects opposite those of the other division (Table 19-2). The primary postganglionic neurotransmitters are acetylcholine for the parasympathetic system and norepinephrine for the sympathetic system. However, sweat glands are an exception because they are innervated by cholinergic (acetylcholine) sympathetic fibers.

AUTONOMIC AFFERENTS

The importance of impulses arising from visceral organs and blood vessels is mainly the initiation of visceral reflexes; most visceral impulses do not reach the level of consciousness. Those autonomic afferent impulses that do reach levels of awareness result in sensations that are vague and poorly localized, e.g., hunger, nausea, fullness of urinary bladder and rectum, and so forth. In certain conditions visceral sensations may become painful.

PRIMARY VISCERAL AFFERENTS

Peripheral nerves carrying autonomic preganglionic and postganglionic fibers to the viscera and blood vessels also contain nerve fibers carrying

1. Preganglionic neurons
   Preganglionic axons:
2. In ventral root
3. In spinal nerve
4. In white communicating ramus
5. Synapsing in same level ganglion
6. Ascending to more cranial ganglion
7. Synapsing in superior cervical ganglion
8. Descending to more caudal ganglion
9. Coursing in splanchnic nerves
10. Synapsing in autonomic plexus ganglia
    Postganglionic axons:
11. In carotid plexus
12. In gray communicating rami to
    all spinal nerves
13. In visceral nerves to thoracic organs
14. In perivascular plexuses

Ganglia:
15. Sympathetic trunk
16. Superior cervical
17. Celiac
18. Superior mesenteric
19. Inferior mesenteric

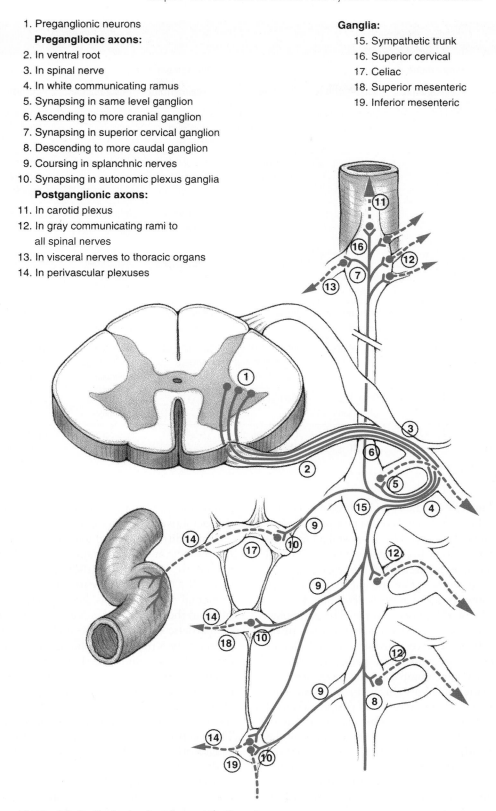

Figure 19-4 Basic circuitry of sympathetic system.

TABLE 19-2 Examples of Visceral Innervation

| Organ | Sympathetic | | | Parasympathetic | | |
	Preganglionic	Postganglionic	Function	Preganglionic	Postganglionic	Function
Iris	C8–T3	Superior cervical ganglion	Dilation of pupil	Edinger-Westphal nucleus	Ciliary ganglion	Constriction of pupil
Parotid gland	T1–T3	Superior cervical ganglion	Secretion reduced and viscid	Inferior salivatory nucleus	Otic ganglion	Secretion increased and watery
Heart	T1–T5	Cervical and upper thoracic ganglia	Increased rate	Dorsal vagal nucleus	Intracardiac ganglia	Decreased rate
Coronary vessels	T1–T5	Cervical and upper thoracic ganglia	Dilation or constriction	Dorsal vagal nucleus	Intracardiac ganglia	Constriction
Bronchi	T2–T5	Upper thoracic ganglia	Dilation	Dorsal vagal nucleus	Pulmonary ganglia	Constriction
Stomach	T6–T10	Celiac ganglion	Inhibition of peristalsis and secretion	Dorsal vagal nucleus	Myenteric and submucosal ganglia	Increased peristalsis and secretion
Sex organs	T10–L2	Inferior hypogastric ganglia	Ejaculation	S2–S4	Cavernous ganglia	Erection
Urinary bladder	T12–L2	Hypogastric ganglia	Contraction of trigone muscle	S2–S4	Vesical ganglion	Contraction of detrusor muscle

visceral impulses in the opposite direction, i.e., toward the brain and spinal cord. These are the autonomic afferents responsible for visceral input. Such afferent fibers come from unipolar neurons located in the spinal and some cranial nerve ganglia.

Various forms of free and encapsulated nerve endings in viscera and in the walls of blood vessels are the receptors for visceral input. The glossopharyngeal nerves; vagus nerves; and second, third, and fourth sacral nerves distribute visceral afferent fibers along parasympathetic paths, whereas the thoracic and upper lumbar spinal nerves distribute visceral afferent fibers through communicating rami to sympathetic nerves and peripheral blood vessels. In general, those fibers associated with reflex control of visceral activity accompany the parasympathetic nerves; those fibers that convey visceral sensations accompany the sympathetic nerves. An exception to this general rule is visceral pain fibers from certain pelvic viscera (sigmoid colon, rectum, neck of the bladder, prostate gland, and cervix of the uterus) that accompany the sacral parasympathetic nerves.

In addition to a vagal route to the brainstem, the thoracic and abdominal viscera send afferent fibers to the spinal cord via the sympathetic trunks (Fig. 19-5). From the heart, coronary vessels, bronchial tree, and lungs, visceral afferent fibers travel in the cardiac and pulmonary nerves to the sympathetic trunk. From the abdominal viscera, afferent fibers travel through the mesenteric and celiac plexuses and the thoracic and lumbar splanchnic nerves to the sympathetic trunk. After following an uninterrupted course, these afferent fibers enter the thoracic and upper lumbar spinal nerves through the white communicating rami. Their cell bodies are located in the dorsal root ganglia of T1 through L2, and their first synapse is in the spinal cord at these segments.

The phrenic nerve contains visceral afferent fibers coming from the pericardium, diaphragm, hepatic ligaments and capsule, pancreas, and

1. Visceral afferent receptors in abdominal organ
2. Perivascular nerves
3. Celiac ganglion
4. Superior mesenteric ganglion
5. Inferior mesenteric ganglion
6. Splanchnic nerves
7. Sympathetic trunk
8. White communicating rami
9. Spinal nerves
10. Cell bodies in spinal (dorsal root) ganglia
11. Dorsal root
12. Synapse in spinal gray
13. Visceral afferent from thoracic organ
14. Superior cervical ganglion

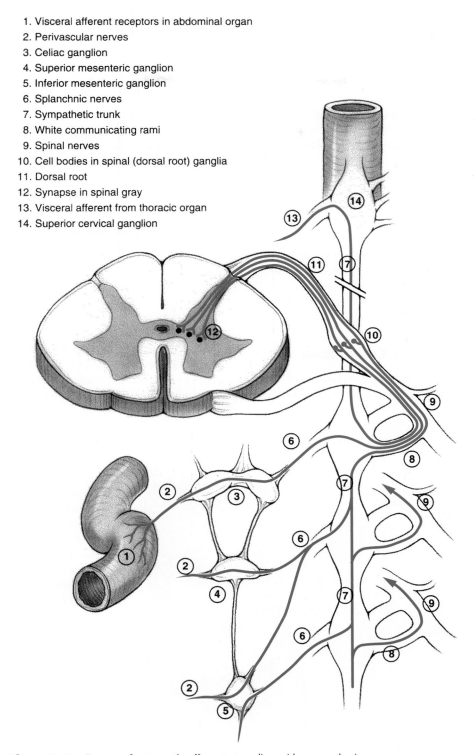

Figure 19-5   Routes of automatic afferents traveling with sympathetic nerves.

suprarenal glands. Visceral afferent fibers from peripheral blood vessels travel centrally in all spinal nerves. The cell bodies of these autonomic afferent components are also unipolar neurons in appropriate dorsal root ganglia.

Receptors in the sigmoid colon, rectum, urinary bladder, proximal part of the urethra, and cervix of the uterus initiate visceral afferent impulses for reflexes and sensations. The visceral afferent impulses from these pelvic viscera also travel centrally by two routes. One route is taken by the fibers that course in the pelvic splanchnic nerves and have their cell bodies located in the dorsal root ganglia of the second, third, and fourth sacral spinal nerves. The other route is through the various hypogastric plexuses, lumbar splanchnic nerves, and sympathetic trunk and its white communicating rami to the cells of origin in the dorsal root ganglia of the lower thoracic and upper lumbar spinal nerves.

BRAINSTEM CENTRAL CONNECTIONS

The solitary tract and solitary nucleus are the only conspicuous brainstem structures that can be iden-

tified with the visceral afferent system. The solitary tract extends from the lower part of the pons to the obex of the medulla and is closely related throughout its course to the solitary nucleus (Fig. 19-6). The primary autonomic afferent fibers in the solitary tract come from the glossopharyngeal nerves and vagus nerves and synapse in the solitary nucleus. Fibers from the solitary nucleus synapse in the reticular formation. From the reticular formation, connections are made with the respiratory center and cardiovascular center, visceral and somatic motor nuclei, and higher centers.

SPINAL CENTRAL CONNECTIONS

Visceral afferent fibers destined for the spinal cord enter through the lateral division of the dorsal root and synapse on cells located in the dorsal horn and intermediate zone (Fig. 19-5). Impulses associated with the initiation of reflexes make secondary connections with visceral or somatic motor neurons of the spinal gray. Visceral impulses destined to reach conscious levels ascend bilaterally in the lateral and posterior parts of the anterolateral quadrants and, on reaching the brainstem, continue through multi-

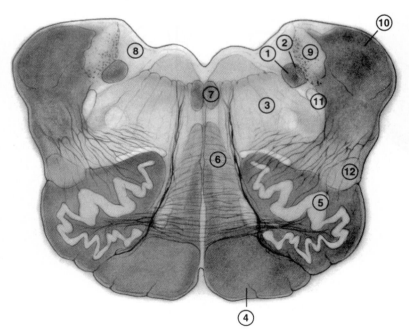

1. Solitary tract
2. Solitary nucleus
3. Medullary reticular formation
4. Pyramid
5. Inferior olivary nucleus
6. Medial lemniscus
7. Medial longitudinal fasciculus
8. Medial vestibular nucleus
9. Spinal (inf.) vestibular nucleus
10. Restiform body
11. Spinal trigeminal nucleus
12. Spinothalamic tract

Figure 19-6   Transverse section of medulla showing central components of autonomic afferents from vagus nerve (inf, inferior).

synaptic pathways in the reticular formation to higher centers. One exception to this route is the path subserving the sensation that urination is imminent. This sensation arises from the urethra and ascends in the dorsal column–medial lemniscus system.

VISCERAL SENSATIONS

True visceral sensations, e.g., heartburn, nausea, hunger, fullness of bladder or bowels, tend to be vague and poorly localized. This vagueness is because of the multisynaptic nature of the central pathways and the meager representation of viscera in the cerebral cortex.

Visceral organs, including the brain and spinal cord, are insensitive to ordinary mechanical and thermal stimuli. Even though handling, cutting, crushing, or burning of viscera occurs during surgical procedures, sensations are not felt. Painful sensations do result from excessive stretch, violent or spasmodic contractions, or decreased blood supply (ischemia). In such conditions the pain may be felt in the region of the organ itself (true visceral pain) or in a cutaneous or even other somatic tissue region (**referred pain**).

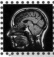

CLINICAL CONNECTION

Pain of visceral origin is not necessarily confined to visceral pathways in its conduction to the spinal cord, because the abdominal wall or the diaphragm may be involved by the disease process. Thus, pain of inoperable carcinoma of the stomach may not be favorably affected by sympathectomy (removal of the sympathetic trunks) because the body wall may be involved. Sympathectomy is, therefore, not a cure-all for visceral pain.

REFERRED PAIN

In pathologic conditions, visceral pain radiates to cutaneous areas and is therefore assumed by the patient to arise mainly or exclusively in surface areas of the body (Fig. 19-7). This kind of pain is called referred pain. It is important to recall that most visceral pain fibers travel with sympathetic nerves and reach the thoracic and upper lumbar spinal nerves through the 14 or 15 pairs of white rami communicating with the sympathetic trunks.

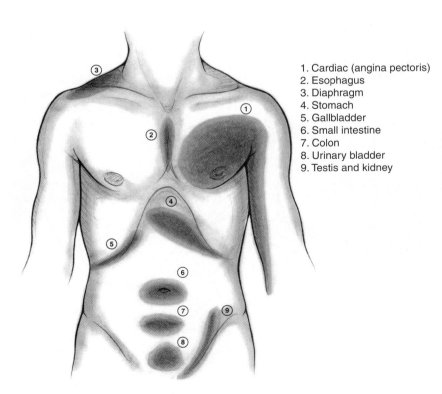

1. Cardiac (angina pectoris)
2. Esophagus
3. Diaphragm
4. Stomach
5. Gallbladder
6. Small intestine
7. Colon
8. Urinary bladder
9. Testis and kidney

Figure 19-7   Common cutaneous areas of referred pain.

Although the region to which the pain is referred may seem unrelated to the pathologic visceral organ, the two loci are part of the same segmental level.

The commonly accepted explanation for referred pain is that within the spinal gray matter the visceral afferent impulses converge on secondary somatic afferent neurons (Fig. 19-8) and lower their threshold of excitation. Thus, an abnormally large volley of visceral afferent impulses causes spinothalamic neurons to fire, resulting in deception of the cerebral cortex.

AUTONOMIC CONTROL CENTERS

Many types of autonomic phenomena have been elicited from various parts of the cerebral hemi-

spheres, e.g., frontal lobe, cingulate gyrus, orbitoinsulotemporal cortex, hippocampus, amygdala, and caudate nucleus. Most of the visceral responses are diffuse and tend to overlap somatic reactions. The autonomic or visceral responses elicited by stimulation in the cerebral hemispheres are funneled through the hypothalamus, the highest center for the regulation of autonomic responses.

In addition to hypothalamic nuclei, other groups of neurons at various levels also strongly influence autonomic activities. In the midbrain, pupillary constriction and lens accommodation centers are located at the levels of the pretectal area and superior colliculus. In the pons, a micturition center rostrally governs the initiation of urination, and pneumotaxic and apneustic centers more caudally influence respiration. Within the medulla are the cardiovascular and the expiratory and inspiratory respiratory centers.

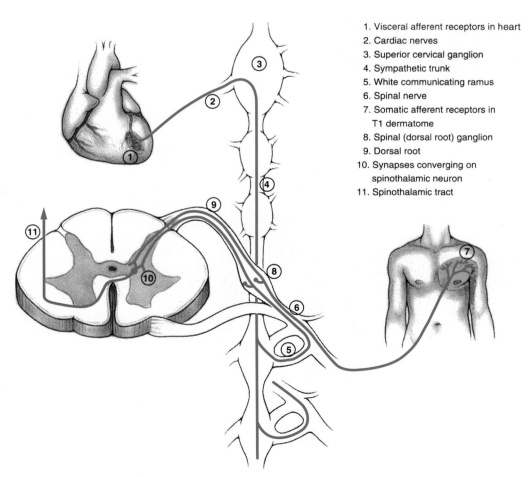

1. Visceral afferent receptors in heart
2. Cardiac nerves
3. Superior cervical ganglion
4. Sympathetic trunk
5. White communicating ramus
6. Spinal nerve
7. Somatic afferent receptors in T1 dermatome
8. Spinal (dorsal root) ganglion
9. Dorsal root
10. Synapses converging on spinothalamic neuron
11. Spinothalamic tract

Figure 19-8 Schematic diagram showing the anatomic basis for visceral referred pain.

Although these various centers receive input from many sources (hypothalamus, cranial nerves, ascending pathways, and so forth), their output is funneled to autonomic efferent and, in many cases, associated somatic neurons (Table 19-3). Examples of such connections are those that control the heart, the urinary bladder, and the sex organs.

CONTROL OF THE HEART

The heart is abundantly supplied by parasympathetic, sympathetic, and afferent nerves (Fig. 19-9).

Visceral afferent impulses arising from the heart travel centrally via the vagus and sympathetic nerves. Those in the vagus have cell bodies located in the nodose ganglion. The cardiac vagal afferent fibers enter the solitary tract and synapse in the solitary nucleus. The cardiac afferent fibers traveling via the sympathetic nerves do so on the left side. Their cell bodies are located in the upper four or five thoracic dorsal root ganglia, and they synapse in the upper thoracic spinal cord segments.

Cardiac control centers are located in the medullary reticular formation. These control centers are influenced mainly by impulses descending from the hypothalamus and by visceral afferent impulses from mechanoreceptors and chemoreceptors located in the walls of the heart, aorta, and carotid arteries. The mechanoreceptors or baro-receptors respond to blood pressure; the chemoreceptors respond to oxygen and carbon dioxide levels in the circulating blood. From these receptors, impulses are carried in the glossopharyngeal and vagus nerves to the solitary tract. After a synapse in the solitary nucleus, these visceral afferent impulses pass to cardiovascular centers in the adjacent reticular formation. Increases in blood pressure elicit vagal responses, and decreases in blood pressure cause sympathetic responses.

Cardiac parasympathetic neurons are located in the medulla in the vicinity of the dorsal vagal nucleus and nucleus ambiguus. The preganglionic fibers travel in the vagus nerves and synapse on ganglion cells in the cardiac plexus and epicardium and along the conducting system of the heart. Postganglionic fibers pass to the sinus and atrioventricular nodes and, to a lesser extent, the atria. The cardiac vagal innervation decreases heart rate and results in **bradycardia**.

Cardiac sympathetic neurons are located in and near the intermediolateral nucleus of the upper six to eight thoracic spinal cord segments. The preganglionic fibers emerge in spinal sympathetic ganglia. Postganglionic fibers travel via the cardiac nerves to the cardiac plexus and are distributed to the sinus and atrioventricular nodes, the atria and ventricles, and the coronary arteries. The cardiac sympathetic innervation increases heart rate and results in **tachycardia.**

TABLE 19-3 Principal Autonomic Centers and Their Output

Function	Location	Output
Vasomotor cardioaccelerator and pressor	Medullary reticular formation	Sympathetic nucleus in spinal cord
Depressor and cardiodecelerator	Medullary reticular formation	Neurons in dorsal vagal nucleus and reticular formation
Respiratory[a]: inspiration and expiration	Medullary reticular formation	Phrenic, intercostal, and abdominal motor neurons
Apneusis and pneumotaxis	Pontine reticular formation	Medullary respiratory centers
Vomiting	Medullary centers	Emetic center, vagal and parasympathetic preganglionic neurons
Micturition: initiation	Pontine reticular formation	Sacral parasympathetic neurons for detrusor contraction and inhibition of Onuf neurons supplying sphincter
Micturition: cessation[a] or prevention[a]	Frontal lobe	Onuf nucleus for contraction of sphincter

[a]Not autonomic.

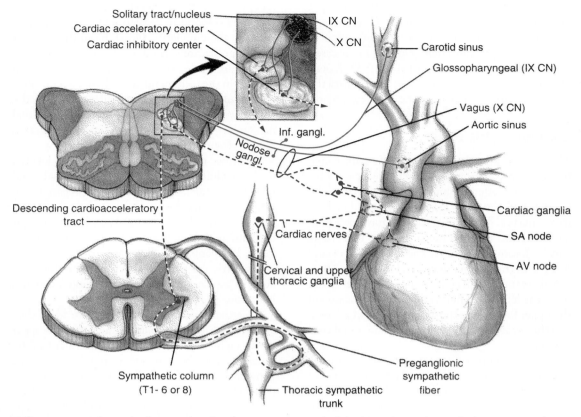

Figure 19-9 Schematic diagram showing the nervous control of the heart (AV, atrioventricular; CN, cranial nerve; gangl, ganglion; inf, inferior; SA, sinoatrial).

The coronary arteries are chiefly controlled by local metabolic factors. Increased metabolism accompanying increased heart rate results in dilation of the coronary arteries and increased blood flow to the heart muscle. Conversely, decreased heart rate results in decreased metabolic rate and constriction of the coronary arteries.

CONTROL OF THE URINARY BLADDER

The urinary bladder and its sphincters are supplied by parasympathetic, sympathetic, somatic motor, and visceral afferent fibers (Fig. 19-10).

Several groups of visceral afferent fibers supply the urinary bladder. Pain and temperature impulses from the mucosa of the fundus travel with the sympathetic nerves and reach the spinal cord via the dorsal roots of T12 and L1. From the mucosa at the neck of the bladder, pain and

temperature impulses travel with the sacral parasympathetic nerves to S2, S3, and S4. The spinothalamic tract then transmits impulses of both groups of pain and temperature fibers to higher centers.

Fullness of the bladder is detected by mechanoreceptors in the bladder wall that send impulses to the spinal cord via the sacral parasympathetic route. The spinothalamic tracts carry "fullness" impulses to higher centers in the thalamus and cerebral cortex. The sensation that micturition is imminent arises from mechanoreceptors in the trigone of the bladder; these visceral afferent impulses travel with the sacral parasympathetic nerves to S2, S3, and S4 and ascend in the dorsal column–medial lemniscus system.

Parasympathetic visceromotor neurons located in S2, S3, and S4 give rise to preganglionic fibers that travel in the pelvic nerve to the hypogastric

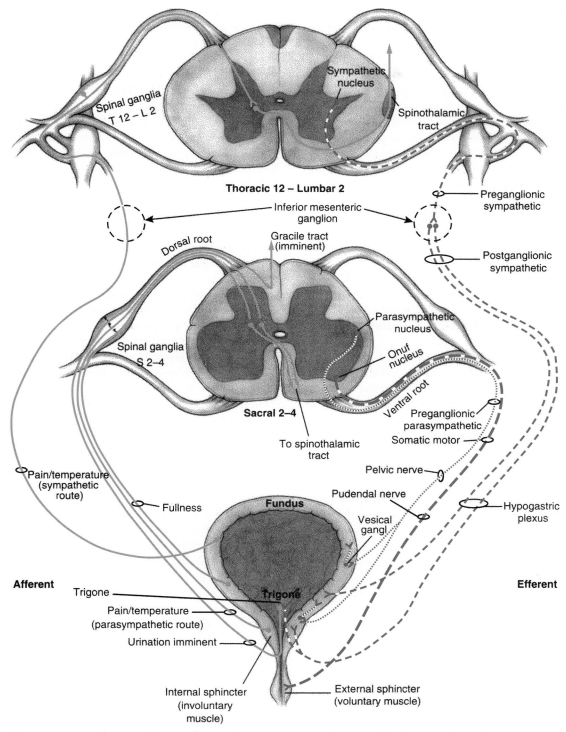

Figure 19-10   Schematic diagram showing the innervation of the urinary bladder (gangl, ganglion).

and then to the vesical plexuses. Vesical ganglion cells give rise to postganglionic parasympathetic fibers that supply the **detrusor muscle** that, on contraction, empties the bladder.

Sympathetic visceromotor neurons in spinal cord segments T11 through L2 give rise to preganglionic fibers that travel in the lumbar splanchnic nerves to the inferior mesenteric ganglion. Postganglionic sympathetic fibers from the inferior mesenteric ganglion reach the bladder via the hypogastric and vesicle plexuses and supply the internal urethral sphincter. During bladder filling, the sympathetic fibers relax the detrusor muscle directly and also indirectly by inhibiting the parasympathetic cells in the vesical ganglia. The sympathetic fibers elicit contraction of the internal urethral sphincter.

Lower motor neurons that make up the Onuf nucleus in S2, S3, and S4 send axons via the internal pudendal nerve and its perineal branch to the skeletal muscle that forms the external urethral sphincter.

Micturition centers are located in the brainstem and cerebral cortex. A cortical center for voluntary control of the initiation and cessation of micturition is located in the superior frontal gyrus on the medial surface of the hemisphere. Two micturition centers are located in the pons. One pontine micturition center sends excitatory impulses to the sacral parasympathetic neurons that elicit contraction of the detrusor muscle. A second pontine micturition center sends excitatory impulses to the lower motor neurons of the Onuf nucleus that supply the external urethral sphincter. During micturition the pontine parasympathetic excitatory center inhibits the other pontine center. Thus, the external urethral sphincter relaxes when the detrusor muscle contracts, and emptying of the bladder occurs.

Reflex bladder control is initiated by visceral afferent impulses from volume and tension receptors in the bladder wall. At low levels of bladder distention, these visceral afferent fibers stimulate the lower motor neurons of the Onuf nucleus, resulting in contraction of the external sphincter. At high levels of bladder distention, visceral afferent impulses stimulate pontine micturition center neurons that inhibit sympathetic and Onuf somatic neurons, resulting in relaxation of the internal and external sphincters, respectively, and elicit parasym-

pathetic activity resulting in contraction of the detrusor and emptying of the bladder. Thus, micturition is controlled by spinopontospinal reflex mechanisms.

Interruption of this reflex results in the so-called **neurogenic bladder.** Two types of neurogenic bladders exist: reflex and nonreflex (Fig. 19-11). The **reflex neurogenic bladder** is of upper motor neuron type; the nonreflex bladder is of lower motor neuron type. The reflex neurogenic bladder may be uninhibited or automatic. The **uninhibited reflex bladder,** which is incontinent but empties fully, results from bilateral lesions of the micturition centers in the frontal lobe. Emptying of the bladder is normal because reflex control of the pontine micturition centers are intact. The **automatic reflex bladder,** which is incontinent and does not empty fully, results from bilateral spinal cord lesions above sacral levels. Emptying of the bladder is incomplete because the spinal reflex pathways that trigger the pontine micturition centers are interrupted. The **nonreflex neurogenic bladder,** which is characterized by severe urinary retention and incontinence, results from bilateral lesions of the sacral spinal cord or the spinal nerve roots in the cauda equina (Fig. 19-11).

CONTROL OF THE SEX ORGANS

The sex organs are innervated by parasympathetic, sympathetic, and visceral afferent fibers. Visceral afferent fibers from the female and male sex organs pass to the spinal cord via sympathetic and sacral parasympathetic routes and have their cell bodies located in the dorsal root ganglia of T10 through L2 and S2 through S4, respectively. An exception to the rule that visceral pain fibers follow the sympathetic nerves occurs in the case of pain from the cervix of the uterus and the prostate. In both cases, pain travels with the parasympathetic nerves and enters the spinal cord at S2 through S4.

The preganglionic parasympathetic fibers arise from S2 through S4, enter the pelvic cavity via the pelvic nerve, and synapse on ganglia in the hypogastric and the uterovaginal or prostatic plexuses. Postganglionic parasympathetic fibers from the uterovaginal ganglia in the female inner-

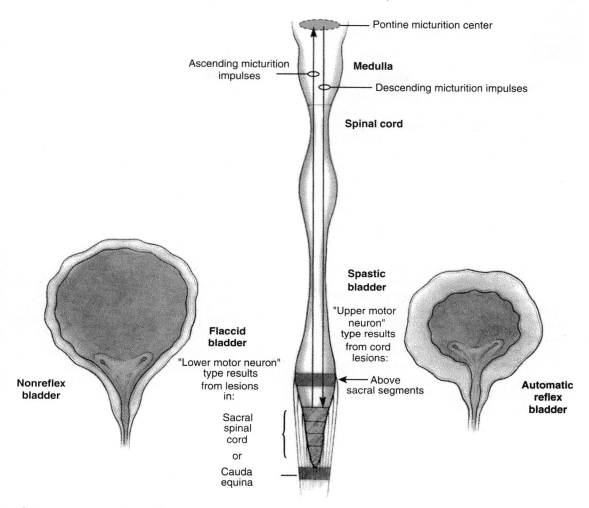

Figure 19-11   Locations of lesions resulting in flaccid and spastic neurogenic bladders.

vate the vaginal glands and erectile tissue of the clitoris. In the male, the postganglionic parasympathetic fibers arise from the cavernous and prostatic ganglia and supply the cavernous or erectile tissue of the penis.

Sympathetic preganglionic fibers arise from T10 through L2 and synapse chiefly in the inferior mesenteric ganglion. Postganglionic sympathetic fibers in the female supply the blood vessels and smooth muscle of the uterus and vagina, whereas

in the male sympathetic postganglionic fibers supply the ductus deferens, prostate gland, and seminal vesicle.

Parasympathetic activity in women produces secretion of vaginal glands and clitoral engorgement; in men parasympathetic impulses are necessary for penile erection. Sympathetic activity in women produces rhythmic contractions of the vagina; in men the sympathetic nerves are necessary for ejaculation.

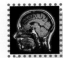

CLINICAL CONNECTION

Two commonly encountered abnormalities associated with the sympathetic system are Horner syndrome, as in the clinical illustration at the beginning of this chapter, and **acute sympathetic shock syndrome.** Horner syndrome is characterized by miosis, ptosis, and anhidrosis (absence of sweating) and may occur as the result of unilateral peripheral or central lesions. The peripheral lesions involve (1) preganglionic fibers chiefly in spinal nerve T1 or in the cervical sympathetic trunk or (2) postganglionic neurons and fibers in the superior cervical ganglion. Central lesions producing Horner syndrome occur chiefly as the result of (1) interrupting the pupillodilator path in the dorsolateral part of the medullary reticular formation or in the cervical spinal cord or (2) destruction of the ciliospinal center in the sympathetic nucleus of C8 and T1.

Acute sympathetic shock syndrome is characterized by bradycardia, hypotension, bilateral Horner syndrome, and difficulties in adjusting to a warm environment because sweating and cutaneous vasodilation cannot be elicited. This syndrome occurs in acute bilateral cervical spinal cord injuries as a result of the interruption of the descending impulses to the sympathetic nuclei. The signs usually subside after several days when reflex regulation of sympathetic activities returns.

Chapter Review Questions

19-1. What are the chief differences between the somatic and autonomic efferent systems?

19-2. Describe the origin of the cranial parasympathetic system.

19-3. Describe the origin of the sacral parasympathetic system.

19-4. Describe the origin of preganglionic sympathetic fibers.

19-5. Name which cranial nerves contain autonomic afferent fibers and describe their connections.

19-6. What are the chief peripheral routes of visceral pain fibers?

19-7. Define and give an explanation for referred pain.

19-8. Where is the site of referral, and what is the anatomic basis of cardiac referred pain?

19-9. Contrast the effects of stimulation of parasympathetic and sympathetic nerves on the heart, urinary bladder, and sex organs.

20

Reticular Formation: Modulation and Activation

A 17-YEAR-OLD HIGH SCHOOL STUDENT lost control while speeding in his automobile and suffered severe head trauma. On arrival at the ER he rapidly became comatose and had a dilated left pupil. CT scan showed a massive left epidural hematoma. Although the hematoma was removed in the OR he never regained consciousness, and now, 6 months later, he has decerebrate posturing and is in irreversible coma.

The reticular formation forms the central core of the brainstem and was so named by 19th century anatomists because histologically it appears as a densely packed intermingling of neuronal cell bodies, axons, and dendrites. It extends throughout the brainstem and contains numerous nuclei, most of which are indistinct. It is located in the central part of the medulla, pons, and midbrain and is surrounded by the various motor, sensory, and visceral nuclei and tracts in the brainstem (Fig. 20-1).

Because of its central location the reticular formation receives input and gives output to all parts of the nervous system. Hence, the reticular formation consists of centers that (1) integrate cranial nerve reflexes, (2) participate in the conduction and modulation of slow pain, (3) influence voluntary movements, (4) regulate autonomic nuclei, (5) are associated with diffuse modulating systems, (6) integrate such basic functions as respiration and sleep, and (7) activate the cerebral cortex.

AFFERENT CONNECTIONS

Input to the reticular formation comes from all parts of the central nervous system (CNS) (Fig. 20-2). Among the more influential sources are the spinal cord, cranial nerves, cerebellum, and forebrain. From the spinal cord comes a massive spinoreticular projection that ascends from the anterolateral quadrants and terminates mainly in the more medial part of the reticular formation at medullary and pontine levels. From the cranial nerves come very strong inputs from the secondary sensory nuclei of the trigeminal, cochlear, and vestibular nerves and a weaker contribution from the glossopharyngeal and vagus nerves (Fig. 20-2).

Input associated with equilibrium and posture, chiefly from the vestibulocerebellum, projects to the reticular formation at medullary levels, whereas input from the spinocerebellum projects chiefly to midbrain and pontine levels.

251

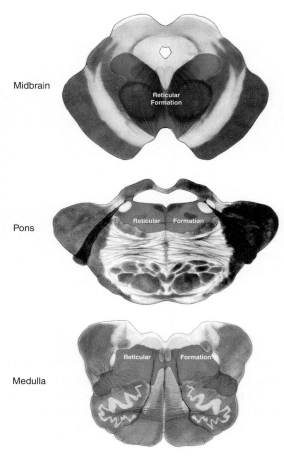

Figure 20-1 Transverse sections of the brainstem showing locations of the reticular formation (shaded).

Impulses descending from the hypothalamus, the thalamus, and the basal ganglia terminate in the midbrain reticular formation. In addition, impulses from the cerebral cortex, mainly the sensorimotor areas, project to the reticular formation at pontine and medullary levels.

EFFERENT CONNECTIONS

The reticular formation has connections with virtually all other nuclei in the brainstem. In addition, efferent fibers from the reticular formation descend into the spinal cord and ascend into the forebrain. The descending fibers form the reticulospinal tracts, which arise at various levels of the reticular formation. The ascending projections arise from all levels of the reticular formation and influence widespread areas of the cerebral cortex.

FUNCTIONS

The reticular formation is associated with cranial nerve activity, the conduction and modulation of slow pain, voluntary movements, autonomic nervous system activity, the distribution of monoaminergic and cholinergic neurotransmitters widely in the CNS, respiration, sleep, and cerebral cortical arousal and wakefulness.

CRANIAL NERVE ACTIVITY

Centers within the reticular formation organize cranial nerve activity at segmental levels (Fig. 20-2).

medulla	swallowing and coughing
	gagging and vomiting
	respiration and circulation
	equilibrium
pons	blinking
	horizontal gaze
	mastication
	auditory reflexes
midbrain	vertical gaze and
	vergence

VOLUNTARY MOVEMENTS

Impulses descending via the pontine and medullary reticulospinal tracts have a strong influence on axial and limb muscles, muscle tone, and myotatic reflexes as described in Chapter 7.

AUTONOMIC NERVOUS SYSTEM ACTIVITY

Impulses from the hypothalamus descend into the reticular formation at midbrain levels and continue into the lateral part of the reticular formation at pontine and medullary levels as described in Chapter 19. Many continue into the spinal cord within the lateral reticulospinal tract. Through reticular formation connections involving the salivatory and vagal nuclei, and also such centers as the pressor, depressor, gastrointestinal, and so forth, salivation, cardiovascular, digestive, and other phenomena are influenced.

SLOW PAIN CONDUCTION AND MODULATION

The role of the reticular formation in the conduction and modulation of slow pain has been described in Chapter 11.

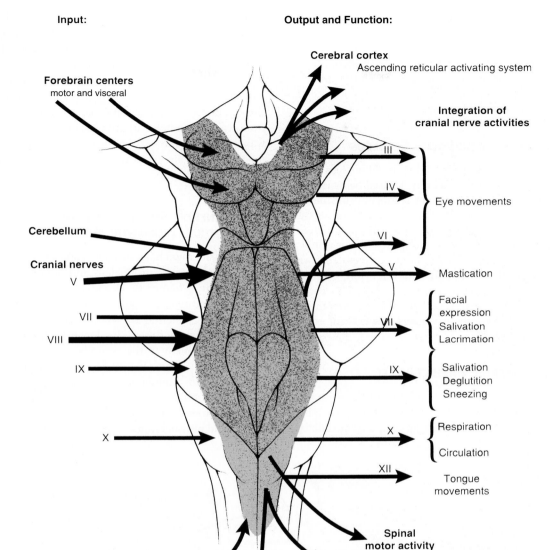

Figure 20-2   Diagram of brainstem reticular formation showing its inputs and outputs. Reticular formation forming central core (shaded area).

DIFFUSE MODULATING SYSTEMS

Several groups of neurons in the brainstem reticular formation form the diffuse modulating systems. Each of these groups is associated with a particular neurotransmitter, which is widely dispersed in various parts of the CNS. Functionally, these systems regulate the excitability of vast numbers of neurons, making them more or less excitable.

There are three major features of these systems: (1) each has a relatively small number of neurons, i.e., 10,000 to 15,000; (2) the axon of each neuron travels a great distance, has innumerable branches, and may influence more than 100,000 widely spread postsynaptic neurons; and

(3) the neurotransmitters are released into the extracellular fluid where they can diffuse and act on many neurons.

Three groups of nuclei in the brainstem (locus ceruleus, raphe, and ventral tegmental) and one in the basal forebrain (basal nucleus of Meynert) chiefly form the diffuse modulating system.

NORADRENERGIC LOCUS CERULEUS

The locus ceruleus is a dark-colored nucleus with melanin-containing neurons located beneath the lateral part of the floor of the rostral pontine fourth ventricle. Its axons are distributed to the cerebral cortex, thalamus, hypothalamus, cerebellar cortex, brainstem, and spinal cord (Fig. 20-3). The noradrenergic projections of the locus ceruleus are involved in the regulation of attention, cortical arousal, and the sleep–wake cycle, as well as learning, memory, anxiety, and mood. Norepinephrine increases brain responsiveness and speeds information processing.

SEROTONERGIC RAPHE NUCLEI

Neurons clustered in the midline of the medulla, pons, and midbrain form the serotonergic raphe nuclei (Fig. 20-4). Those near the pontomedullary junction are the nucleus raphe magnus, which projects to the spinal cord for the modulation of slow pain (see Chapter 11). Those in the rostral pons and midbrain project to the thalamus, to limbic system structures such as the hippocampus, amygdala, accumbens and septal nuclei, and to the cerebral cortex. The serotonergic projections from the raphe nuclei are involved in the sleep–wake cycle and are also implicated in control of mood and certain types of emotional behavior, especially aggression.

DOPAMINERGIC SUBSTANTIA NIGRA AND VENTRAL TEGMENTAL AREA

The compact nigra has massive dopaminergic projections to the caudate nucleus and putamen as described in Chapter 8. Degeneration of these dopaminergic neurons results in Parkinson disease. The ventral tegmental area is located posteromedial to the compact nigra. Its dopaminergic neurons project chiefly to the accumbens, amygdala, and prefrontal cortex (Fig. 20-5). The relationship of increased dopaminergic activity in the accumbens nucleus elicited by psychostimulant drugs like amphetamines and cocaine coincides with the reward and pleasure functions of this nucleus.

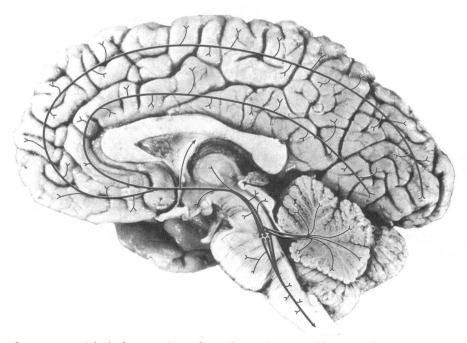

Figure 20-3   Principal connections of noradrenergic axons of locus ceruleus.

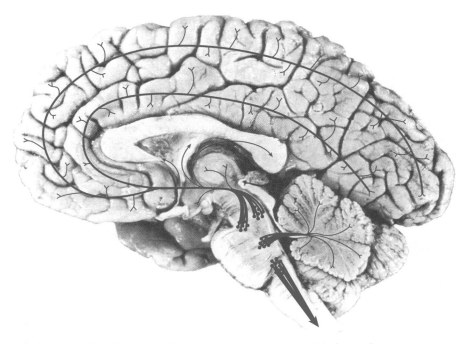

Figure 20-4 Principal connections of serotonergic axons of raphe nuclei.

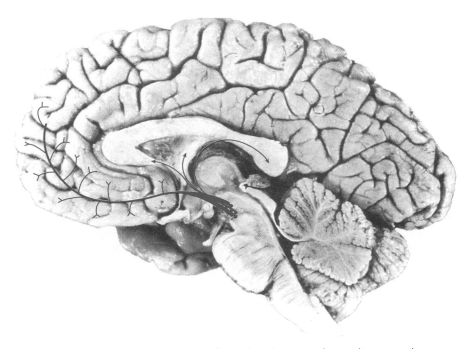

Figure 20-5 Principal connections of dopaminergic axons of ventral tegmental area.

CHOLINERGIC BRAINSTEM AND BASAL FOREBRAIN SYSTEM

Cholinergic neurons in the pons and midbrain project to the thalamus and regulate the excitability of thalamic nuclei. Cholinergic neurons in the basal nucleus of Meynert (Fig. 20-6), located in the anterior perforated substance, project to widespread areas of the cerebral cortex and play a major role in cortical excitability, memory, and learning. The degeneration of those neurons in Alzheimer patients may account for their impaired cognitive functioning.

RESPIRATION

Although often considered a function of the autonomic nervous system, respiration is actually a viscerosomatic reflex that may be influenced by various centers in the brainstem and forebrain. The lower motor neurons or final common paths for inspiration are located in the spinal cord. Those at the C3 and C4 levels innervate the diaphragm via the phrenic nerve and those at the T1 to T10 levels innervate the intercostal muscles via the intercostal nerves. The rhythmic activation of the inspiratory lower motor neurons is controlled by the **respiratory center** located bilaterally in the ventrolateral medulla at the caudal part of the fourth ventricle. This center receives input, chiefly from chemoreceptors, carried centrally in the glossopharyngeal and vagus nerves to the solitary nucleus, which integrates their input and then projects to the ventrolateral respiratory center. The **pneumotaxic center** located in the dorsolateral tegmentum of the rostral pons inhibits the inspiratory phase of respiration. Although respiration as well as circulation, digestion, and other autonomic phenomena may be momentarily influenced by stimulation of the cingulate gyrus, the hypothalamus seems to be the chief forebrain center that can influence respiration regularly. It does so via projections descending through the periaqueductal gray and adjacent tegmentum of the midbrain.

In comatose patients, abnormal patterns of respiration correlate with the loss of function at various levels of the CNS (Fig. 20-7). Bilateral dysfunction of structures deep in the cerebral hemispheres or in the diencephalon results in **Cheyne-Stokes** respiration, in which hyperpnea alternates with apnea (no breathing). Impairment of the deep periaqueductal gray and adjacent paramedian reticular formation in the midbrain or isthmus of the pons results in **central neurogenic hyperventilation,** a sustained, rapid, deep hyperpnea. Injury of the

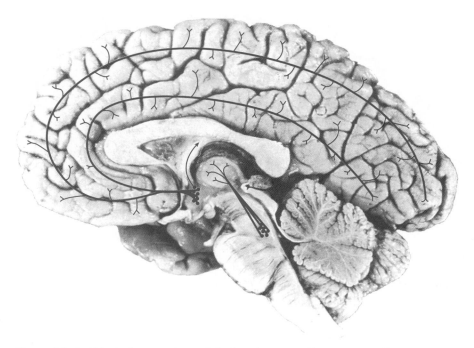

Figure 20-6 Principal connections of cholinergic axons of brainstem and basal nuclei.

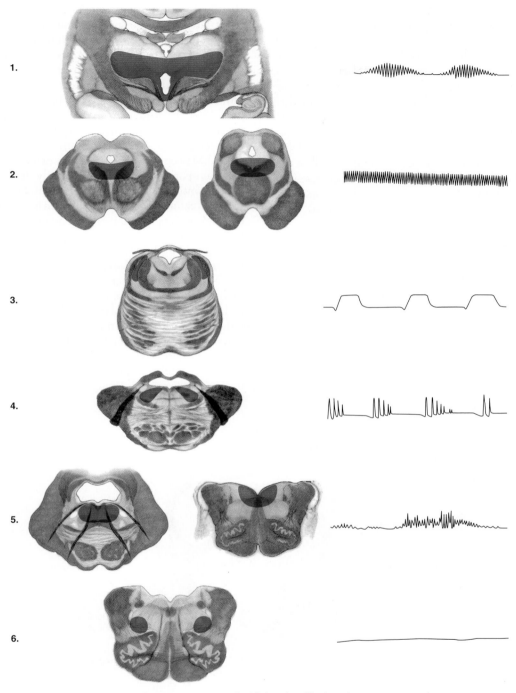

Figure 20-7 Respiratory patterns associated with levels of lesions in comatose patients.
1. Deep forebrain—Cheyne-Stokes
2. Midbrain—central neurogenic hyperventilation
3. Rostral pons—apneustic breathing
4. Midpons—cluster breathing
5. Caudal pons or rostral medulla—ataxic breathing
6. Respiratory centers in mid-medulla—respiratory arrest

dorsolateral tegmentum at rostral pontine levels results in **apneustic breathing,** which consists of prolonged inspiration alternating with prolonged expiration. **Cluster breathing** in which there are three or four rapid, deep breaths alternating with periods of apnea may occur with damage at mid-pontine levels. Impairment of the dorsomedial reticular formation in the caudal pons or rostral medulla results in **ataxic breathing,** in which respiration is irregular and of uneven depths. Finally, bilateral lesions in the ventrolateral medulla at the level of the respiratory centers or of their descending projections in the caudal medulla or rostral cervical spinal cord result in **respiratory arrest.**

SLEEP

Sleep is a complex and highly organized phenomenon that is regulated chiefly by centers in the pontine reticular formation. Two major stages exist: **rapid eye movement (REM)** and **nonrapid eye movement (NREM)** sleep. In addition to the rapid conjugate eye movements in REM sleep, it is characterized by decreased tone in virtually all muscles except the external ocular muscles and

the diaphragm; muscle twitches; fluctuations of heart rate, blood pressure, respiration, and body temperature; miosis; penile erection and clitoral engorgement; dreaming; and an electroencephalographic (EEG) pattern similar to that of the waking state. In addition to the absence of rapid eye movements in NREM sleep, it is characterized by decreased neuronal activity, reduced body movements, decreased heart rate and blood pressure, and a sleep-state EEG pattern.

REM sleep is regulated chiefly by neurons at the midbrain-pontine junction, particularly the dorsolateral pontine reticular formation ventrolateral to the locus ceruleus (Fig. 20-8). This area is extremely complex and appears to include individual populations of neurons that facilitate the various activities occurring during REM sleep. Bilateral destruction of this area results in the loss of REM sleep.

NREM sleep is generated by groups of neurons in the anterior hypothalamic nucleus, preoptic area, and the medulla, particularly the dorsal medullary reticular formation and the solitary nucleus. The anterior hypothalamic nucleus and preoptic area are very active during NREM sleep and inactive during REM sleep and wakefulness. This anterior hypothalamic sleep center is thought to facilitate NREM

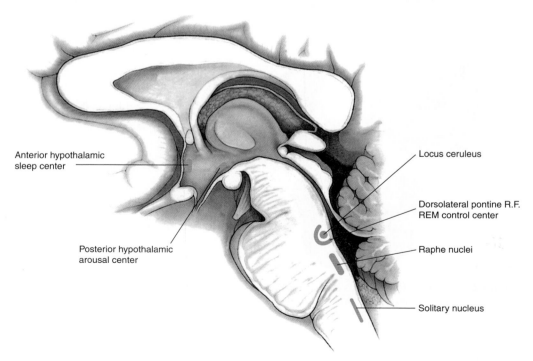

Figure 20-8 Centers and nuclei associated with sleep (R.F., reticular formation; REM, rapid eye movement).

sleep by inhibiting arousal centers in the posterior hypothalamus. Bilateral lesions of the anterior hypothalamic sleep center result in insomnia.

The role of other groups of neurons in the brainstem and forebrain in controlling sleep is not well established. For instance, noradrenergic neurons in the locus ceruleus and serotonergic neurons in the raphe nuclei are active during wakefulness. Cholinergic neurons in the basal forebrain and dorsolateral pontine reticular formation are active in REM sleep and wakefulness. Dopaminergic neurons in the hypothalamus and brainstem are active in sleep and wakefulness. Thus, the actual circuitry regulating sleep is extremely complex. However, it seems well established that the anterior hypothalamus induces sleep, the posterior hypothalamus is associated with arousal, the dorsolateral reticular formation at the junction of the pons and midbrain elicits REM sleep, and the raphe and solitary nuclei are active during NREM sleep.

AROUSAL AND WAKEFULNESS

Activation of the cerebral cortex, as occurs in arousal and wakefulness, is entirely dependent on the influence of the reticular formation on the cerebral cortex via the **ascending reticular activat-**

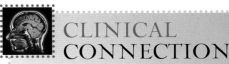

CLINICAL CONNECTION

N arcolepsy is characterized as sudden and spontaneous episodes of sleep at any time during the day. Unlike normal sleep, which begins with the NREM phase, narcolepsy begins with the REM phase.

Sleep apnea is the absence of breathing for a considerable period of time, i.e., a minute or more during sleep. It occurs with upper airway obstructions or deficient central respiratory mechanisms. It occurs repetitively and the victim awakens each time, so that it results in sleepiness when awake as a result of the loss of sleep.

ing system (ARAS). In the absence of the ARAS, stimulation of the somatosensory, auditory, visual and, in fact, any or all of the sensory pathways cannot awaken the cerebral cortex. Numerous nuclei in the brainstem reticular formation contribute to the ARAS (Fig. 20-9). Included in these are the monoaminergic cell groups in the raphe nuclei, locus ceruleus, and ventral tegmental area, as well as cholinergic neurons in the dorsolateral pontine tegmentum. These ARAS components funnel through the paramedian midbrain reticular formation and divide into dorsal and ventral routes in the diencephalon. The dorsal route projects to

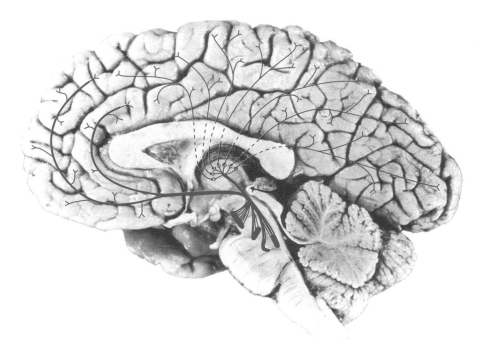

Figure 20-9   Projections of the ascending reticular activating system.

relay nuclei and to intralaminar and other nuclei that have widespread cortical connections. The ventral route enters the lateral hypothalamic zone and is joined by projections from other neurons in the hypothalamus and basal forebrain. Lesions in the medulla or pons do not affect arousal and wakefulness. However, paramedian tegmental lesions in the rostral midbrain interrupt the ARAS and result in coma.

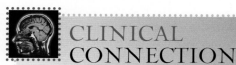

CLINICAL CONNECTION

Unilateral intracranial masses such as large epidural or subdural hematomas may result in uncal herniation, whereby the uncus becomes wedged between the free edge of the tentorium and the midbrain. This causes the midbrain to shift to the opposite side, resulting in stretching of the oculomotor nerve ipsilateral to the space-occupying mass. Because pupilloconstrictor fibers are on the surface of the oculomotor nerve, pupillary dilation ipsilateral to the mass is an early sign of uncal herniation. Continued compression of the midbrain and its blood supply results in interruption of the ARAS. As the ARAS becomes more compromised, drowsiness followed by coma occurs. If the ARAS becomes irreparably damaged, irreversible coma results as exemplified in the case history at the beginning of the chapter.

Chapter Review Questions

20-1. What are the chief cranial nerve, spinal cord, and forebrain inputs to the reticular formation?

20-2. What are the chief functions of the reticular formation outputs to the cranial nerves, spinal cord, and forebrain?

20-3. Alterations in which basal forebrain nucleus are associated with decreased cerebral cortical cholinergic activity in Alzheimer disease?

20-4. The pleasure induced by psychostimulants such as amphetamine or cocaine is associated with increased activity of what neurotransmitter in which limbic system center?

20-5. Bilateral lesions at which CNS levels result in respiratory arrest?

20-6. Which parts of the hypothalamus are associated with sleep and arousal?

20-7. Which part of the brain is chiefly associated with REM sleep?

20-8. A head trauma patient with third nerve signs who now has become semicomatose may be suffering damage in which part of the CNS?

Summary of the Cranial Nerves: Components and Abnormalities

COMPONENTS AND LESIONS

The cranial nerves consist of 12 pairs of nerves attaching to the brain (Fig. 21-1) and emerging from the cranial cavity to provide sensory, motor, and visceral innervation to structures chiefly in the head and neck, but also in the thorax and abdomen. Whereas the spinal nerves contain four functional types of fibers, i.e., general somatic afferents and efferents and general visceral afferents and efferents, the cranial nerves contain additional components. The functional components of the cranial nerves and their classifications and distributions are given in Table 21-1.

TABLE 21-1 Functional Components and Distribution for Cranial Nerve Fibers

Type	Distribution
Afferent	
General somatic (GSA)	Skin, skeletal muscle, joints, bone
General visceral (GVA; autonomic afferents)	Visceral organs
Special somatic (SSA)	Retina, auditory and vestibular receptors
Special visceral (SVA)	Gustatory and olfactory receptors
Efferent	
General somatic (GSE)	Skeletal muscle from somites
General visceral (GVE; autonomic efferents)	Smooth muscle and glands
Special somatic (SSE; special visceral [SVE])	Skeletal muscle from branchial arch mesoderm

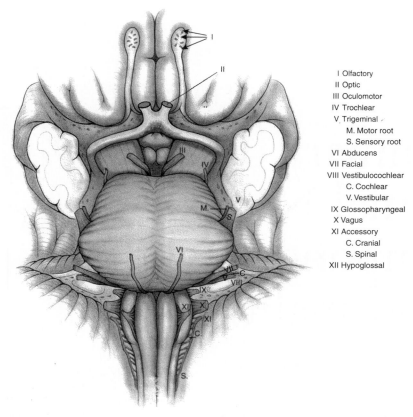

I Olfactory
II Optic
III Oculomotor
IV Trochlear
V Trigeminal
    M. Motor root
    S. Sensory root
VI Abducens
VII Facial
VIII Vestibulocochlear
    C. Cochlear
    V. Vestibular
IX Glossopharyngeal
X Vagus
XI Accessory
    C. Cranial
    S. Spinal
XII Hypoglossal

Figure 21-1   The cranial nerves. See Table 21-1 for components and distributions.

TABLE 21-2   Special Sensory Cranial Nerves: Olfactory, Optic, and Vestibulocochlear

Nerve	Function	Origin	Peripheral Distribution	Central Connections	Signs
I Olfactory	Olfaction or smell	Olfactory epithelium	Superior nasal concha and nasal septum	Olfactory bulb	Loss of sense of smell (anosmia)
II Optic	Vision	Retinal ganglion cells	Retinal bipolar cells	Lateral geniculate nuclei	Blindness
	Light reflex (afferent limb)	Retinal ganglion cells	Retinal bipolar cells	Pretectal nuclei	Absence of pupillary constriction bilaterally on testing blind eye
VIII Vestibular	Balance	Vestibular ganglion	Maculae of utricle and saccule	Vestibular nuclei	Dysequilibrium
	Vestibulo-ocular reflex (afferent limb)	Vestibular ganglion	Cristae of semicircular ducts	Vestibular nuclei	Absence of vestibulo-ocular reflex (VOR)
Cochlear	Hearing	Spiral ganglion	Spiral organ	Cochlear nuclei	Deafness

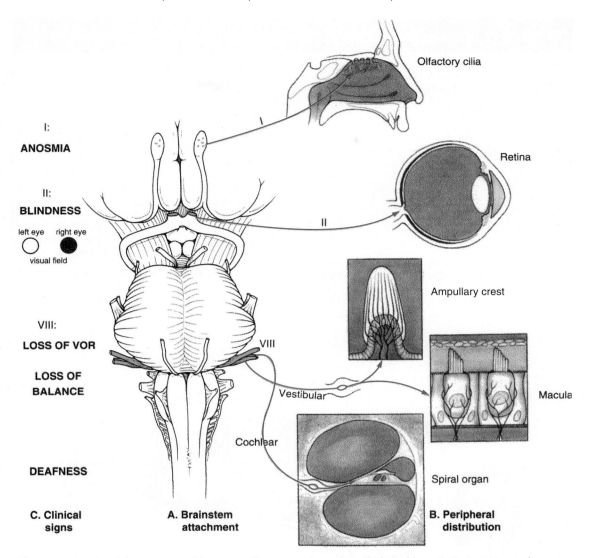

Figure 21-2 Special sensory cranial nerves: olfactory, optic, and vestibulocochlear. **A.** Brainstem attachment. **B.** Peripheral distribution. **C.** Clinical signs (VOR, vestibulo-ocular reflex).

TABLE 21-3   Ocular Motor Nerves: Oculomotor, Trochlear, and Abducens

Nerve	Function	Origin	Peripheral Distribution	Signs
III Oculomotor	Eye movements	Oculomotor nucleus	Medial, superior, inferior recti, inferior oblique muscles	Ophthalmoplegia with eye turned down and out
	Elevation of eyelid	Oculomotor nucleus	Superior palpebral levator	Ptosis
	Pupillary constriction and accommodation	Edinger-Westphal nucleus	Ciliary ganglion; postganglionics to sphincter of pupil and ciliary muscles	Mydriasis; loss of accommodation of lens
IV Trochlear	Eye movements	Trochlear nucleus (contralateral)	Superior oblique muscle	Diplopia: extorsion of eye; weakness in depression of adducted eye
VI Abducens	Eye movements	Abducens nucleus	Lateral rectus muscle	Diplopia: medial deviation; abductor paralysis

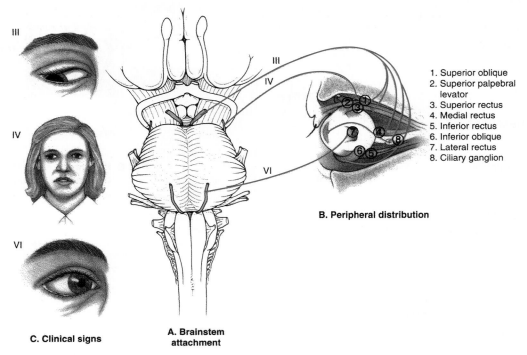

1. Superior oblique
2. Superior palpebral levator
3. Superior rectus
4. Medial rectus
5. Inferior rectus
6. Inferior oblique
7. Lateral rectus
8. Ciliary ganglion

B. Peripheral distribution

C. Clinical signs

A. Brainstem attachment

Figure 21-3   Ocular motor nerves: oculomotor, trochlear, and abducens. **A.** Brainstem attachment. **B.** Peripheral distribution. **C.** Clinical signs (right III, IV, and VI nerves).

TABLE 21-4 Trigeminal Nerve

Nerve	Function	Origin	Peripheral Distribution	Central Connections	Signs
V Trigeminal	Mastication	Motor trigeminal nucleus	Masseter, temporalis, pterygoids, mylohyoid, tensor palatini, anterior belly of digastric		Weakness of jaw; ipsilateral deviation of opened jaw
	Dampens tympanic membrane	Motor trigeminal nucleus	Tensor tympani		Insignificant
	Sensations	Trigeminal ganglion	Face, anterior scalp, oral and nasal cavities, orbit	Principal and spinal trigeminal nuclei	Facial hemianesthesia
	Proprioceptive reflexes	Mesencephalic trigeminal nucleus	Muscles of mastication, periodontal membrane, temporomandibular joint	Motor trigeminal nucleus	Insignificant

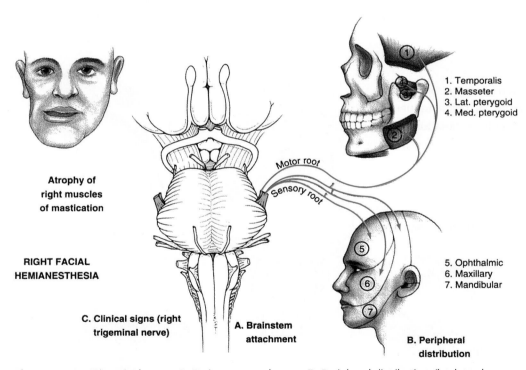

Atrophy of right muscles of mastication

1. Temporalis
2. Masseter
3. Lat. pterygoid
4. Med. pterygoid

Motor root

Sensory root

RIGHT FACIAL HEMIANESTHESIA

5. Ophthalmic
6. Maxillary
7. Mandibular

C. Clinical signs (right trigeminal nerve)

A. Brainstem attachment

B. Peripheral distribution

Figure 21-4 Trigeminal nerve. **A.** Brainstem attachment. **B.** Peripheral distribution (lat, lateral; med, medial). **C.** Clinical signs.

TABLE 21-5 Facial Nerve

Nerve	Function	Origin	Peripheral Distribution	Central Connections	Signs
VII Facial	Facial expression	Facial nucleus	Facial muscles, stylohyoid, posterior belly of digastric		Facial paralysis; loss of corneal reflex
	Dampens stapes	Facial nucleus	Stapedius		Hyperacusis
	Secretion	Superior salivatory nucleus	Pterygopalatine ganglion: secretomotor to lacrimal and nasal glands		Loss of lacrimation
			Submandibular ganglion: secretomotor to submandibular and sublingual glands		Dry mouth
	Taste	Geniculate ganglion	Taste buds in anterior two-thirds of tongue	Solitary nucleus	Loss of taste in ipsilateral anterior tongue

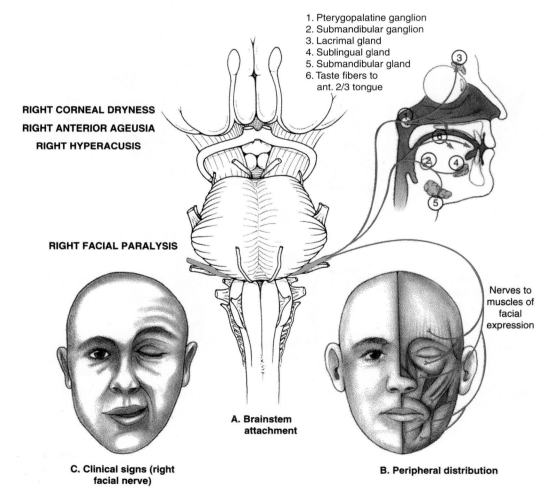

1. Pterygopalatine ganglion
2. Submandibular ganglion
3. Lacrimal gland
4. Sublingual gland
5. Submandibular gland
6. Taste fibers to ant. 2/3 tongue

RIGHT CORNEAL DRYNESS
RIGHT ANTERIOR AGEUSIA
RIGHT HYPERACUSIS

RIGHT FACIAL PARALYSIS

Nerves to muscles of facial expression

A. Brainstem attachment

C. Clinical signs (right facial nerve)

B. Peripheral distribution

Figure 21-5 Facial nerve. **A.** Brainstem attachment. **B.** Peripheral distribution (ant, anterior). **C.** Clinical signs.

TABLE 21-6	**Glossopharyngeal Nerve**				
Nerve	**Function**	**Origin**	**Peripheral Distribution**	**Central Connections**	**Signs**
IX Glossopharyngeal	Elevate pharynx during swallowing	Nucleus ambiguus	Stylopharyngeus and superior pharyngeal constrictor		Dysphagia
	Salivation	Inferior salivatory nucleus	Otic ganglion: secretomotor to parotid		Insignificant
	Taste	Inferior (petrosal) ganglion	Posterior third of tongue	Solitary nucleus	Loss of taste in tongue posteriorly
	General sensations	Superior and inferior ganglia	Posterior oral cavity, tonsillar region, auditory tube, middle ear	Spinal trigeminal nucleus	Anesthesia, loss of gag reflex (afferent limb)
	Chemoreceptor and baroreceptor reflexes (afferent limbs)	Inferior ganglion	Carotid bulb and sinus	Solitary nucleus	Loss of carotid sinus reflex (if bilateral lesion)

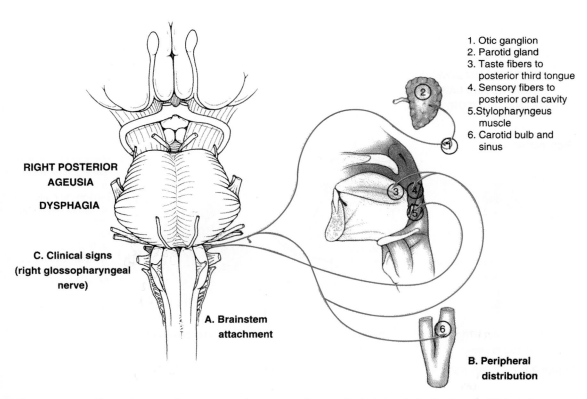

1. Otic ganglion
2. Parotid gland
3. Taste fibers to posterior third tongue
4. Sensory fibers to posterior oral cavity
5. Stylopharyngeus muscle
6. Carotid bulb and sinus

RIGHT POSTERIOR AGEUSIA

DYSPHAGIA

C. Clinical signs (right glossopharyngeal nerve)

A. Brainstem attachment

B. Peripheral distribution

Figure 21-6 Glossopharyngeal nerve. **A.** Brainstem attachment. **B.** Peripheral distribution. **C.** Clinical signs.

TABLE 21-7   Vagus Nerve

Nerve	Functions	Origin	Peripheral Distribution	Central Connections	Signs
X Vagus	Swallowing and vocalization	Nucleus ambiguus	Palatal muscles, pharyngeal constrictors, vocal muscles		Dysphagia, weak and hoarse voice, sagging of palatal arch, contralateral deviation of uvula
	Cardiac depressor, bronchoconstrictors, GI motility and secretion	Dorsal motor nucleus of vagus	Terminal ganglia in cardiac, pulmonary, enteric plexuses		Insignificant if unilateral
	Taste	Inferior (nodose) ganglion	Epiglottal and palatal regions	Solitary nucleus	Insignificant
	Sensations	Inferior (nodose) ganglion	Epiglottis, larynx, respiratory tree, GI tract	Solitary nucleus	Hemianesthesia of pharynx and larynx, loss of cough reflex (afferent limb)
	Chemoreceptor and baroreceptor reflexes	Inferior (nodose) ganglion	Aortic bulb and sinus	Solitary nucleus	Insignificant if unilateral
	Sensations	Superior (jugular) ganglion	External ear and auditory canal	Spinal trigeminal nucleus	Anesthesia of external auditory canal

GI, gastrointestinal.

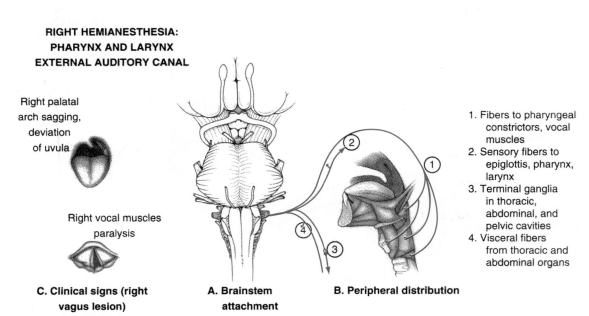

RIGHT HEMIANESTHESIA:
PHARYNX AND LARYNX
EXTERNAL AUDITORY CANAL

Right palatal
arch sagging,
deviation
of uvula

Right vocal muscles
paralysis

1. Fibers to pharyngeal
   constrictors, vocal
   muscles
2. Sensory fibers to
   epiglottis, pharynx,
   larynx
3. Terminal ganglia
   in thoracic,
   abdominal, and
   pelvic cavities
4. Visceral fibers
   from thoracic and
   abdominal organs

C. Clinical signs (right
vagus lesion)

A. Brainstem
attachment

B. Peripheral distribution

Figure 21-7   Vagus nerve **A.** Brainstem attachment. **B.** Peripheral distribution. **C.** Clinical signs.

TABLE 21-8   Accessory and Hypoglossal Nerves

Nerve	Function	Origin	Peripheral Distribution	Signs
XI Accessory	Swallowing and vocalization	Nucleus ambiguus (cranial accessory)	Pharyngeal and vocal muscles (with vagus)	Insignificant
	Head and shoulder movements	Spinal accessory nucleus in C1–C5 or C6	Sternomastoid and trapezius muscles	Weakness in turning head toward opposite side and shrugging shoulder
XII Hypoglossal	Tongue movements	Hypoglossal nucleus	Styloglossus, hyoglossus, genioglossus, and intrinsic tongue muscles	Unilateral atrophy, ipsilateral deviation on protrusion, fasciculations

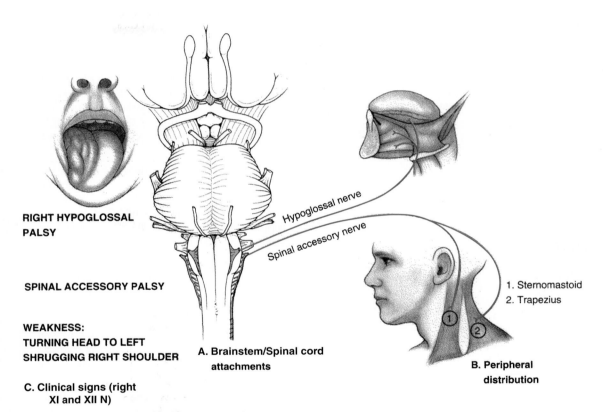

RIGHT HYPOGLOSSAL PALSY

SPINAL ACCESSORY PALSY

WEAKNESS: TURNING HEAD TO LEFT SHRUGGING RIGHT SHOULDER

Hypoglossal nerve

Spinal accessory nerve

1. Sternomastoid
2. Trapezius

A. Brainstem/Spinal cord attachments

B. Peripheral distribution

C. Clinical signs (right XI and XII N)

Figure 21-8   Accessory and hypoglossal nerves. **A.** Brainstem attachments. **B.** Peripheral distribution. **C.** Clinical signs (N, nerve).

TABLE 21-9   Cranial Nerve Components and Distributions

Nerve	Cells of Origin	Central Connections	Peripheral Distribution	Function	Symptoms and Signs of Damage
I Olfactory	Bipolar cells in olfactory epithelium (special sensory)	Olfactory bulb	Cilia at surface of olfactory epithelium in superior nasal concha and upper third of nasal septum	Smell	Anosmia
II Optic	Ganglion cells of retina (special sensory)	Lateral geniculate nuclei	Bipolar cells of retina	Vision	Blindness
		Superior colliculus and pretectal nuclei		Pupillary reflexes ~~and accommod~~	Absence of light reflexes on shining light in blind eye
III Oculomotor	Oculomotor nucleus (somatic motor)		Medial, superior, and inferior recti, inferior oblique, and levator palpebrae superioris	Moves the eye and elevates upper eyelid	Ophthalmoplegia with eye deviated down and out, severe ptosis
	Edinger-Westphal nucleus of oculomotor complex (visceral motor)		Ciliary ganglion; postganglionics via short ciliary nerves to sphincter of pupil and ciliary muscle	Pupil constriction and accommodation of lens – near vision	Mydriasis; loss of pupillary light and accommodation reflexes in ipsilateral eye
IV Trochlear	Trochlear nucleus (somatic motor)		Superior oblique muscle	Extorsion; depression of adducted eye ∟moves eyeball	Diplopia, head tilt to unaffected side; weakness in depression of ipsilateral adducted eye
V Trigeminal	Trigeminal ganglion (general sensory)	Spinal trigeminal nucleus (caudal part) and principal trigeminal nucleus	Anterior scalp, face, mucous membranes of nose and mouth, teeth, contents of orbit, tympanic membrane, supratentorial meninges	Somatosensations – sensation to face – 3 parts V1 V2 V3	Loss of facial sensations and corneal reflex on stimulation ipsilaterally
	Motor trigeminal nucleus (branchial motor)		Masseter, temporalis, pterygoids, mylohyoid, tensors tympani and	Mastication – chewing – only V3	Weakness and wasting of muscles of mastication;

(continued)

TABLE 21-9   Cranial Nerve Components and Distributions *(Continued)*

Nerve	Cells of Origin	Central Connections	Peripheral Distribution	Function	Symptoms and Signs of Damage
			palatini, anterior belly of digastric		deviation of opened jaw to ipsilateral side
	Mesencephalic trigeminal nucleus (general sensory)		Muscles of mastication, periodontal membrane, temporomandibular joint, and external ocular muscles	Proprioceptive reflexes	Insignificant
VI Abducens	Abducens nucleus (somatic motor)		Lateral rectus muscle	Abduction of eye — *eye muscle*	Diplopia, esotropia (convergent strabismus) and abductor paralysis of ipsilateral eye
VII Facial	Facial nucleus (branchial motor)		Facial muscles, buccinator, stapedius, stylohyoid, posterior belly of digastric, platysma, occipitalis	*blinking* — Facial expression, articulation, winking, ingestion of food and drink · *tears - keeps nose moist*	Paralysis of ipsilateral upper and lower facial muscles
	Superior salivatory nucleus (visceral motor)		1. Major petrosal nerve to nerve of pterygoid canal to pterygopalatine ganglion; post-ganglionics via maxillary nerve to lacrimal gland and mucosal glands of nasal cavity and palate	Nasal and lacrimal secretions	Loss of lacrimation
			2. Chorda tympani to lingual nerve to submandibular ganglion; post-ganglionics to submandibular, sublingual and lingual glands	Salivary secretion	Decreased salivation; dry mouth
	Geniculate ganglion (special sensory)	Solitary nucleus (rostral part)	Taste buds in anterior two-thirds of tongue	Taste	Loss of taste in anterior two thirds of tongue ipsilaterally

(handwritten notes) ↳ tearing – keeps noise moist – saliva secretion – involved w/ taste – anterior 2/3 of tongue

TABLE 21-9   Cranial Nerve Components and Distributions *(Continued)*

Nerve	Cells of Origin	Central Connections	Peripheral Distribution	Function	Symptoms and Signs of Damage
	(general sensory)	Spinal trigeminal nucleus (caudal part)	Posterior auricular region, external auditory meatus, tympanic membrane	Somatosensations	Insignificant
VIII Vestibulocochlear	Vestibular ganglion (special sensory)	Vestibular nuclei and cerebellum	Hair cells of ampullary crests in semicircular ducts and maculae of saccule and utricle	Equilibrium	Vertigo, dysequilibrium, and nystagmus
	Spiral ganglion (special sensory)	Dorsal and ventral cochlear nucleus	Hair cells of spiral organ (of Corti)	Hearing	Neural deafness
IX Glossopharyngeal	Nucleus ambiguus (rostral part) (branchial motor)		Stylopharyngeus and superior pharyngeal constrictor	Elevates pharynx	Slight dysphagia
	Inferior salivatory nucleus (visceral motor)		Tympanic plexus to minor petrosal nerve to otic ganglion– postganglionics via auriculotemporal nerve to parotid gland	Salivary secretion	Partial dry mouth
	Inferior (petrosal) ganglion (special sensory)	Solitary nucleus (rostral part)	Taste buds in posterior third of tongue	Taste	Loss of taste in posterior third of tongue ipsilaterally
	(general sensory)	Spinal trigeminal nucleus	Anterior surface epiglottis, root of tongue, border of soft palate, uvula, tonsil, pharynx, auditory tube, middle ear	Somatosensations	Anesthesia of tonsillar region and loss of gag reflex from ipsilateral stimulus
	(visceral sensory)		Carotid sinus and bulb	Reflexes	Insignificant
X Vagus	Nucleus ambiguus (branchial motor)		Palate, pharyngeal constrictors and intrinsic muscles of larynx	Deglutition and phonation	Dysphagia, hoarseness, and paralysis of soft palate with deviation of velum and uvula to contralateral side

(handwritten margin notes)

IX + X work together speaking + swallowing

~ used in speaking + swallowing

—sensory supply to area around tonsills
—gagging

—if lose sensation to this nerve will die b/c nerve controls much of organs in chest/trunk

(continued)

TABLE 21-9   Cranial Nerve Components and Distributions *(Continued)*

Nerve	Cells of Origin	Central Connections	Peripheral Distribution	Function	Symptoms and Signs of Damage
	Dorsal motor nucleus of vagus and region of nucleus ambiguus (visceral motor)	*sends sensory input to organs heart + lungs*	Cardiac nerves and plexus to ganglia of heart; pulmonary plexuses to ganglia of respiratory tree; esophageal, gastric, celiac, superior and inferior mesenteric plexuses to myenteric and submucous ganglia of digestive tract down to transverse colon	Cardiac depressor, broncho-constrictor, GI tract peristalsis and secretion	Insignificant
	Inferior (nodose) ganglion (special sensory)	Solitary nucleus (rostral part)	Taste buds in region of epiglottis	Taste	Insignificant
	(visceral sensory)	Solitary nucleus	Posterior surface of epiglottis, pharynx, larynx, trachea, bronchi, esophagus, stomach, small intestine, ascending and transverse colon	Visceral sensations and reflexes *– visceral afferents – input from organs*	Anesthesia of pharynx and larynx ipsilaterally
			Aortic sinus and bulb	Reflexes	
	Superior (jugular) ganglion (general sensory)	Spinal trigeminal nucleus (caudal part)	External ear and meatus	Somatosensations	Anesthesia of ipsilateral external auditory meatus
XI Accessory (cranial part) *– part of vagus so X*	Nucleus ambiguus (caudal part) (branchial motor)		Communicates with vagal branches to muscles of pharynx and larynx	Deglutition and phonation	Insignificant
XI spinal part *accessory nerve*	Motoneurons of spinal accessory nucleus in C1–C5 or C6 (somatic motor)		Sternomastoid and trapezius muscles	Movements of head and shoulder	Weakness in shrugging ipsilateral shoulder and turning head to opposite side

GI, gastrointestinal.

TABLE 21-9   Cranial Nerve Components and Distributions (Continued)

Nerve	Cells of Origin	Central Connections	Peripheral Distribution	Function	Symptoms and Signs of Damage
XII Hypoglossal	Hypoglossal nucleus (somatic motor)		Styloglossus, hyoglossus, genioglossus and intrinsic muscles of tongue	Movements of tongue	Wasting of ipsilateral tongue muscles and deviation to ipsilateral side on protrusion

Chapter Review Questions

21-1.   Damage to which cranial nerve is associated with each of the following?

a. weak and hoarse voice accompanied by sagging of the left soft palate
b. weakness in depression of the adducted right eye
c. on protrusion the tongue deviates to the left side
d. right facial hemianesthesia
e. absence of ocular movements and nystagmus on irrigating the left external auditory meatus with cold or warm water
f. esotropia and paralysis of abduction of the right eye
g. loss of taste on the posterior third of the left side of the tongue

21-2.   Name the cranial nerves and interneurons involved in the following reflexes:

a. blinking on irritating the cornea with a wisp of cotton
b. pupillary constriction on increased light intensity in either eye
c. gagging on stimulation of tonsillar region
d. slowing of heart rate on applying pressure on the eyeball
e. lacrimation and salivation on pinching the tongue
f. contraction of the masseter muscle on a short downward tap to the chin
g. vomiting on putting a finger down the throat

The Blood Supply of the Central Nervous System: Stroke

A 55-YEAR-OLD MAN, a heavy smoker with diabetes and a history of atherosclerotic coronary disease, suffered several episodes of complete visual loss in his left eye, described as though someone pulled a shade over his orbit. Associated with this visual loss was numbness and tingling in the right hand and fingers, drooping of the right side of the face, and significant difficulty in producing words. All of these symptoms occurred without warning and cleared completely within 20 minutes. The patient's neurologic examination was normal, and the only positive finding was a loud bruit over his left carotid artery. An angiogram demonstrated severe atherosclerotic blockage at the proximal internal carotid artery (ICA) and a carotid endarterectomy was performed. No further transient ischemic episodes were experienced.

The neurons of the central nervous system (CNS), unlike the primary cells of most organ systems, are very dependent on aerobic metabolism. When deprived of blood flow for only 20 seconds, the brain is reduced to a state of unconsciousness; if circulation is not reestablished in 4 to 5 minutes, this state is usually irreversible. The brain itself makes up approximately 2% of the body weight (1500 g) but uses 15% of the total cardiac output (5 L/min) and consumes 20% (50 mL/min) of the total available oxygen. This enormous blood flow and oxygen consumption demand an extensive yet smoothly functioning delivery system, the cerebrovascular system.

Different areas of the cerebrum and spinal cord receive different amounts of blood depend-ing on metabolic activity. Under most circumstances, the more metabolically active gray matter has a greater flow than the white matter (75 versus 25 mL/100 g/min). In addition, certain neurons in the CNS (i.e., selected layers of the hippocampus and the cerebellar and cerebral cortices) display a selective vulnerability to oxygen loss such that they are affected first in states of acute **hypoxia.**

The cerebrovasculature autoregulates to maintain a constant amount of blood flow to the neuraxis despite fluctuations in systemic blood pressure. The larger extracerebral vessels possess a readily identifiable adventitial plexus of nerves, but autoregulation persists even after their complete removal; unlike the peripheral vascular system, the

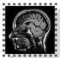

CLINICAL CONNECTION

Total cerebral blood flow averages approximately 750 mL/min. This 750 mL is supplied by the two carotid arteries and the basilar artery, each contributing approximately 250 mL/min. The total intracranial blood volume is 100 to 150 mL at any instant; thus, the intracranial circulating pool turns over five to seven times each minute. Average cerebral blood flow (CBF) is 55 mL/100 g of brain tissue per minute. If CBF falls to less than 30 to 35 mL/100 g/min ischemia occurs; if CBF falls below 20 mL/100 g/min infarction occurs. Extended flows below 15 mL/100 g/min inevitably result in massive infarction.

sympathetic and parasympathetic influences on cerebrovascular tone are quite limited.

Cerebral autoregulation is closely related to local metabolic processes, and many metabolites affect cerebral blood flow. The most important metabolites that affect cerebral blood flow are the local concentrations of oxygen and carbon dioxide. Hypoxia or **hypercarbia** or both result in cerebral vasodilation and increased cerebral blood flow, whereas **hypocarbia** results in vasoconstriction and diminished blood flow.

CLINICAL CONNECTION

Clinically, the effects of oxygen and carbon dioxide on cerebrovascular tone can be manipulated in patients with elevated intracranial pressure. One of the common treatments of elevated intracranial pressure is hyperventilation. Hyperventilation lowers the P_{CO_2} and elevates the P_{O_2}, causing cerebral vasoconstriction and diminished cerebral blood flow, thereby resulting in secondary lowering of the intracranial pressure.

Intracranial arteries differ considerably in histologic composition from those found elsewhere in the body. The intima of intracranial vessels possesses a well-developed internal elastic membrane (IEM), which is actually thicker than that found in extracranial vessels. The media (composed of muscle and elastica), however, is much less prominent than that of extracranial arteries. The adventitia is thin and contains no paravas-

cular supporting tissue, no external elastic lamina, and no vasa vasorum. Histologically, intracranial veins are thin-walled structures consisting mostly of collagen with minimal elastic tissue, little muscle, and no valves.

CLINICAL CONNECTION

In primates, small discontinuities of the media occur at the points where larger intracranial arteries branch. In these areas the adventitia actually abuts the IEM. Clinically, these so-called media gaps relate to the location of saccular aneurysms formed as the IEM is damaged by progressive atherosclerosis. With the congenital absence of the media and with developmental damage to the IEM, the vessel wall is supported by only the endothelium and adventitia. This weak support progressively balloons to form an aneurysm.

The intracranial extracerebral vessels are contained within the subarachnoid space (Fig. 1-4). As these vessels and their branches penetrate the brain, they become intracerebral. A small perivascular extension of the subarachnoid space is formed alongside these penetrating vessels. This **Virchow-Robin space** extends from the general subarachnoid space and gradually thins as the vessel penetrates deep into the brain substance.

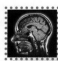

CLINICAL CONNECTION

Disease processes in the subarachnoid space such as subarachnoid hemorrhage and meningitis may gain entrance into the brain tissue itself as they fill the perivascular spaces surrounding the penetrating vessels.

THE BLOOD–BRAIN BARRIER

The concept of a selective barrier between the intravascular space and the brain is suggested by the result of dyes (such as trypan blue) being introduced into the bloodstream. Most of the body tissues including the meninges are stained, but not the brain. The blood-brain barrier selectively prevents the penetration of certain substances into the cerebral space. The selective permeability of the blood–

brain barrier rests along the capillary endothelium (Fig. 1-5). The tight junctions and nonfenestrated composition of the capillary endothelium impede the passage of many substances.

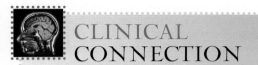

CLINICAL CONNECTION

In certain areas of the brain, circumventricular organs such as the neurohypophysis, the area postrema, the pineal, the subcommissural and subfornical organs, the optic recess, and the median eminence have a fenestrated capillary endothelium that allows these areas to stain after intravascular dye administration. Similarly, in infants the capillary endothelium is immature and fenestrated, allowing substances such as bilirubin to enter. Elevation of bilirubin in the neonate may lead to staining in the basal ganglia, thalamus, and ependyma, a condition called **kernicterus.**

Physiologically, the passage of substances across the blood–brain barrier depends on their molecular size, lipid miscibility, and degree of ionic dissociation. Many drugs that are useful in the treatment of systemic disorders are ineffective in identical CNS disorders on account of their inability to cross the blood–brain barrier. The astrocytic foot processes control the intracerebral volume by regulating the quantity of substances such as sodium, water, and glucose that enter this space. Disruptions of the astrocytic foot processes generally result in leakage of fluid into the brain with the development of **cerebral edema.** This condition occurs commonly with trauma and tumors.

CEREBRAL VASCULATURE

The anterior and posterior parts of the brain receive blood from the carotid and vertebral arteries, respectively (Fig. 22-1). Hence, two cerebral

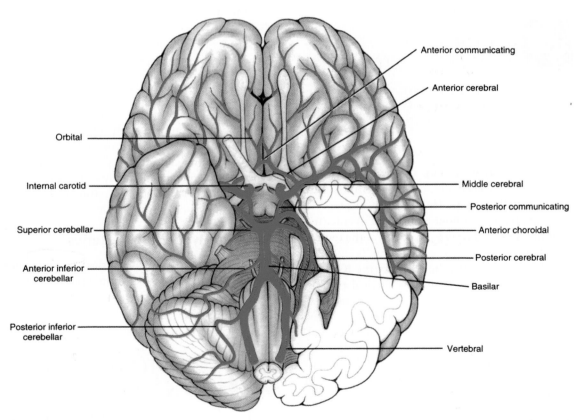

Figure 22-1 Major cerebral arteries on base of brain. On the left, the cerebellar hemisphere and ventral part of the temporal lobe have been removed.

circulatory systems are described: an anterior or carotid system and a posterior or vertebral-basilar system.

ANTERIOR OR CAROTID SYSTEM

The common carotid artery begins on the right as the brachiocephalic trunk bifurcates into the common carotid and the subclavian arteries. The left common carotid artery branches from the arch of the aorta at its highest point. Each common carotid artery lies within the carotid sheath, with the internal jugular vein lateral and the vagus nerve dorsal (lying between the artery and vein). Near the upper border of the thyroid cartilage, the common carotid artery bifurcates into the internal (ICA) and external carotid arteries. The carotid sinus and carotid body, which influence blood pressure and respiratory regulation, respectively, are located at the bifurcation and extend along the proximal few millimeters of the ICA.

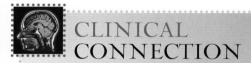

CLINICAL CONNECTION

Clinically, the carotid bifurcation is a common site of atherosclerotic narrowing and the subsequent production of cerebral ischemia and stroke.

From the bifurcation, the external carotid artery proceeds medially to divide into its many extracranial branches, whereas the ICA proceeds posterolaterally (without branching) to enter the carotid canal in the petrous portion of the temporal bone.

Radiographically, the course of the ICA can be subdivided into four segments: cervical, petrous, cavernous, and cerebral. The cervical segment extends from the common carotid bifurcation to the point where the artery pierces the carotid canal. The petrous segment is contained within the carotid canal of the petrous portion of the temporal bone. This portion of the artery has several small branches to the inner ear. The cavernous segment is contained within the cavernous sinus and extends from the point the artery leaves the carotid canal to the point at which it enters the dura near the anterior clinoid process.

CLINICAL CONNECTION

The angiographic shape of the ICA as it winds its way through the petrous canal and the cavernous sinus is termed the **carotid siphon.** The cavernous segment is not actually bathed in the venous blood of the sinus but is surrounded by sinus endothelium and supported by numerous trabeculae. Several prominent branches, including the tentorial (which supplies the tentorium), the inferior hypophysial (which supplies the posterior lobe of the pituitary gland), and the cavernous (which supplies the surrounding dura), are located along this portion of the vessel. As the ICA leaves the cavernous sinus, it pierces the dura and becomes for the first time an intracranial vessel (cerebral segment).

The cerebral segment is the terminal portion of the ICA and ends as the internal carotid bifurcates into the anterior and middle cerebral arteries (MCA; Fig. 22-1). Other major branches of the cerebral segment include the ophthalmic artery, the superior hypophysial arteries, the posterior communicating artery, and the anterior choroidal artery.

Ophthalmic Artery

The ophthalmic artery leaves the ICA beneath the optic nerve and enters the orbit through the optic foramen with the optic nerve (Fig. 22-2). It gives rise to the central artery of the retina and eventually communicates freely with the external carotid artery via its lacrimal, ethmoidal, supraorbital, supratrochlear, and nasal branches.

Superior Hypophysial Arteries

The superior hypophysial arteries exit from the internal carotid arteries to form a plexus around the pituitary stalk (Fig. 22-3).

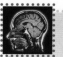

CLINICAL CONNECTION

The capillaries of these vessels aid in the formation of the hypophysial-portal system that supplies the anterior lobe of the pituitary gland (Fig. 18-3).

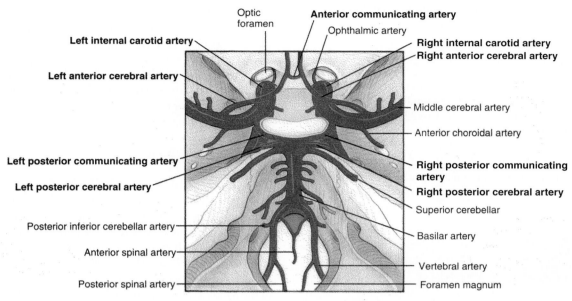

Figure 22-2   The cerebral arterial circle of Willis (bold) and other major cerebral arteries as observed on the floor of the cranial cavity.

Posterior Communicating Artery

The posterior communicating artery leaves the dorsolateral surface of the ICA just before its terminal branching and joins the proximal portion of the posterior cerebral artery, thus connecting the anterior and posterior circulations (Figs. 22-1, 22-2).

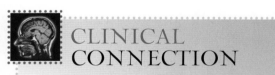

CLINICAL CONNECTION

Clinically, one of the most frequent sites for aneurysm formation is where the posterior communicating artery arises from the ICA.

Anterior Choroidal Artery

The anterior choroidal artery usually arises from the internal carotid just proximal to its bifurcation. Sometimes, however, it arises from the MCA, the posterior communicating artery, or the bifurcation of the middle and anterior cerebral arteries. The anterior choroidal artery crosses the optic tract and passes toward the medial surface of the temporal lobe (Figs. 22-1, 22-3). The penetrating branches of the anterior choroidal artery supply the hippocampal formation, the amygdaloid nucleus, and the

ventral and entire retrolenticular part of the posterior limb of the internal capsule. In addition, the anterior choroidal artery supplies the **choroid plexus** of the inferior horn of the lateral ventricle (Fig. 22-1).

Anterior Cerebral Artery

The anterior cerebral artery (ACA) is divided by the anterior communicating artery into proximal or precommunicating (A-1) and distal or postcommunicating (A-2) segments.

A-1 SEGMENT   The A-1 segment begins at the carotid bifurcation and passes over the optic tract and chiasm to reach the anterior communicating artery (Figs. 22-1 to 22-3). Along its course, branches supply portions of the anterior hypothalamus.

RECURRENT ARTERY OF HEUBNER   The recurrent artery of Heubner is conspicuous by its large size. It arises from either the distal part of the A-1 segment or the proximal part of the A-2 segment and courses laterally along the A-1 segment to join the lateral striate arteries as they enter the anterior perforated substance (Fig. 22-3). The recurrent artery supplies the ventral parts of the head of the caudate nucleus, the anterior pole of the putamen, the anterior part of the globus pallidus, and the anterior limb of the internal capsule as far dorsal as the top of the globus pallidus.

ANTERIOR COMMUNICATING ARTERY

The anterior communicating artery joins the two anterior cerebral arteries with the A-1 segments of these vessels located proximally and the A-2 segments distally (Figs. 22-1 to 22-3). Anatomically, the anterior communicating artery is seldom a distinct vessel but more often constitutes a complex network or web of vessels. Small perforators from the anterior communicating artery supply the genu of the corpus callosum, septum pellucidum, and septal nuclei.

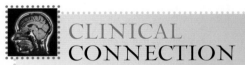

CLINICAL CONNECTION

The anterior communicating artery forms an important potential source of blood flow between the two hemispheres, particularly when one ICA occludes. In addition, the anterior communicating artery is another one of the frequent sites of saccular aneurysm formation.

POSTCOMMUNICATING OR A-2 SEGMENT The A-2 segment of the ACA begins at the anterior communicating artery (Figs. 22-1 to 22-3). Proximal branches of the A-2 segment include the orbital artery (Fig. 22-1), which supplies the gyrus rectus and olfactory bulb and tract, and the frontopolar artery, which supplies the anterior part of the superior frontal gyrus. The A-2 segment ends by bifurcating into the callosomarginal artery and the pericallosal trunk near the genu of the corpus callosum (Fig. 22-4).

CALLOSOMARGINAL ARTERY The callosomarginal artery follows the course of the callosomarginal sulcus, supplying anterior, middle, and posterior frontal branches to the superior frontal gyrus (Fig. 22-4). It ends as the paracentral artery to the paracentral lobule. All of these branches anastomose with prerolandic and postrolandic branches of the MCA as they turn onto the convexity of the hemisphere.

PERICALLOSAL TRUNK ARTERY The pericallosal trunk artery is regarded as a continuation of the ACA. It passes posteriorly in close rela-

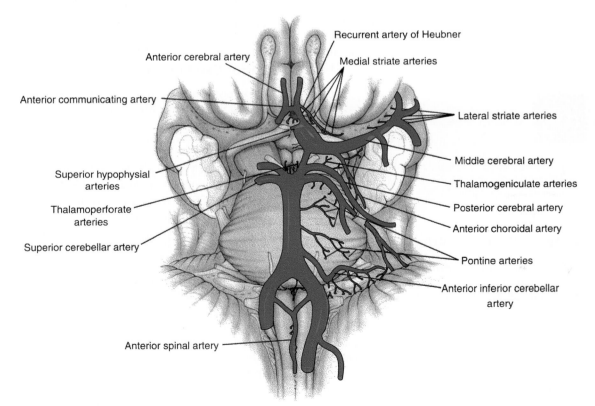

Figure 22-3 Perforation zones for major penetrating arteries on base of brain.

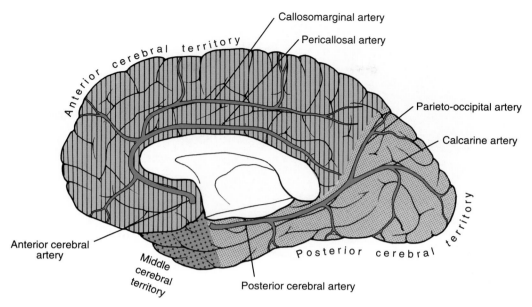

Figure 22-4   Major arterial territories on the medial surface of the hemisphere.

tion to the corpus callosum, supplying penetrating vessels to the corpus callosum, septum pellucidum, and fornix. Terminal branches include the precuneal artery, which supplies the precuneus, and the posterior callosal artery, which supplies the splenium of the corpus callosum (Fig. 22-4).

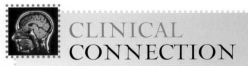

CLINICAL CONNECTION

A stroke in the cortical distribution of one ACA results in sensorimotor deficit in the opposite foot and leg. Urinary incontinence and contralateral frontal lobe signs may also be observed.

Middle Cerebral Artery

The MCA is the largest branch of the ICA. It is the cerebral artery most often occluded. It is divided into a proximal (M-1) segment and a distal (M-2) segment by the MCA bifurcation.

M-1 SEGMENT   The proximal portion of the MCA is related to the lowest portion of the insula as the artery travels to reach the lateral or **sylvian fissure.** From this segment, 10 to 15 penetrating

vessels, the lateral striate arteries or the lenticulostriate arteries, arise and supply the dorsal part of the head and the entire body of the caudate nucleus, most of the lentiform nucleus, and the internal capsule above the level of the globus pallidus. Like the recurrent artery of Heubner, these penetrating arteries run a recurrent course back along the M-1 segment to penetrate the lateral two-thirds of the anterior perforated substance (Fig. 22-3).

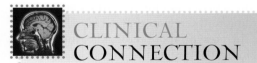

CLINICAL CONNECTION

Clinically, the lenticulostriate vessels are the most common site of spontaneous hypertensive hemorrhage in individuals with long-standing hypertension.

The other M-1 segment branches include the anterior temporal artery, which supplies the most anterior portion of the temporal lobe, and the orbitofrontal artery, which supplies the lateral portions of the orbital surface of the frontal lobe.

M-2 SEGMENT   The bifurcation of the MCA is located at the base of the insula and it forms the

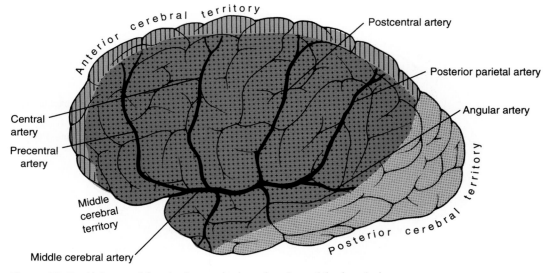

Figure 22-5   Major arterial territories on the lateral surface of the hemisphere.

M-2 segment, which consists of the superior and inferior trunks. These trunks travel deep in the lateral (sylvian) fissure along the insula. At the insula, branches travel along the frontal and temporal opercula to exit the lateral fissure and proceed along the convexity of the hemisphere. Generally, the superior trunk supplies branches to the frontal and parietal lobes, and the inferior trunk supplies the temporal and occipital lobes (Fig. 22-5). The angiographic shape of the superior and inferior trunks and their branches is called the **middle cerebral candelabra.** The branches of both the superior and inferior trunks are named according to the region they supply. These include the precentral or prerolandic, the central or rolandic, the postcentral or postrolandic, the anterior and posterior parietal, the angular, the posterior temporal, and the posterior occipital arteries. The precentral, central, postcentral, anterior and posterior parietal, and angular arteries leave the lateral fissure and supply most of the cerebral convexity, anastomosing with the branches of the ACA near the anterior and dorsal margins of the convexity. The posterior temporal and posterior occipital branches supply most of the temporal and occipital convexity, anastomosing with branches of the posterior cerebral artery at the posterior and ventral margins of the hemisphere.

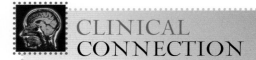

CLINICAL CONNECTION

A stroke in the cortical distribution of the MCA results in a severe sensorimotor deficit in the contralateral face and upper limb. With dominant hemisphere involvement, global aphasia also results; with nondominant hemisphere involvement, the neglect syndrome or amorphosynthesis results.

POSTERIOR OR VERTEBRAL-BASILAR SYSTEM

Vertebral Arteries

The vertebral arteries are the first branches of the subclavian arteries. They generally enter the transverse foramina of cervical vertebra (CV) 6 and travel upward through the transverse foramina of the other cervical vertebrae to reach the superior margin of CV1, where they pierce the atlanto-occipital membrane. They then enter the cranial cavity through the foramen magnum ventral to the hypoglossal nerves, travel along the anterior or lateral surfaces of the medulla, and join to form the basilar artery near the pontomedullary junction (Fig. 22-1).

After entering the cranial cavity, each vertebral artery gives rise to a posterior spinal artery that descends along the posterolateral aspect of the spinal cord. The vertebral arteries, 1 to 2 cm

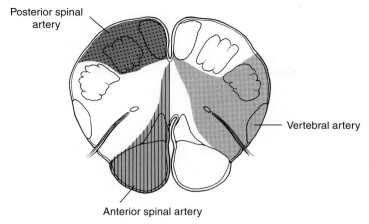

Figure 22-6   Arterial territories in the caudal medulla.

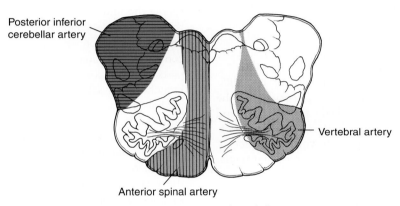

Figure 22-7   Arterial territories in the rostral medulla.

before joining to form the basilar artery, give rise to their largest branches, the posterior inferior cerebellar arteries (PICA).

The PICA curve around the medulla ventral to the roots of cranial nerves (CN) IX, X, and XI. The PICA reach the region of the cerebellar tonsil and proceed along the posterior inferior cerebellar surface (Fig. 22-1). Multiple penetrating vessels supplying the posterolateral medulla arise from the PICA as they curve around this region (Figs. 22-6, 22-7). Other branches supply the choroid plexus of the fourth ventricle before the PICA terminate as inferior vermian and tonsillar-hemispheric branches, which supply all of the posterior and inferior parts of the cerebellum.

Immediately before the vertebral-basilar junction, anterior spinal arteries arise from both vertebral arteries and join almost immediately to form a single anterior spinal artery that runs along the anterior median fissure of the spinal cord (Figs. 22-2, 22-3).

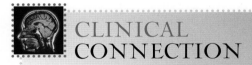

CLINICAL CONNECTION

A stroke in the distribution of the vertebral artery (or the PICA) results in an ipsilateral loss of pain and temperature sensations in the face, contralateral loss of pain and temperature sensation in the limbs, trunk, and neck, an ipsilateral Horner syndrome, hoarseness, dysphagia, nystagmus, vertigo, diplopia, ipsilateral ataxia, and ipsilateral loss of taste. This combination of signs is the **lateral medullary** or **Wallenberg syndrome.**

Basilar Artery

The basilar artery begins near the pontomedullary junction and travels in the shallow median groove on the ventral surface of the pons to end at the midbrain. At the midbrain it divides into the posterior cerebral arteries (PCA) (Figs. 22-1 to 22-3). As the basilar artery travels along the pons, it supplies multiple penetrating vessels to the pons itself. These vessels penetrate the pons as paramedian, short circumferential, and long circumferential arteries (Fig. 22-8). Symmetric large branches arising at about the middle of the basilar artery are called the anterior inferior cerebellar arteries (AICA) (Figs. 22-1, 22-3). Similar large paired vessels arising just proximal to the termination of the basilar artery are called the superior cerebellar arteries (SCA; Figs. 22-1 to 22-3).

The AICA emerge from the basilar artery and travel along the course of VII CN and VIII CN (Fig. 22-3). At times, these vessels may actually enter the internal auditory meatus for a short distance, but ultimately they reach the anterior and inferior portions of the cerebellum, their principal area of supply. The labyrinthine or internal auditory arteries may arise from the AICA or directly from the basilar artery.

Just proximal to the bifurcation of the basilar artery into the PCA, the basilar artery gives off the SCA. These vessels encircle the midbrain and end by dividing into hemispheric and superior vermian branches that supply the superior aspects of the cerebellum and most of the cerebellar nuclei and superior cerebellar peduncles (Fig. 22-8).

Posterior Cerebral Arteries

The PCA begin at the basilar bifurcation near the tip of the dorsum sellae. A short distance after arising, the PCA anastomose with the posterior communicating arteries (Figs. 22-1 to 22-3), thus connecting the anterior and posterior cerebral circulations. Each of the PCA swings around the anterior aspect of the oculomotor nerve, passes laterally along the surface of the cerebral crus to reach the dorsal surface of the free margin of the tentorium, and then proceeds posteriorly along the inferomedial surface of the temporal lobe (Figs. 22-1, 22-3).

The PCA give rise to brainstem and cortical branches. The chief brainstem branches are named according to their areas of supply as follows: thalamoperforate, medial posterior choroidal, and quadrigeminal, which arise medial to the anastomosis with the posterior communicating artery and supply the midbrain (Figs. 22-9, 22-10); and the thalamogeniculate, lateral posterior choroidal, and peduncular, which arise lateral to the posterior communicating anastomosis and supply the lateral parts of the posterior diencephalon. Cortical branches arise as the PCA courses along the inferomedial surface of the temporal lobe to reach the occipital lobe, and they supply the hippocampus and the medial and inferior surfaces of the temporal and occipital lobes. The PCA ends by forming the parieto-occipital and calcarine arteries found in the respective sulci (Fig. 22-4). The calcarine artery supplies the primary visual area. The cortical branches of the PCA extend slightly onto the lateral surfaces of the temporal and occipital lobes where they anastomose with branches of the MCA.

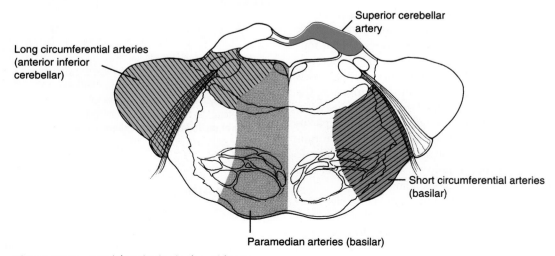

Figure 22-8 Arterial territories in the midpons.

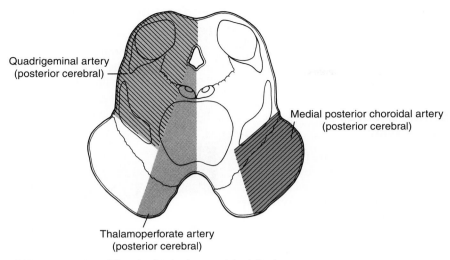

Quadrigeminal artery
(posterior cerebral)

Medial posterior choroidal artery
(posterior cerebral)

Thalamoperforate artery
(posterior cerebral)

Figure 22-9 Arterial territories in the caudal midbrain.

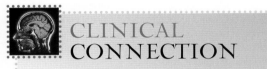

CLINICAL CONNECTION

A stroke in the cortical distribution of the posterior cerebral artery results in a contralateral homonymous hemianopsia. With dominant (usually left) hemisphere involvement, reading and writing abnormalities also result.

THE CEREBRAL ARTERIAL CIRCLE OF WILLIS

The **cerebral arterial circle,** described by Sir Thomas Willis in 1664, consists of the larger cerebral vessels and their interconnections located on the ventral surface of the brain. The arteries of the **circle of Willis** (Fig. 22-2) include anterior communicating, left anterior cerebral, left internal carotid, left posterior communicating, left posterior cerebral, basilar, right posterior cerebral, right posterior communicating, right internal carotid, and right anterior cerebral. A perfectly symmetric circle of Willis in which each component vessel is of the same caliber occurs only in a minority of instances. More commonly, one or more of the arteries (most frequently the anterior cerebral, posterior cerebral, anterior communicating, or posterior communicating) are, to some degree, atrophic.

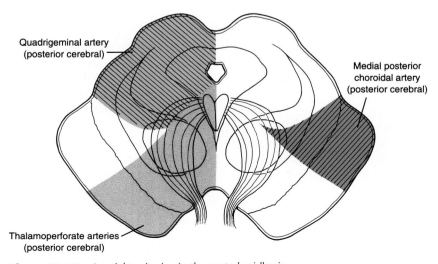

Quadrigeminal artery
(posterior cerebral)

Medial posterior
choroidal artery
(posterior cerebral)

Thalamoperforate arteries
(posterior cerebral)

Figure 22-10 Arterial territories in the rostral midbrain.

The function of the cerebral arterial circle of Willis is debated, but it probably serves as a potential vascular shunt, assisting in the development of collateral circulation to the brain should one of the proximal vessels (such as the carotid or basilar) become temporarily or permanently occluded.

Developmental Changes in the Circle of Willis

During embryologic development, the internal carotid arteries supply blood to the anterior, middle, and posterior cerebral arteries, the latter via a large posterior communicating artery. With development, however, the distal posterior cerebral supply comes from the basilar artery through the proximal posterior cerebral artery as the posterior communicating artery atrophies. In most people, the result of this atrophy is an anterior circulation (consisting of the anterior and middle cerebral arteries supplied by the carotid arteries) and a posterior circulation (consisting of the posterior cerebral arteries supplied by the vertebral-basilar trunk). However, in 20% of the population, the embryologic circulation persists, with one or both posterior cerebral arteries being supplied mainly by the anterior circulation through persistently large posterior communicating arteries.

In instances in which one or more of the primary pathways for blood flow is lost, the maintenance of cerebral blood flow depends on collateral sources. The circle of Willis is one of the most important sources of collateral circulation to the brain, but its effectiveness depends on the size of each component. Other collateral pathways exist in connections between the anterior (carotid) and posterior (basilar) circulations (such as the primitive trigeminal, otic, and hypoglossal arteries). These vessels generally disappear with development. Other prominent sources of collateral flow include anastomoses between the external carotid and the internal carotid and vertebral arteries. Clinically, these collaterals are most frequently seen in patients who have occlusive disease of a carotid or vertebral artery in the neck. In these instances, it is not uncommon to find the intracranial portions of the occluded vessels supplied via the ophthalmic branch of the carotid artery or via the muscular branches of the vertebral artery from the external carotid ramifications about the orbit and in the neck. Similar anastomoses between the meningeal vessels and the vessels on the surface of the cerebrum may be seen.

Perforating Central Branches

The branches of the cerebral arterial circle of Willis that penetrate the ventral surface of the brain are called the perforating, penetrating, central, or ganglionic branches and are divided into four groups: medial striate, lateral striate, thalamoperforate, and thalamogeniculate (Fig. 22-3).

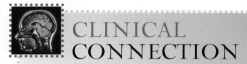

CLINICAL CONNECTION

Collateralization through perforating vessels is generally not seen. Border zones or **watershed areas,** however, occur between major cerebral vessel territories, i.e., between the anterior and middle cerebral arteries and between the middle and posterior cerebral arteries. In these regions anastomoses exist that can provide collateral circulation via vasodilation in response to proximal vessel occlusion. On the other hand, these regions are more sensitive to overall reduction in cerebral blood flow. Hence, watershed areas are susceptible to ischemic injuries after cardiac arrest.

MEDIAL STRIATE ARTERIES   The medial striate arteries arise chiefly from the A-1 segment of the ACA, although some may arise from the most proximal part of the A-2 segment, the anterior communicating artery, or the most terminal part of the ICA. Collectively referred to as the medial striate arteries, they enter the brain in the medial third of the anterior perforated substance. The largest and most lateral of these arteries to enter the brain is the recurrent artery of Heubner (Fig. 22-3). The medial striate arteries are the principal sources of the blood supply to the supraoptic and preoptic regions of the hypothalamus and to the ventral part of the head of the caudate nucleus and the adjacent parts of the anterior limb of the internal capsule and putamen.

LATERAL STRIATE ARTERIES   The lateral striate arteries usually arise entirely from the M-1 segment of the MCA, although sometimes a few may come from the initial part of the ACA (Fig. 22-3). They are frequently called the lenticulostriate arteries, and they enter the brain in the lateral two-thirds of the anterior perforated substance. The lateral striate arteries supply the dorsal part of the head of the caudate nucleus, most

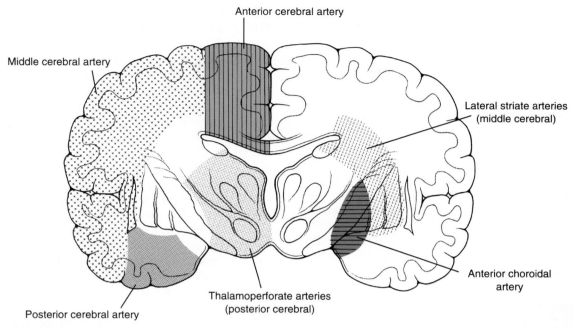

Anterior cerebral artery

Middle cerebral artery

Lateral striate arteries
(middle cerebral)

Anterior choroidal
artery

Thalamoperforate arteries
(posterior cerebral)

Posterior cerebral artery

Figure 22-11   Arterial territories of diencephalon and hemisphere.

of the putamen and adjacent part of the globus pallidus, and the dorsal part of the posterior limb of the internal capsule (Fig. 22-11).

As mentioned previously, these vessels are the most common sites of spontaneous hemorrhage in individuals with long-standing hypertension. For this reason, collectively they are called the "artery of cerebral hemorrhage."

THALAMOPERFORATE ARTERIES   Thalamoperforate arteries arise along the posterior communicating artery and the posterior cerebral artery proximal to the point at which these two vessels join. These penetrating arteries enter the brain in the posterior perforated substance (Fig. 22-3). The more anterior vessels supply the tuberal region of the hypothalamus and the anteromedial part of the thalamus, including the anterior and medial dorsal nuclei (Fig. 22-11). The more posterior vessels supply the mamillary region of the hypothalamus, the subthalamus, the adjacent parts of the thalamus, and the medial parts of the rostral midbrain tegmentum and cerebral crus (Figs. 22-9, 22-10).

THALAMOGENICULATE ARTERIES   The thalamogeniculate arteries arise from the posterior cerebral artery distal to its anastomosis with the posterior communicating artery, and penetrate

the brain at the geniculate bodies. They supply the most posterior parts of the thalamus, including the ventral lateral and ventral posterior nuclei and the medial three-fourths of the metathalamic nuclei.

SPINAL CORD VASCULATURE

The spinal cord is supplied by paired posterior spinal arteries and a single larger anterior spinal artery. In addition, multiple radicular vessels arise segmentally from cervical, intercostal, lumbar, and sacral arteries. The anterior and posterior spinal arteries are not of sufficient caliber to maintain circulation throughout the entire spinal cord. Hence, they rely to a great extent on the radicular component.

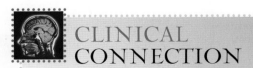

CLINICAL CONNECTION

The largest radicular artery is the so-called artery of Adamkiewicz, which generally enters the spinal cord in the lower thoracic or upper lumbar area. Clinically, this area of the spinal cord is susceptible to vascular insult should this radicular artery be compromised.

The anterior spinal artery descends along the surface of the cord at the anterior median fissure and supplies from five to nine sulcal arteries to each spinal cord segment. Each sulcal artery passes to the bottom of the anterior median fissure, where it swings right or left to enter the spinal cord and supply that side. In addition to the sulcal arteries, the anterior spinal artery supplies coronal arteries that course laterally along the surface of the cord to anastomose with similar branches from the posterior spinal arteries. The latter are located in the posterolateral sulci and also give rise to penetrating branches that accompany the posterior roots into the spinal cord. The sulcal and coronal branches of the anterior spinal artery supply the anterior two-thirds of the spinal cord, whereas the penetrating and coronal branches of the posterior spinal arteries supply the posterior third (Fig. 22-12).

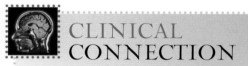

CLINICAL CONNECTION

A stroke in the distribution of the anterior spinal artery results in the development of total motor paralysis and dissociated sensory loss below the level of the lesion. The sensory loss, if dissociated (loss of pain and temperature but no involvement of position and vibration sense), is caused by sparing of the dorsal columns supplied by the posterior spinal arteries.

VEINS OF BRAIN AND SPINAL CORD

Unlike systemic veins, cerebral veins are without valves and muscle tissue. The venous system of the brain is divided into a superficial and a deep portion (Figs. 22-13, 22-14). The superficial veins are larger and more numerous than the corresponding cortical arteries and tend to lie alongside the arteries in the cerebral sulci. The superficial venous system empties into the more superficially located sinuses, especially the superior sagittal, inferior sagittal, and transverse sinuses, via anastomotic or draining veins. The most prominent anastomotic veins are the superficial middle cerebral vein draining into the cavernous or sphenoparietal sinus, the great anastomotic vein (of Trolard) draining into the superior sagittal sinus, and the posterior anastomotic vein (of Labbé) draining into the transverse sinus.

The deep venous system consists of the great vein (of Galen), the internal cerebral veins, the basal vein (of Rosenthal), and their tributaries including the transcerebral veins, which drain the white matter, and the subependymal veins, which drain the periventricular structures.

The great vein (of Galen) is located beneath the splenium of the corpus callosum and receives the paired internal cerebral veins, the two basal veins (of Rosenthal), and drainage from the medial and inferior parts of the occipital lobe. The internal

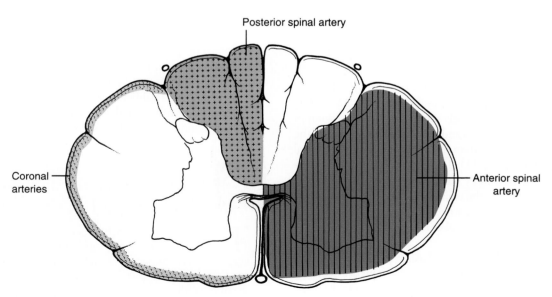

Figure 22-12   Arterial territories in the spinal cord.

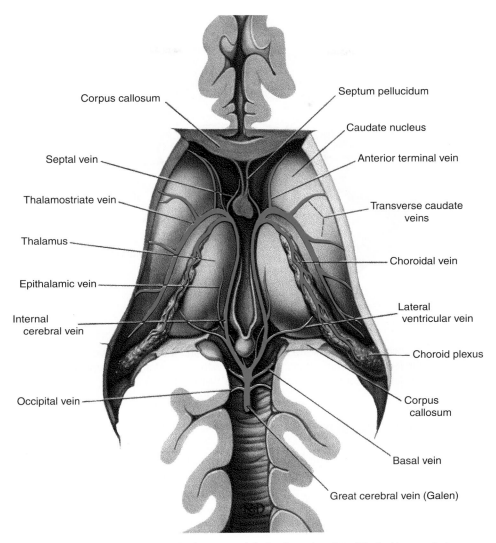

Corpus callosum

Septal vein

Thalamostriate vein

Thalamus

Epithalamic vein

Internal
cerebral vein

Occipital vein

Septum pellucidum

Caudate nucleus

Anterior terminal vein

Transverse caudate
veins

Choroidal vein

Lateral
ventricular vein

Choroid plexus

Corpus
callosum

Basal vein

Great cerebral vein (Galen)

Figure 22-13 The internal cerebral veins and their tributaries. (Modified with permission from Carpenter MB, Sutin J. Human Neuroanatomy. Baltimore: Williams & Wilkins, 1983.)

cerebral veins lie in the roof of the third ventricle. Large tributaries include the thalamostriate veins (draining the thalamus and striatum), choroidal veins (from the choroid plexus of the lateral ventricle), and septal veins (from the septum pellucidum).

The basal vein (of Rosenthal) begins near the anterior perforate substance, encircles the cerebral crus, and ends at the great vein (of Galen). Basal vein drainage includes the medial and inferior surfaces of the frontal and temporal lobes, the insular and opercular cortices, and regions of the hypothalamus and midbrain.

The venous drainage of the spinal cord is concentrated in a dense plexus of veins located in the epidural space (Batson internal vertebral venous plexus).

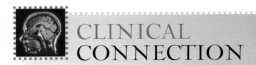

CLINICAL
CONNECTION

This valveless spinal maze of veins communicates freely with sacral, lumbar, and intercostal veins, thus providing an open pathway for tumor and infection metastases.

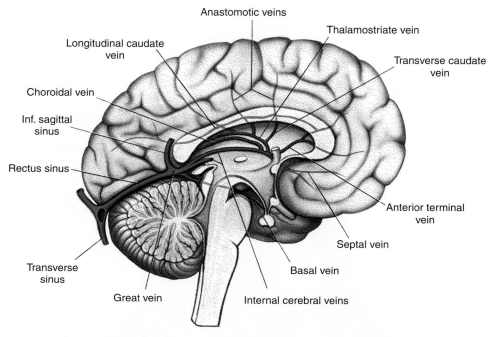

Anastomotic veins

Thalamostriate vein

Longitudinal caudate vein

Transverse caudate vein

Choroidal vein

Inf. sagittal sinus

Rectus sinus

Anterior terminal vein

Septal vein

Transverse sinus

Basal vein

Great vein

Internal cerebral veins

Figure 22-14 Midsagittal view of the internal cerebral veins showing the relationship of the great vein to the rectus sinus (inf, inferior). (Modified with permission from Carpenter MB, Sutin J. Human Neuroanatomy. Baltimore: Williams & Wilkins, 1983.)

Chapter Review Questions

22-1. What are the chief morphologic features of cerebral arteries?

22-2. What is the anatomic substrate of the blood–brain barrier?

22-3. Describe the arterial circle of Willis.

22-4. What is the arterial supply of the spinal cord?

22-5. List the arterial supply of each of the following:
  a. Broca speech area
  b. lower limb sensorimotor cortex
  c. visual cortex
  d. posterior limb of internal capsule
  e. dorsolateral part of rostral medulla
  f. anterior and lateral funiculi of spinal cord

The Cerebrospinal Fluid System: Hydrocephalus

A 6-MONTH-OLD INFANT is brought to the emergency room with elevated temperature (103°F) and irritability. On arrival, the child suffers a generalized convulsion and becomes somnolent. A spinal tap demonstrates turbid cerebrospinal fluid with elevated white blood cells and diminished glucose. A gram-positive organism is identified. After a course of antibiotics the child makes a complete recovery. Three months later, the infant returns with developmental delay, an increasing head circumference, and bulging anterior fontanelle. A computed tomography (CT) scan shows ventriculomegaly. A ventriculoperitoneal shunt is inserted. At 12 months, there is complete restoration of normal milestones.

Cerebrospinal fluid (CSF) circulating in the ventricles and the surrounding subarachnoid space of the brain provides protective cushioning for the brain against the forces associated with surface contact pressure and sudden movement.

THE VENTRICULAR SYSTEM

The ventricular system consists of a lateral ventricle in each hemisphere, a third ventricle in the diencephalon, and a fourth ventricle in the hindbrain between the cerebellum, pons, and rostral medulla. The cerebral aqueduct, in the midbrain, connects the third and fourth ventricles.

LATERAL VENTRICLES

The lateral ventricles (left and right) are divided into five identified parts: anterior or frontal horn, body or central part, atrium or trigone, posterior or occipital horn, and inferior or temporal horn (Fig. 23-1).

Anterior or Frontal Horn

The segment of the lateral ventricle anterior to the interventricular foramen (of Monro) is called the anterior or frontal horn. Medially, it is bounded by the septum pellucidum, fornix, and genu of the corpus callosum. Laterally, the head of the caudate bulges into the frontal horn. The floor of the frontal horn is formed by the rostrum of the corpus callosum.

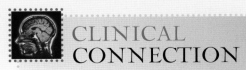

CLINICAL CONNECTION

Clinically, the frontal horns are devoid of choroid plexus, making them an excellent place for the positioning of spinal fluid diversion systems (shunts).

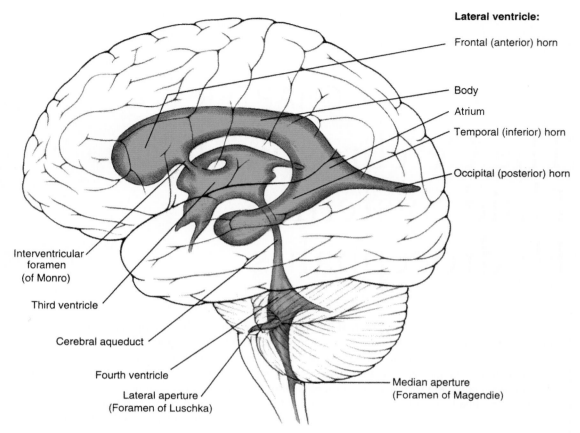

Figure 23-1　The ventricles and their locations in the brain. Left lateral view.

Body

The body or central part of each lateral ventricle extends from the foramen of Monro to the splenium of the corpus callosum. Like the frontal horn, the septum pellucidum continues as the medial border of the ventricular body, and the ventricular roof remains bounded by the corpus callosum. Laterally, the ventricular body is adjacent to the body of the caudate nucleus, and its floor is formed by the thalamus with the fornix, choroid plexus, and thalamostriate vein visible on the surface from medial to lateral.

Atrium

The atrium or trigone is the most expanded part of the lateral ventricle and is triangular in shape. Anteriorly, it is related to the fornix and pulvinar. The atrium contains an abundant tuft of choroid plexus, the **glomus** or **choroid enlarge-**

ment, along its anterior wall, which is continuous with the choroid plexus of the body and temporal horn.

Posterior or Occipital Horn

The posterior or occipital horn is within the occipital lobe and is the most variable part of the ventricular system. Medially, the calcar avis, formed by the calcarine fissure, bulges into the occipital horn. Like the frontal horn, the occipital horn is also devoid of choroid plexus.

Inferior or Temporal Horn

The inferior or temporal horn is within the temporal lobe. It extends to within 3 cm of the temporal pole. Its roof is formed by the tapetum of the corpus callosum. Medially, it is bounded by the tail of the caudate nucleus and the hippocampus, and it contains choroid plexus in its superior-medial aspect.

INTERVENTRICULAR FORAMEN (OF MONRO)

The interventricular foramen is the passageway between each lateral ventricle and the single third ventricle. Bordering the interventricular foramen are the anterior tubercle or nucleus of the thalamus, septum pellucidum, column of the fornix, and thalamostriate vein. Passing through the interventricular foramen is the choroid plexus.

THIRD VENTRICLE

The third ventricle is bordered bilaterally by the thalamus dorsally and hypothalamus ventrally (Fig. 4-2). Sometimes a connection between the thalami, the interthalamic adhesion or mass intermedia, bridges across the third ventricle. Anteriorly, the third ventricle is bounded by the lamina terminalis with the anterior commissure dorsal and the optic recess ventral. The floor of the third ventricle is formed by the infundibular recess and tuber cinereum with the mamillary bodies posteriorly. The roof of the third ventricle is formed by the tela choroidea, which contains the internal cerebral veins and choroid plexus. Posteriorly, suprapineal and infrapineal recesses are formed above and below the pineal gland with the posterior commissure inferior. The third ventricle drains into a tubular canal, the cerebral aqueduct (of Sylvius).

CEREBRAL AQUEDUCT OF SYLVIUS

The cerebral aqueduct is located within the midbrain and connects the third and fourth ventricles. Its length is 1.5 to 1.8 cm, and its diameter is 1 to 2 mm. It is arched in a slightly dorsal direction.

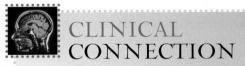

CLINICAL CONNECTION

Clinically, the cerebral aqueduct is the narrowest part of the ventricular system. **Obstructive hydrocephalus** caused by aqueductal blockage commonly occurs here.

FOURTH VENTRICLE

The fourth ventricle is a single midline cavity whose rhomboid-shaped floor is formed by the pons and rostral medulla. It expands posteriorly in an inverted kite shape, with its roof bounded by the superior and inferior medullary vela and the superior cerebellar peduncles. Choroid plexus is attached to the inferior medullary velum and extends laterally through the lateral apertures (**foramina of Luschka**) into the subarachnoid space at the origin of cranial nerves (CN) IX and X. The lateral borders of the fourth ventricle are the three cerebellar peduncles. A median aperture, the **foramen of Magendie,** empties into the vallecula, an anterior extension of the cisterna magnum.

SUBARACHNOID SPACE AND CISTERNS

The subarachnoid space is continuous across the cerebral and cerebellar convexities and along the spinal cord. Extracerebral arteries and veins and cranial nerves are suspended in this space by web-like arachnoid trabeculations. In vivo, this space is distended with CSF, which bathes and nourishes the structures contained within. The subarachnoid cisterns are expansions of the subarachnoid space, occurring primarily along the ventral surface of the brainstem and basal forebrain. The CSF in the cisterns provides support and buoyancy for cerebral vessels and cranial nerves.

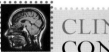

CLINICAL CONNECTION

Under normal circumstances, no real CSF barrier exists across the ependymal surface of the ventricles or across the pial-glial membranes, so that the cerebral extracellular (interstitial) space communicates freely with the CSF circulation.

The subarachnoid cisterns (Fig. 23-2) are readily identifiable in vivo because they are filled with CSF. In the cadaveric brain they are difficult to observe because they have collapsed.

The cisterna magna is the largest of the cisternal compartments. It is located posterior to the medulla and caudal to the cerebellum. Its forward projection between the cerebellar tonsils is the vallecula, into which the median aperture empties.

The pontomedullary cistern lies ventral to the pons and the medulla, between these structures and the clivus. It contains the basilar artery and its branches.

The lateral cerebellomedullary cistern is located lateral to the rostral medulla and surrounds CN IX, X, and XI.

A

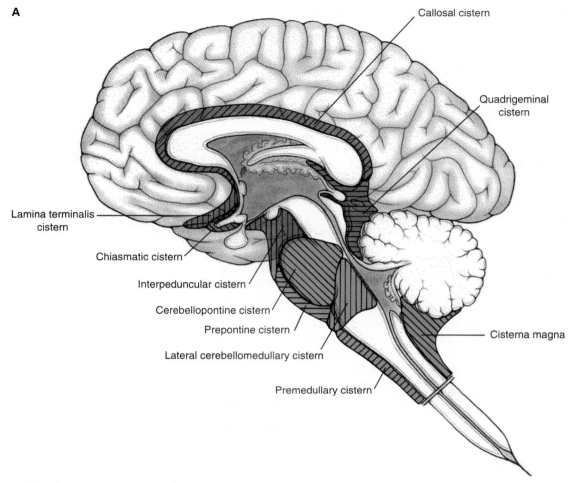

Figure 23-2 **A.** The subarachnoid cisterns at or near the median plane. (*continued*)

The cerebellopontine (CP) cistern is located in the CP angle and surrounds CN V, VII, and VIII. It is immediately beneath the tentorium and lateral to the petrous ridge.

The quadrigeminal cistern overlies the tectum of the midbrain and contains the vein of Galen. Anteriorly it is bounded by the pineal gland and the pulvinar, superiorly by the splenium of the corpus callosum, posteriorly by the free edge of the tentorium, and inferiorly by the central lobule of the cerebellum.

The interpeduncular cistern straddles the interpeduncular fossa. It is triangular in shape and bounded anteriorly by the membrane of Liliequist, an unusually tough arachnoidal trabecula between the interpeduncular cistern and chiasmatic cistern.

The crural cistern is a lateral and dorsal expansion of the interpeduncular cistern that separates the cerebral peduncles from the parahippocampal gyri.

The ambient cistern joins the interpeduncular and crural cisterns to the quadrigeminal cistern. It lies adjacent to the tentorial edge and contains the posterior cerebral artery and CN IV and VI.

The chiasmatic cistern surrounds the optic chiasm and the pituitary stalk, the carotid cistern surrounds the cerebral segment of the carotid artery, and the olfactory cistern surrounds the olfactory tract in the olfactory sulcus.

The lamina terminalis cistern is immediately adjacent to the lamina terminalis. It contains the anterior cerebral and anterior communicating arteries.

The sylvian cistern fills the lateral or sylvian fissure and contains the middle cerebral artery and its branches. The callosal cistern lies immediately

B

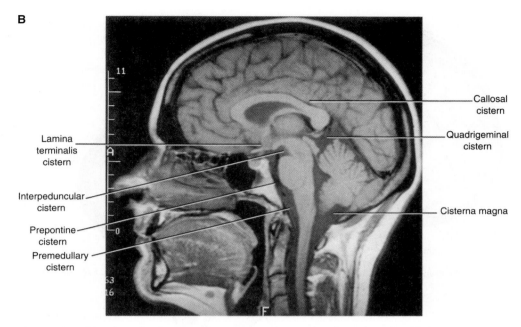

Figure 23-2 (*Continued*)   **B.** Magnetic resonance image showing subarachnoid cisterns at or near the median plane.

adjacent to the corpus callosum and contains the pericallosal arteries.

CHOROID PLEXUS

The vast majority of CSF is secreted by the choroid plexus contained within the lateral, third, and fourth ventricles through an energy-dependent secretory process. Some CSF is produced by the flow of brain extracellular fluid across the ependymal lining of the ventricular system. As a result of these two methods of formation, CSF can be considered a plasma ultrafiltrate that serves a role in maintaining a constant chemical milieu for neurons.

CLINICAL CONNECTION

Total (normal) CSF volume is approximately 150 mL, with 75 mL in the cisterns, 50 mL in the subarachnoid space, and 25 mL in the ventricles. CSF is formed at the rate of about 0.5 mL/min (450 to 600 mL/day). Thus, the total pool of CSF undergoes replacement between three and four times a day.

CEREBROSPINAL FLUID CIRCULATION

Cerebrospinal fluid circulates within the ventricles of the brain and within the cranial and spinal subarachnoid space (Fig. 23-3). It is produced in the lateral, third, and fourth ventricles and exits the ventricular system through the three openings in the fourth ventricle: the median aperture and paired lateral apertures (Fig. 23-1). After exiting the ventricular system, CSF enters the cisterns around the lower and upper brainstem. From the cisterns, CSF then flows along the convexity of the cerebrum to its absorption site in the **arachnoid granulations** chiefly along the superior sagittal sinus (Fig. 23-3).

CEREBROSPINAL FLUID TAP

CSF can be sampled from a number of locations. Most commonly a CSF tap is done in the lower back via a puncture of the dural sac into the lumbar subarachnoid space (Fig. 2-3). Lumbar punctures should be performed below the LV2 lumbar spinous process, the commonest level of spinal cord termination at the conus medullaris. Other reservoirs of CSF can also be accessed, including the lateral ventricle (ventriculostomy), cervical

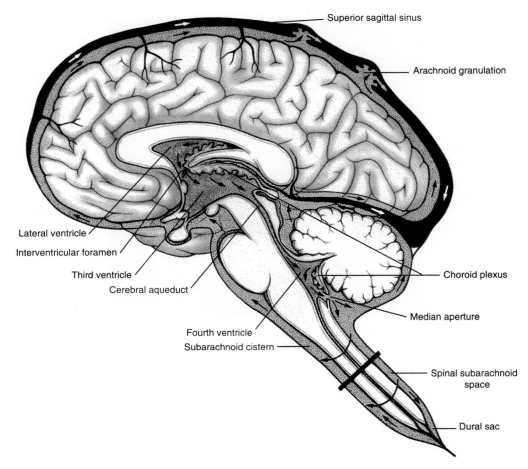

Figure 23-3 Cerebrospinal fluid circulation. Cerebrospinal fluid produced in the choroid plexus of the lateral and third ventricles flows through the aqueduct, fourth ventricle, and outlet foramina into the subarachnoid cisterns. Through the cisterns the fluid passes into the subarachnoid space up over the convexities toward the superior sagittal sinus for the final absorption through the arachnoid villi.

subarachnoid space (lateral C1–2 puncture), and cisterna magna (cisternal tap).

The chemical content of normal CSF relates to its location in the CSF pathway. For example, ventricular CSF contains approximately 15 mg/100 mL protein and about 75 mg/100 mL glucose, whereas lumbar CSF contains approximately 45 mg/100 mL protein and about 60 mg/100 mL glucose. Normally, few if any cells are found in the CSF regardless of its removal site.

HYDROCEPHALUS

Obstruction of the CSF pathway can result in the stagnation of flow and the development of hydrocephalus. By current definition hydrocephalus implies a dilation of one or more parts of the ventricular system owing to an abnormal collection of CSF. This is meant to exclude the ventricular dilation that commonly occurs after cerebral atrophy as seen in dementia. The sites of hydrocephalus formation relate to the part of

CLINICAL CONNECTION

CSF is normally a clear, colorless fluid. Changes in CSF appearance often give clues as to the disease process: red—blood from recent hemorrhage; turbid—pus from infectious process; yellow—excessive protein from stagnation of flow or blood breakdown.

the CSF pathway involved in the disease process. In general, two types of hydrocephalus occur: obstructive and communicating. **Obstructive hydrocephalus** refers to any disease process that restricts CSF flow within or from the ventricular system. Thus, a blockage located anywhere along the ventricular pathways (such as at the interventricular foramen of Monro, at the aqueduct, or at the outlet foramina of the fourth ventricle) produces obstructive hydrocephalus with enlargement of those ventricles proximal to the obstruction. Any disruption of flow after the CSF has exited the ventricular system, on the other hand, is referred to as **communicating hydrocephalus.** Communicating hydrocephalus occurs with obstructions in the cisternal pathways, along the subarachnoid space, or at the arachnoid villi.

INTRACRANIAL PRESSURE

Pressure within the intracranial-spinal space (ICP) is normally less than 100 mm H_2O. ICP is determined by the volumes of brain tissue, CSF, blood, and other compressible tissue within the rigid cranial vault. An increase in the size of any single component (e.g., brain swelling, CSF collection, vasodilation) results first in a diminishment in the size of the other components (compensatory), but then in an increase in ICP.

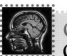

CLINICAL CONNECTION

Headaches, nausea, vomiting, changes in level of consciousness, extraocular muscle palsies, papilledema, and head enlargement (in infants) are associated with elevated ICP.

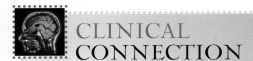

CLINICAL CONNECTION

Obstructive hydrocephalus is commonly associated with congenital malformations such as aqueductal stenosis or with tumors that protrude into the ventricular pathway, thereby obstructing flow. Communicating types of hydrocephalus usually result from processes that occur in the cisternal or subarachnoid space such as hemorrhage or infection. Regardless of its cause and site, the diagnosis of hydrocephalus is readily discernible by cranial CT and magnetic resonance imaging.

Chapter Review Questions

23-1.   What are the functions of CSF?

23-2.   Name the parts of the lateral ventricle and give their locations.

23-3.   Describe the flow of CSF from its formation to its absorption.

23-4.   Contrast the noncommunicating and communicating types of hydrocephalus.

Development of the Nervous System: Congenital Anomalies

The development of the central nervous system is a multistep process far more complicated than that for any other organ system in the human body. Late in the third week of embryogenesis the nervous system arises from the outermost layer of the three cell layers of the gastrula, the **ectoderm.** The dorsal midline of the ectoderm is induced to form the **neural plate** by diffusible signals from surrounding tissues, particularly the underlying notochord. During neurulation the neural plate is transformed into first **neural folds** and then, with closure, the **neural tube** (Fig. 24-1). Derivatives of the neural plate give rise to neurons, macroglia (astrocytes and oligodendrocytes), and ependymal cells. Microglia do not have a neuroectodermal origin, but rather arise from mesenchymal cells.

The **neural crest** arises from cells at the lateral margin of the neural plate that remain separated from the neural tube. Neural crest cells migrate away from the neural tube and become neurons and supporting cells in cranial and spinal sensory ganglia and postganglionic autonomic ganglia in the peripheral nervous system and the meninges surrounding the brain and spinal cord.

NEURULATION

The neural tube gives rise to the central nervous system (CNS). Closure of the neural tube begins in the future cervical region of the spinal cord and continues rostrally and caudally. Closure of the neural tube anteriorly at the anterior neuropore occurs at 24 days of gestation, and closure at the posterior neuropore occurs 2 days later. Rostrally the neural tube enlarges as the brain with the formation of three primary brain vesicles, the prosencephalon (forebrain), the mesencephalon (midbrain), and the rhombencephalon (hindbrain; Fig. 24-2). Later in development the forebrain divides into the telencephalon (cerebral hemispheres) and diencephalon, whereas the hindbrain becomes the metencephalon (pons and cerebellum) and myelencephalon (medulla oblongata). A persistent cephalic flexure of the neural tube at the junction between the mesencephalon and the rhombencephalon results in the future change in axial orientation of the forebrain. Caudal to the myelencephalon the neural tube becomes the spinal cord. The lumen of the neural tube forms the ventricular system in the brain, but becomes the constricted and nonpatent central canal in the spinal cord.

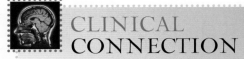

CLINICAL CONNECTION

Failure of the neural tube to close results in dysraphic defects occurring most commonly at the anterior and posterior neuropores. Anencephaly resulting from failure of the anterior neuropore to close in turn results in a malformed brain exposed by the lack of a bony cranium and continuous with the skin of the scalp. This condition is always fatal. Defects in the closure of the posterior neuropore result in different disorders. Commonly the vertebral arches fail to develop and fuse, resulting in spina bifida. Spina bifida may be accompanied by a protrusion of a meningeal sac containing cerebrospinal fluid (meningocele) or, if the sac contains neural tissue, a meningomyelocele. A significant percentage of neural tube birth defects can be prevented by maternal use of folic acid before and during pregnancy.

NEUROGENESIS, GLIOGENESIS, AND POLARITY OF THE CNS

Initially the neural tube is composed of a layer of pseudostratified columnar neuroepithelial cells. Cell division away from the dorsal and ventral midline of the neural tube results in the formation of three layers: a **ventricular** layer adjacent to the lumen where cell division occurs, a **marginal** layer farthest from the lumen formed predominantly by cell processes, and the **mantle** or **intermediate** layer between the ventricular and marginal layers to be occupied by postmitotic neurons and glia. At first, the processes of the neuroepithelial cells extend from the lumen to the external surface of the neural tube. Mitotic cell division occurs in the ventricular layer, and the nuclei of the daughter cells migrate outward to the marginal layer where DNA synthesis occurs, after which they return to the ventricular zone for another round of cell division.

A common progenitor gives rise to all CNS cells except microglia. **Neuroblasts** are generated first and migrate permanently away from the ventricular zone into the mantle layer and differentiate into neurons. Later, **glioblasts** give rise to cells that migrate into the marginal and mantle layers and differentiate into astrocytes and oligoden-

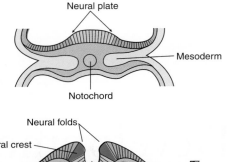
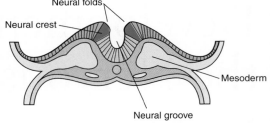
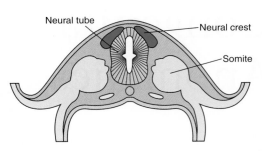

Figure 24-1 The central nervous system develops from specialized neural ectoderm (color) that folds and forms the neural tube. The peripheral nervous system develops from the neural crest located at the lateral edge of the neural ectoderm external to the neural tube.

droglia. Lastly, ependymal cells are generated and remain in the ventricular layer to later line the central canal in the spinal cord and ventricles in the brain. Because of the continued addition of new neuroblasts the dorsal and ventral parts of the mantle layer increase in thickness, forming the **alar** and **basal** plates, respectively (Fig. 24-3). A longitudinal groove on the lateral wall of the neural tube, the **sulcus limitans,** separates the alar and basal plates.

The dorsal and ventral midlines of the neural tube form the roof plate and floor plate, respectively. The roof and floor plates do not contribute directly to neurogenesis. Rather, specialized glial cells, acting together with the underlying mesodermal cells and the notochord

3 Primary brain vesicles

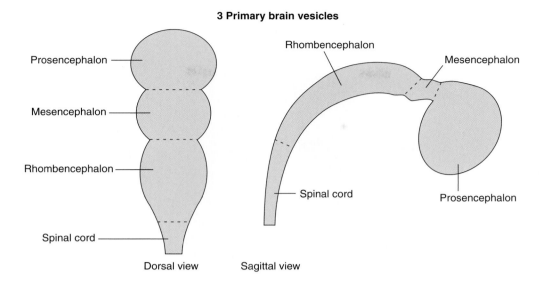

Prosencephalon

Mesencephalon

Rhombencephalon

Spinal cord

Dorsal view

Rhombencephalon

Mesencephalon

Spinal cord

Prosencephalon

Sagittal view

5 Secondary brain vesicles

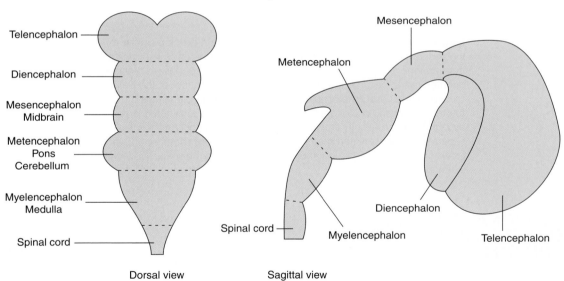

Telencephalon

Diencephalon

Mesencephalon
Midbrain

Metencephalon
Pons
Cerebellum

Myelencephalon
Medulla

Spinal cord

Dorsal view

Mesencephalon

Metencephalon

Diencephalon

Spinal cord

Myelencephalon

Telencephalon

Sagittal view

Figure 24-2   The brain develops from the rostral part of the neural tube with the initial formation of three expansions of the primary brain vesicles. Later these vesicles differentiate into five secondary vesicles, each of which gives rise to the major brain subdivisions seen in the adult.

in the floor plate and with the overlying epidermal ectoderm in the roof plate, are responsible for the dorsal and ventral patterning of the alar and basal plates. Concentration gradients of diffusible tropic factors from the floor plate and surrounding mesenchyme and different proteins from the roof plate and adjacent ectoderm direct the phenotypic determination of neurons in the alar and basal plates.

The morphologic and functional specification of neural cells along the rostral-caudal axis of the neural tube is determined by expression of genes different from the dorsal-ventral patterning genes. The development of distinctive caudal to rostral subdivisions of the neural tube, with increasing structural complexity, reflects the segmental gene expression and resultant actions with restricted caudal to rostral boundaries.

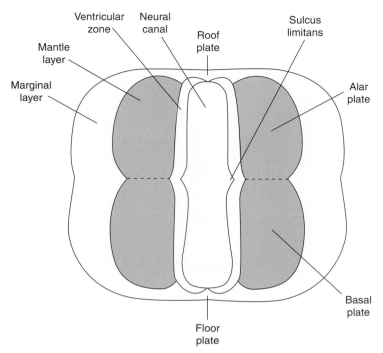

Figure 24-3 All parts of the central nervous system develop similar to the general pattern seen best in the spinal cord. Neurons and glia originate from an inner ventricular zone and migrate along the specialized radially oriented glia to become located in the incipient gray matter of the alar (sensory) and basal (motor) plates. The sulcus limitans separates the future sensory and motor areas. The marginal layer is constituted largely by cellular processes. In progressively more rostral subdivisions the separation of sensory and motor areas becomes more complex, and at levels of the mesencephalon and more rostral levels the sulcus limitans is not evident.

NEURONAL MIGRATION, SELECTIVE AGGREGATION, AND DIFFERENTIATION

Adult CNS neurons are mostly organized in morphologically and functionally related nuclei (spinal cord, brainstem, and diencephalon) or layers (tectum, cerebral cortex, and cerebellar cortex). Migrating neurons are guided from the ventricular layer to distant locations by contact guidance and tropic signaling. Specialized **radial glia** extend processes perpendicularly from the ventricular germinal epithelium to the outer edge of the developing brain. The formation of nuclei within the brainstem, diencephalon, and basal forebrain is complex and may involve both radial migration and circumferential movements around the edges or through the developing brain. Spatially adjacent parts of the developing neural tube give rise to morphologically and functionally different nuclei. Based on time of birth of neurons, different tropic factors determine the migration routes for the neurons forming these nuclei.

AXONAL GROWTH, TRACT FORMATION, AND MYELINATION

Axons of projection neurons must grow considerable distances, past numerous inappropriate targets, before reaching their appropriate synaptic targets. Axonal growth is guided by molecular signals on cell surfaces or in the extracellular matrix or by freely diffusing molecules. Signaling molecules may be either chemoattractants or chemorepellants. Chemoattractants provide a tropic signal for growing axons to follow. Chemorepellants repulse growing axons from entering incorrect targets or from growing past the intended target. At the leading edge of an elongating axon is a growth cone with motile fingerlike filopodial extensions with embedded receptors that actively sample the environment for molecular signals. Following appropriate molecular pathways, new membrane is added to the leading edge of the growing axon, which is adherent to the underlying substrate. Later, growing axons can fasciculate with these early growing pioneer axons, thereby forming axonal tracts in the CNS. Myelination of CNS axons begins around the 16th week of gestation and continues until about 3 years of age.

SYNAPTOGENESIS

Upon reaching an appropriate synaptic target growing axons must then recognize specific neurons in order to develop synaptic connections. Synaptogenesis requires a chemical interaction between the growth cone and the target muscle or neuron. Transformation of the growth cones begins with the release of signaling molecules that act on the target cell and the clustering of receptor proteins at the site of contact. In return the target cell signals back to the growth cone to begin differentiation into the presynaptic element.

The development of synaptic connections is not precise in either number or location. Many developing synapses are transient and are eliminated with continued maturation of the CNS. Impulse activity plays a critical role in synapse elimination, serving to refine and increase the precision of connections. More active contacts are strengthened at the expense of less active ones. Target neurons appear to control the retraction of presynaptic axon terminals by removing receptors from the postsynaptic membrane.

PROGRAMMED CELL DEATH OR APOPTOSIS

Common to the development of the central and peripheral nervous systems is the overproduction of neurons and the subsequent elimination of the surfeit number by programmed cell death (apoptosis). Estimates are that about half the neurons produced during development are *normally* eliminated by programmed cell death. Experimental studies have shown that trophic factors help regulate the number of surviving neurons to match the needs for connectivity.

DEVELOPMENT OF THE CENTRAL NERVOUS SYSTEM

SPINAL CORD

In the developing spinal cord the mantle layer gives rise to the gray matter and the marginal layer becomes the surrounding white matter. The fundamental morphologic and functional organization of the spinal cord is determined early in the developing neural tube. Neuroblasts in the alar plate develop into sensory neurons in the dorsal horn of the spinal cord, whereas neuroblasts in the basal plate differentiate into motor neurons in the ventral horn and the preganglionic sympathetic (T1 to L2) and parasympathetic (S2 to S4) neurons in the lateral horn and intermediate zone. The mantle layer between the alar and basal plates gives rises to the intermediate zone. The central processes of neuroblasts in the dorsal root ganglia grow into the spinal cord at the dorsal horns. The peripheral processes of the dorsal root ganglion neurons join with the outgrowing axons in the ventral roots from motor neurons in the ventral horn to form the spinal nerves. Developmental relationships between spinal cord segments and the cutaneous area innervated by neurons in the attached dorsal root ganglion and the muscle fibers innervated by motor axons in the ventral root create the segmental dermatomes and myotomes seen in the adult (Fig. 11-2).

BRAIN

The fundamental processes that occur in the development of the neural tube forming the spinal cord continue in the brain but follow a much more modified plan from caudal to rostral divisions.

The Rhombencephalon and Mesencephalon Form the Brainstem

The lumen of the neural tube forming the rhombencephalon enlarges, forming the fourth ventricle. This expansion forces the alar plates to move to a location dorsolateral to the basal plates. The sulcus limitans, which disappears in the spinal cord, persists on the floor of the fourth ventricle, separating sensory nuclei laterally from motor nuclei medially. The presence of structures derived from branchial arches, in addition to the somites, results in additional functional subdivisions of the alar and basal plates that form longitudinally oriented columns of nuclei in the brainstem. The basal plate gives rise to (1) medial somatic motor nuclei (medullary hypoglossal nucleus, pontine abducens nucleus, and mesencephalic trochlear and oculomotor nuclei) that innervate tongue and eye musculature derived from somatic mesoderm, (2) intermediate visceral motor or secretory nuclei (dorsal motor vagal and inferior salivatory nuclei in the medulla, the superior salivatory nucleus in the pons, and the Edinger-Westphal nucleus in the midbrain) that provide parasympathetic preganglionic innervation of visceral motor ganglia in the head, thorax, and abdomen, and (3) lateral nuclei (nucleus ambiguus in the medulla and facial and trigeminal motor nuclei in the pons) that innervate muscles that develop from branchial arch mesoderm.

The alar plates gives rise to (1) the trigeminal somatosensory nuclei in the pons and medulla, receiving primary input from the head; (2) the solitary nucleus that receives general visceral input from the abdomen and thorax and special visceral input (taste) from the tongue; and (3) the special somatic vestibular and cochlear nuclei. The dorsolateral edges of the metencephalic alar plates bend medially, giving rise on each side to a specialized area called the rhombic lip. Parts of the cerebellum that will form the roof of the fourth ventricle develop from the rostral part of the rhombic lip. From the caudal part of the rhombic lip neurons arise and migrate circumferentially to form nuclei located in the ventral brainstem.

In the mesencephalon the lumen of the neural tube gradually becomes reduced in size, forming the cerebral aqueduct. The marginal zone of the basal plate enlarges with the ingrowth of developing axons from the cerebral cortex and forms the cerebral crus on the ventral surface on each side of the mesencephalon. The alar plates give rise to the tectum on the dorsal surface of the mesencephalon, which later forms the superior and inferior colliculi on each side and the substantia nigra just posterior to the cerebral crus.

Cerebellum

The cerebellum develops from the rhombic lips and the caudal part of the mesencephalon. The most

rostral part of the rhombic lips and the medial mesencephalon are close together and fuse early, forming the anterior part of the cerebellum. More caudally the rhombic lips are initially widely separated, but with continued development expand medially and fuse at the midline. The cerebellar anlage begins to be divided by transverse oriented fissures. The posterolateral fissure appears first, followed by the primary fissure, which together establish the subdivision of the cerebellum into the anterior, posterior, and flocculonodular lobes. Later, secondary fissures subdivide the lobes into lobules.

The three-layered cerebellar cortex develops in an outside to inside direction (Fig. 24-4A). The earliest generated neurons will form the cerebellar nuclei just above the fourth ventricle. Next, the principal cell type in the cerebellar cortex, the Purkinje neurons, arise and migrate radially away from the germinal epithelium through the incipient cerebellar nuclei toward the surface. Later, cortical interneurons follow behind and migrate past the Purkinje cells to form an outer molecular layer. A second wave of neurogenesis originating away from the ventricular germinal epithelium and located at the edge of the rhombic limp gives rise to neuroblasts that migrate circumferentially onto the surface of the cerebellum, where they form a secondary or external germinal layer. Cell division in this external layer gives rise to immature neurons that migrate inward along radial glial processes to form the deepest of the cortical layers, the internal granule cell layer. As these granule neurons migrate inward, they leave behind a trailing process that becomes axons in the molecular layer that signal the continued differentiation of the Purkinje cells.

Prosencephalon

The most rostral primary brain vesicle, the prosencephalon, gives rise to the diencephalon (between brain) and the telencephalon (end brain), which forms the cerebral hemispheres.

DIENCEPHALON Progressing from the brainstem to the diencephalon, the organizational structure of the neural tube changes further, with the basal and floor plates disappearing. The lumen of the neural tube in the diencephalon forms the third ventricle. Diencephalic nuclei develop from the alar and roof plates. Medial swellings of the diencephalic alar plates are divided by a longitudi-

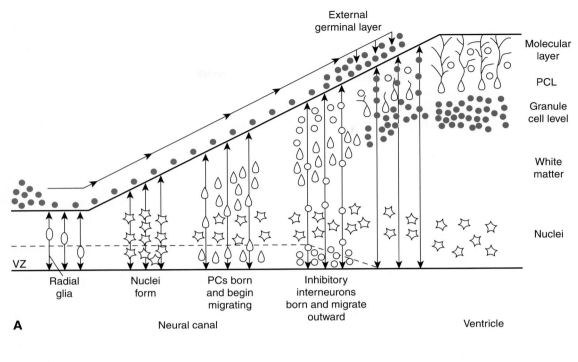

External
germinal layer

Molecular
layer

PCL

Granule
cell level

White
matter

Nuclei

VZ

Radial
glia

Nuclei
form

PCs born
and begin
migrating

Inhibitory
interneurons
born and migrate
outward

A   Neural canal   Ventricle

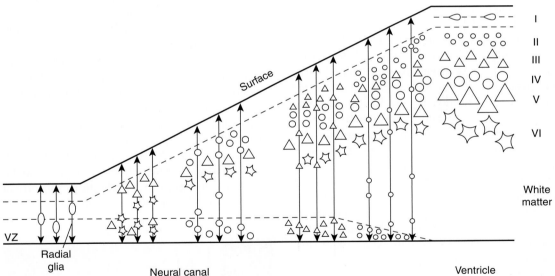

Surface

I

II

III

IV

V

VI

White
matter

VZ

Radial
glia

Neural canal   Ventricle

B

Figure 24-4 Development of the layers in the cerebellar cortex (**A**) and cerebral cortex (**B**) follows different mechanisms. In the cerebellum an earlier wave of ventricular neurogenesis gives rise to neurons that migrate radially outward to the surface. This is followed later by a second wave of neurogenesis in a lateral germinal zone from which neural precursor cells migrate onto the surface, where they divide and migrate inward to form the granule layer. In the cerebral cortex all neurons arise from the ventricular zone (VZ) and migrate radially outward to the surface. The oldest neurons are located in the deeper layers of the cortex and the younger neurons are located in progressively more superficial cortical layers (PCs, Purkinje cells; PCL, Purkinje cell layer).

nal hypothalamic sulcus into the dorsal part, which will become the thalamus, and a ventral part, which will develop into the subthalamus laterally and the hypothalamus medially. Earlier-formed alar plate neurons migrate to what will be the lateral thalamic and subthalamic nuclei, and later-formed neurons will form progressively more medial thalamic nuclei and hypothalamic nuclei. The formation of the diencephalic nuclei, especially in the thalamus, results in the narrowing of the third ventricle, and frequently the thalami fuse in the midline, forming the massa intermedia or interthalamic adhesion. The roof plate develops into the epithalamus or pineal gland.

Two structures develop away from the diencephalon. From the floor of the third ventricle an infundibular stalk evaginates downward to make contact with an upward expanding Rathke's pouch. These two structures fuse and form the pituitary gland or hypophysis. The anterior hypophysis or adenohypophysis forms from Rathke's pouch, whereas the posterior part of the hypophysis or neurohypophysis develops from the infundibular stalk through which axons grow down from the hypothalamus.

From the ventral part of the diencephalon an optic vesicle extends toward the surface of the ectoderm. This vesicle remains attached to the diencephalon by the optic stalk in which is a luminal extension of the third ventricle. An expanded tip of the optic vesicle invaginates, eventually becoming the neural retina of the eye. The optic vesicle contacting the surface ectoderm results in the formation of a lens placode from which the remaining internal components of the eye develop. Mesenchyme surrounding the optic stalk and disc differentiate into the coverings of the eye. It is important to remember that the retina is a derivative of the neuroectoderm and as such an extension of the CNS. Developing axons from the retina will grow back to the diencephalon through the optic stalk, forming the optic nerves, chiasm, and tracts.

TELENCEPHALON The rostral end of the neural tube gives rise to the telencephalon. From the lateral sides of the neural tube outpockets develop with extensions from the lumen of the neural tube. These cavities will form the lateral ventricles in the cerebral hemispheres and will remain connected to the diencephalic third ventricle via the interventricular foramen of Monro

on each side. The telencephalon is composed of the cortex forming the cerebral hemispheres and nuclei buried in the cerebral hemisphere and surrounded, except on the ventral surface, by white matter.

The cerebral cortex is layered and develops in an inside-outside direction (Fig. 24-4B). The phylogenetically newest part of the cortex, which constitutes the bulk of cortical gray matter, is the six-layered neocortex. Waves of immature neurons migrate outward along radial glia processes to a cortical plate. The earliest generated cortical neurons form what will be the deeper layers of the cortex (layers V and VI). At this time the axons of these neurons are developing their axonal projections to subcortical areas. Neurons generated later follow successively along the radial glia and form progressively more superficial cortical layers. The morphologic and functional organization of the cerebral cortex in vertically oriented columns is owing to the vertically direct migration of neurons by the radial glia. The relatively consistent formation of cortical folds (gyri) separated by shallow fissures (sulci) within the lobes of the cerebral hemispheres is the result of differential production and migration of cortical neurons.

The prodigious growth of the cerebral hemispheres results in their covering the diencephalon, mesencephalon, and cerebellum. The hemispheres become connected to each other by commissures of growing axons between the two sides, the largest of which is the corpus callosum. The hemispheres are connected to the other parts of the CNS by axonal pathways growing from the thalamus to the cerebrum and from the cerebrum to subcortical structures by the large internal capsule.

CLINICAL CONNECTION

Defects in neurogenesis, neuronal migration, or postmigratory differentiation can result in the abnormal development of the cerebral cortex. When gyri fail to develop the cortex is smooth or lissencephalic in appearance. Atypically large (pachygyria) or small (microgyria) gyri also occur with abnormal cortical development. Other developmental disorders result in the abnormal positioning of migrating cortical neurons to inappropriate layers or confined to the subcortical white matter.

Chapter Review Questions

24-1. The CNS develops from what layer of the gastrula?

24-2. Which develops from the neural crest?

24-3. What developmental defect results in anencephaly?

24-4. What is the importance of the notochord in the development of the CNS?

24-5. What specialized glia are critically important for guiding migratory neurons?

24-6. Generally, in early development there is an overproduction of neurons whose number is pared down by apoptosis during continued maturation. What underlies the selective death of the surfeit neurons?

24-7. How is neuronal migration in the cerebellar cortex different from that in the cerebral cortex?

24-8. What is the name of the condition in which cortical gyri fail to develop?

CHAPTER 25

Aging of the Nervous System: Dementia

FOR SEVERAL YEARS a relatively healthy 80-year-old widow who lives alone changed from being socially active and very independent of her children to her condition now, in which she becomes frequently confused about relatively minor events and has significant problems remembering recent conversations she's had with her children. Lately she started confabulating stories in an attempt to explain why she does not remember something. During the last 12 months quarterly appointments with her geriatrician have demonstrated her scores on the Mini Mental Status Exam to be progressively declining.

There exists a biologic clock in the nuclei of cells. Aging, the process of ever-increasing and accumulating genetic mutations coupled with an ever-declining capability of cell divisions, is ongoing throughout life, but typically is not manifested until more senior years. All organ systems show age-related changes. During normal aging of the brain there is an accumulation of lipofuscin, lysosomally degraded intracellular proteins resulting in the accumulation of lipoproteinaceous pigments. Age-related changes in the brain are typically manifested behaviorally by a progressive decline in memory and cognitive abilities, including learning, comprehension, visual and auditory acuity, analytical skills and problem solving, speed of voluntary and reflexive movements, and possibly abnormal behavioral changes. There is great variation as to the age of onset, the temporal progression, and severity of dysfunction in individuals. **Senile dementia** is a clinical syndrome defined by the Diagnostic and Statistical Manual (DSM IV) of the American Psychiatric Association that is characterized by the loss of memory coupled with a cognitive deficit such as language, problem solving, and impaired social and occupational functioning. Dementia can be irreversible or reversible.

TYPES OF SENILE DEMENTIA

ALZHEIMER DISEASE

The most prevalent form of irreversible senile dementia is Alzheimer disease. Alzheimer disease affects approximately 7% of individuals older than 60 and 40% of individuals older than 80. Alzheimer disease can appear earlier in life in individuals with a familial history of early-onset dementia.

The cause for Alzheimer disease is unknown, and corresponding risk factors predictive of the disorder are imprecise. Other than a brain biopsy, there is not a diagnostic test for Alzheimer disease; rather, the disorder can only be confirmed at autopsy by the presence of characteristic light microscopic pathologic changes in the brain. These neurohistologic

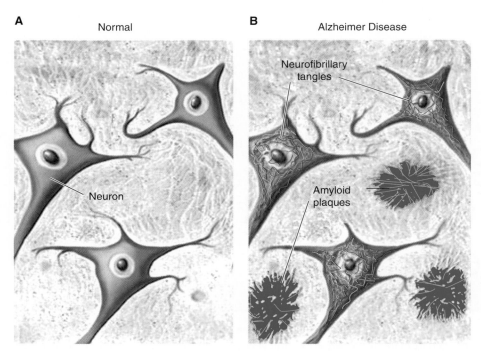

A Normal   **B** Alzheimer Disease

Figure 25-1   Neuropathologic changes in the brain from a patient with Alzheimer disease. **A.** Normal neurons. **B.** Senile plaque of amyloid protein surrounding an intact neuron. The surrounded neuron will eventually degenerate as the result of the amyloid deposit. Neurofibrillary tangles are densely packed in a neuron's soma and processes. This neuron will degenerate as the result of the abnormal accumulation of these fibrils.

changes include observations of abnormal protein deposits (Fig. 25-1) and the degeneration of neurons in specific parts of the brain (Fig. 25-2). Preceding the death of neurons abnormalities in the cell's cytoskeleton appear. **Neurofibrillary tangles** of the microtubule binding protein tau form in the soma and proximal dendrites of neurons. These cytoskeletal protein tangles initially impede cellular metabolism and axoplasmic transport, leading to impaired synaptic function and eventually to neuronal death. After the death of neurons the insoluble neurofibrillary tangles remain in the extracellular space as evidence of their cells' demise.

Extracellular deposits of another protein result in the formation of **amyloid senile plaques** in the neuropil (Fig. 25-1B) and walls of cerebral blood vessels. Amyloid protein is derived from a larger amyloid precursor protein synthesized in the endoplasmic reticulum and inserted in the membrane of dendrites, axons, and cell bodies of neurons. The function of the amyloid precursor protein is unknown. The extracellular domain of the amyloid precursor protein is cleaved, resulting in the

formation of the amyloid plaques. Senile plaques are frequently associated with abnormal neurons, astrocytic processes, and activated microglia. It is assumed that the amyloid protein is toxic to surrounding structures.

Neurofibrillary tangles and senile plaques are not uniformly distributed in the cortex. Neurofibrillary tangles are densest in the parahippocampal gyrus, the entorhinal cortex, and the temporal pole. There is a relatively low density of tangles in the primary motor and sensory cortices. Less pervasive than neurofibrillary tangles, senile plaques are most common in the temporal and posterior parietal lobes.

Neuron Loss

By 80 years of age the brain normally has decreased in weight by about 15%. This shrinkage is caused in part by diminished protein syntheses in older neurons but, in itself, is not correlated with senescence. Part of the decrease may be attributable to shrinkage in the size of neurons, particularly larger

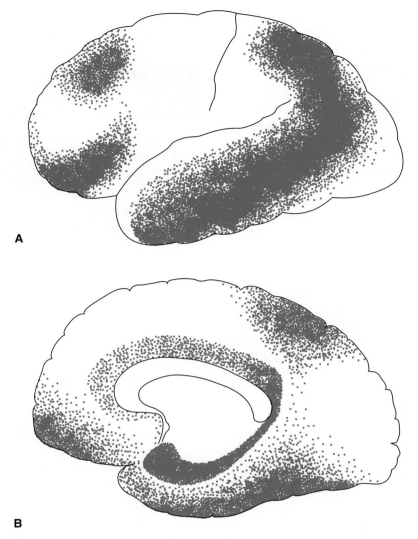

A

B

Figure 25-2 Representative drawings of the lateral (**A**) and medial (**B**) surfaces of the cerebral hemispheres to indicate the distribution and relative density of neurodegenerative changes (neuronal death, neurofibrillary tangles, and senile plaques) occurring in Alzheimer disease. The intensity of the shading from light to dark reflects progressively increased neuropathologic disease.

cells like cortical pyramidal neurons, coincident with atrophy of the dendritic spines and branches. Coincident with shrinkage of dendrites is a 15 to 20% loss of synapses. In demented individuals the decrease in synaptic contacts is much greater.

Specific types of neurons in regionally restricted parts of the brain degenerate in Alzheimer disease. This is characterized by a "thinning" of the gyri and a widening of the sulci. Thus, the combination of dendritic shrinkage and neuronal death results in morphologic changes character-

ized as **brain atrophy**. In the prefrontal, posterior parietal, and temporal lobes pyramidal neurons selectively degenerate (Fig. 25-2), contributing to alterations in mood, sleeping patterns, awareness of the external environment, and memory. Supranormal degeneration of cholinergic neurons in the basal nucleus of Meynert and noradrenergic neurons in the locus ceruleus probably contribute to the memory impairment and impaired attention as well. Degeneration of neurons in the amygdala and anterior thalamic nucleus underlie abnormal behaviors. At this time there is no efficacious therapeutic treatment for Alzheimer disease.

VASCULAR AND OTHER DEMENTIAS

The second leading cause of dementia in the elderly is attributable to cerebrovascular disease and accounts for 10 to 20% of all cases of senile dementia. Vascular dementia results from multiple sublethal infarcts that occur during a temporally protracted period in spatially widespread areas of the cerebrum that cumulatively result in memory impairment and behavioral abnormalities. Unlike Alzheimer disease, vascular dementia has an uneven distribution of deficits and frequently can be associated with identifiable cerebrovascular disease and focal brain damage as manifested, for example, by unilateral pyramidal system signs. Hypertension is the single most predictive risk factor for vascular dementia. Other causes include diabetes mellitus, tobacco and alcohol use, cardiac arrhythmias, and other heart-related diseases. Being able to identify the risk factors associated with vascular dementia allows for preventive therapeutic strategies to include treatment for hypertension, smoking cessation, control of diabetes, and other treatment regimens.

Individuals can also suffer from a variable combination of Alzheimer and vascular dementia with both vascular disease and degenerative changes in the cerebrum. Other forms of irreversible dementia are of subcortical origin such as occurs in patients with Parkinson or Huntington disorders and some hereditary spinocerebellar ataxias. Dementia resulting from chronic alcoholism is irreversible, but not progressive if alcohol consumption is curtailed. Reversible causes of dementia include toxic drug interactions, electrolyte imbalances, infections, and metabolic and endocrine disorders.

CLINICAL CONNECTION

Experimental findings, principally in aged rats, strongly support the maxim "use it or lose it." Similar to skeletal muscles, which atrophy as the result of denervation inactivity, the structure of aging central nervous system neurons appears to be tightly linked to work and mental stimulation and activity. Rats housed under environmentally austere conditions, not unlike institutionalized senior citizens, experience the loss of synapses and dendritic spines on cortical neurons. Conversely, when similarly aged rats, not unlike senior neuroanatomists, are maintained in environmentally enriched housing, there is a significant increase in synaptic contacts (plasticity). The preservation of mental capacity has also been shown to be linked to diet, weight, and exercise.

Chapter Review Questions

25-1. What are the hallmark neuropathologic changes seen in the postmortem brains of Alzheimer patients?

25-2. What is the most common cause of senile dementia?

25-3. Magnetic resonance imaging of the brain of a patient with atrophy of the brain would reveal what neuropathologic changes?

25-4. Where do most neuropathologic changes occur in the aging cerebral cortex?

26

Recovery of Function of the Nervous System: Plasticity and Regeneration

TWO ADULT MEN involved in an automobile accident suffered nervous system injuries. In one patient the PNS was damaged, and in the other patient the lesion was in the CNS. Although some neurologic abnormalities were different in the two patients, they both had paralysis of the fingers in the right hand. The families of the patients inquired about the possibility of functional recovery.

For more than a century and a half the soma or cell body of the neuron was considered the trophic center because of the concentration of organelles that metabolically support the entire neuron. All dendrites and the axon are absolutely dependent for their nourishment and survival on active transport mechanisms that move essential nutrients from the soma into axons and dendrites. Intraaxonal transport is bidirectional with different components transported at different rates and directions. Organelles and vesicles needed for synaptic transmission are generally moved by fast anterograde axonal transport (100 to 400 mm/day), whereas homeostasis of axonal structure is largely supported by slow anterograde axonal transport (1 to 2 mm/day) of cytoskeletal and axolemmal proteins and essential metabolites needed for oxidative phosphorylation and glycolysis. Retrograde transport (100 to 200 mm/day) returns from the axonal terminal waste products of normal metabolism and tropic signals from target structures.

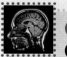

CLINICAL CONNECTION

In addition to normal trophic signaling from the periphery, retrograde transport may have a deleterious effect on neurons with the incorporation and transport of pathogenic proteins and viruses such as tetanus toxin, rabies, and polio. Alternatively, anterograde transport can move the herpes zoster virus centrifugally and result in shingles.

WALLERIAN OR ANTEROGRADE AXONAL DEGENERATION IN THE PERIPHERAL NERVOUS SYSTEM

Axons degenerate directly as the result of traumatic injury or indirectly as the result of toxins, inflammation, metabolic and myelin disorders, and ischemia. Wallerian or anterograde axonal degeneration occurs from the site of injury distally to the terminals (Fig. 26-1). Axotomy, the separation of an axon into proximal and distal segments, triggers a cascade of events all along the axon distal to the injury site and locally in the axon just proximal to the injury site. Within hours after severing an axon the proximal axonal segment seals itself by calcium-mediated fusing of intraaxonal vesicles with the opened axolemma membrane, resulting in the formation of a progressively smaller opening followed by closure and the reestablishment of ionic balances. Axoplasmic transport and action potential propagation continue in the distal axon segment during a relatively short postinjury latent period. Distally, there is a proximal to distal depletion of the metabolic substrates for mitochondrial energy production necessary for the maintenance of ionic gradients. Depressed ATP production eventually results in the change in membrane permeability in the distal axon segment, starting first at the site of injury and continuing over time distally. The loss of ionic gradients allows water to enter the axon, resulting in swelling and, more deleterious, the influx of sodium and calcium ions. The rise in intraaxonal calcium is both necessary and sufficient to trigger the physical degeneration of the axon. Elevated intraaxonal calcium activates photolytic enzymes, which mediate the breakdown of the cytoskeleton followed by the axolemma. The onset of axonal degeneration is closely followed by the fragmentation of the surrounding myelin into progressively smaller droplets. Macrophages are activated within several days of the injury by the release of bioactive molecules from the Schwann cells. The macrophages degrade the myelin sheath and phagocytize the proteolipid debris. The rapid removal of myelin debris in a peripheral nerve is essential for later recovery and necessary for activating mitogenesis of Schwann cells and removal of myelin-associated proteins, which can block axonal regrowth. Although axonal degeneration is always followed by degeneration of surrounding myelin, the reverse in not necessarily the case. Demyelinating peripheral neuropathies do not trigger axonal degeneration. Rather the axons remain anatomically and functionally intact, and attempts to remyelinate are undertaken.

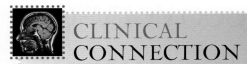

CLINICAL CONNECTION

Recent experimental findings in mice with a mutation characterized phenotypically as Wallerian-like degeneration slow (*Wlds*) have begun to challenge the concept that interrupted axonal transport leading to mitochondrial dysfunction and an increase in intraaxonal calcium immediately trigger axonal degeneration in the injured distal segment. Transected axons in *Wlds* mice continue to propagate action potentials up to 2 weeks after injury, and the physical breakdown of the axon can be prolonged for a similar period of time. The activation of astrocytes, macrophages, and microglia is also delayed and prolonged in mice carrying the *Wlds* mutation. Interestingly the *Wlds* mutation does not appear to rescue neuronal cell bodies from dying after axotomy. Although it appears that the *Wlds* protein can promote axonal survival by yet undefined mechanisms, there is tremendous potential for this discovery to lead to important therapeutic advances in treating damaged axonal tracts and nerves.

FUNCTIONAL RECOVERY AFTER AXONAL INJURY IN THE PERIPHERAL NERVOUS SYSTEM

Axons in the peripheral nervous system (PNS) can regenerate after injury. From a bulbous expansion of the proximal axon sprouts form within several hours, but this is an abortive process as the sprouts lack the necessary support from the cell body for continued growth and quickly degenerate. Successful axonal regeneration depends on the neuronal cell body surviving axotomy.

THE AXON REACTION

Within hours after axotomy, ultrastructural changes are observed in the cell bodies of axotomized

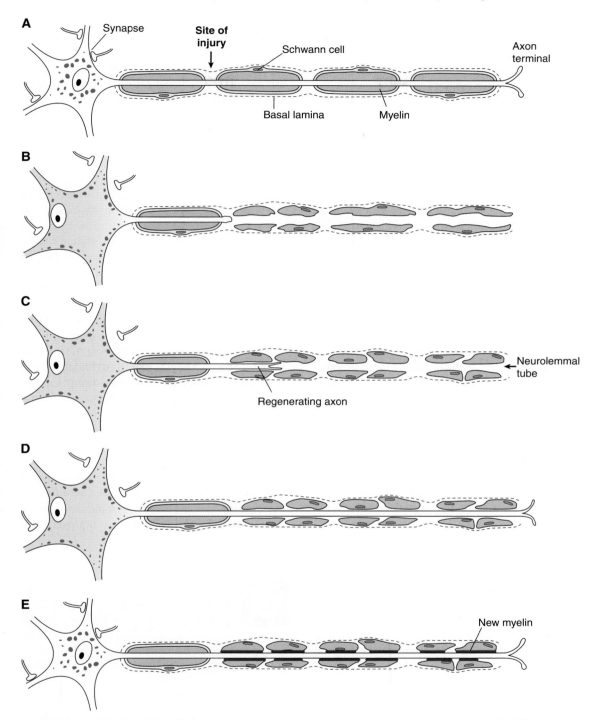

Figure 26-1   Sequela of morphologic changes after injury to a myelinated PNS axon. **A.** Normal cell body and myelinated axon. **B.** Axon reaction characterized by chromatolysis, swelling, and eccentric nucleus in cell body and Wallerian or anterograde degeneration of axon and its myelin. **C.** Growth sprout initially regenerating into neurolemmal tube formed by Schwann cells. **D.** Axon regenerating to effector site. **E.** Return to normal: functional regeneration.

neurons. Several days later characteristic neurohistologic changes are evident that collectively constitute the **axon reaction** (Fig. 26-1B). These changes include the movement of the nucleus to an eccentric location adjacent to the cell membrane and often directly across from the axon hillock. Secondary to altered ionic pump properties and resultant changes in membrane permeability, the soma swells. Most characteristic is the dissolution of the dense clumps of rough endoplasmic reticulum or Nissl bodies leading to **chromatolysis** or loss of basophilic staining. There is an increase in the size of the nucleolus. Finally, synaptic boutons disconnect from the dendrites and soma of the now dysfunctional neuron.

There are a number of determinants for survival of an axotomized neuron: proximity of injury site to the cell body and the correlated loss of axoplasm, proportion of surviving collateral projections providing access to target-derived trophic factors, and finally, age of the patient with evidence that damage in the young is more deleterious than in the old. If the threshold for continued degeneration has not been crossed, axotomized neurons will attempt to regenerate their axon from the site of injury distally.

AXONAL REGENERATION IN THE PNS

Sustained regrowth of an axon starts from the proximal end of a severed stump and continues with the addition of new axonal membrane at the leading edge of the regenerating axon. Growth cones, not unlike those in development, search for molecular signals to guide them toward their targets. Schwann cells are critical elements for successful regeneration. Beginning 3 to 4 days after injury, mitogens released by invading macrophages trigger the division of Schwann cells along the length of the nerve segment. Chemoattractants or **tropic** substances released by Schwann cells provide guidance signals for regrowing axons to extend distally.

The degree of functional regeneration largely depends on the type of injury. The greatest chance for functional regeneration occurs after compressive or ischemic nerve injury in which the neurolemmal tube and basal lamina remain virtually intact as occurred in the patient in the case history at the beginning of this chapter with a PNS com-

pression injury to the median and ulnar nerves. Regenerating axons grow into the tube they originally occupied. The strength of attraction of tropic signals is concentration dependent. When regenerating axons are challenged to grow across an injury site where the proximal and distal nerve stumps are spatially separated, the chances for functional recovery become diminished and largely depend on the distance between the two nerve ends. In clean-cut types of injury, e.g., a razor blade or sharp knife, the proximal and distal stumps can be aligned and surgically sutured together. Ideally the cut ends of the larger nerve fascicles can be approximated and oriented such that the regenerating axons have a greater chance to grow into their original neurolemmal tube. Functional recovery is least likely after nerve injuries such as gun shots, in which a relatively long segment of nerve is obliterated. Under these conditions strategies to surgically repair the injury can include the approximation and suturing of the proximal and distal nerve stumps by positioning and fixating the limb to bring the two surfaces together. Other treatments to bridge the gap between proximal and distal nerve stumps include the grafting of nerve segments harvested from a different nerve from the patient or connecting the two segments with a biodegradable tube through which regenerating axons are grossly guided to the distal stump. In all cases it is critical to bring the proximal and distal nerve stumps within several millimeters of each other because the diffusion of sufficient concentrations of tropic signals from Schwann cells in the distal stump is limited by this distance.

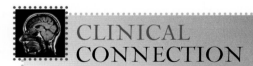

CLINICAL CONNECTION

A neuroma can develop at the site of peripheral nerve injury when regenerating sensory axons fail to reenter neurolemmal tubes. Blindly ending sensory axons can be activated by nonphysiologic stimuli resulting in the transmission of painful sensations to the CNS. This phenomenon is considered the basis for phantom limb pain.

It was once generally thought that regenerating axons would grow into any vacant distal neurolemmal tube. Recent findings indicate that neurolemmal tubes that surrounded motor or sensory axons selectively attract the same type of regenerating axons.

Axons regenerate 1 to 2 mm/day, the rate of slow axoplasmic transport. On reaching the distal end of the neurolemmal tube and the effector muscle or gland for a motor axon, or a receptor for a sensory axon, functional connections are reestablished. Once reconnected, trophic signals are conveyed retrogradely to the cell body where, over time, the morphologic organization of the cell returns to normal and the disengaged synapses reestablish functional connections with the soma and dendritic membrane (Fig. 26-1E). The regenerated axon also becomes remyelinated. If the connection of the regenerated axon is inappropriate, i.e., a motor axon with a sensory receptor or vice versa, the trophic signal returning to the cell body is recognized as inappropriate and the cell and its axons will degenerate. Schwann cells surrounding inappropriately connected regenerated axons or hollow neurolemmal tubes will degenerate with time.

FUNCTIONAL RECOVERY AFTER AXONAL INJURY IN THE CENTRAL NERVOUS SYSTEM

After injury, central nervous system (CNS) axons undergo anterograde axonal degeneration for the same reasons as axons in the PNS. Axotomized central neurons similarly undergo retrograde axon reaction, and continued survival or eventual death is based on proximity of the lesion to the cell body, sustaining collaterals, and age. However, unlike in the PNS, functional regeneration does not occur after damage to CNS axons. Injured CNS axons have the intrinsic capacity to regenerate, but a number of extrinsic factors preclude functional reinnervation. Spinal cord injury best illustrates these constraints. At the site of spinal injury reactive astrocytes divide or enlarge to form an impenetrable physical barrier or glial scar around the injury site to protect degeneration and inflammatory reactions from spreading into undamaged areas, as well as to reestablish the blood-brain barrier. The reactive astrocytes also produce proteoglycans that act as a chemical barrier that is inhibitory to axonal

regrowth. Spinal trauma can result in the formation of a central cavity surrounded by a rim of intact tissue or alternatively a complete separation of the spinal cord. In either type of injury there is a significant gap that regenerating axons must bridge to grow to distant targets. Finally, three proteins in the oligodendroglial membrane of myelinated central axons interact with a single receptor (Nogo) on the leading edge of regenerating axonal growth cones. These myelin proteins trigger the immediate collapse of the growth cones, thereby inhibiting axonal regeneration.

If regenerating axons were induced to grow past a glial scar, across or around a cavity or separation, and through the nonpermissive substrate of CNS myelin, the final obstacle would be for the axons to reach their appropriate target neurons. Unlike in the PNS where regenerating axons are guided to their destinations by the neurolemmal tubes formed by Schwann cells and the basal lamina and where each Schwann cell is dedicated to a single axon, in the CNS there are no neurolemmal tubelike guidance channels, and oligodendroglia myelinate many different axons.

Although there are significant impediments for any functionally meaningful CNS axonal regeneration, experimental findings are encouraging that show that exogenous trophic factors, stems cells, Schwann cells, and gene therapy can promote, in a limited manner, central axonal regeneration.

CNS PLASTICITY

It was thought for many years that once central axonal connections formed during development they remain immutable throughout life. Basic research during the past 40 years in animals and more recent functional imaging studies in humans have shown the nervous system to be very modifiable or plastic. **Plasticity** in both neuronal morphology and electrical responsiveness occurs with normal changes in the internal milieu of the nervous system, with external changes in environment, and with behavioral adaptations, as well as with injury to the CNS. Functional plasticity occurs in diverse CNS systems and can include changes in hypothalamic nuclei during pregnancy and lactation, in the motor system at multiple levels with the learning of new motor skills during practice and training, and in sensory systems in response to novel external stimuli. Connectional plasticity can be simple changes in synaptic efficacy such as that which occurs presynaptically in short-term facilitation and post-tetanic potentiation, or occurs postsynaptically with long-term potentiation and long-term depression. Morphologic changes can include presynaptic remodeling of axonal terminal arbors or postsynaptic distal dendrites or dendritic spines.

LESION-INDUCED PLASTICITY

As neurogenesis in the adult is very restricted, limited to the birth of new primary neurons in the olfactory mucosa and new granule cells in the hippocampus, and CNS axonal regeneration does not occur, it may be surmised that the partial functional recovery that occurs after CNS trauma or stroke is the result of **lesion-induced plasticity.** The extent of central plasticity is age and systems dependent.

DEVELOPMENTAL PLASTICITY

One form of developmental plasticity seen after early CNS lesions is the persistence of normally transient neurons and connections. Surfeit or exuberant connections develop along with axonal circuits that normally persist into the adult. When these latter connections are damaged, the normally transient axonal projections can persist and maintain synaptic input to target neurons. As the result of ongoing growth-related gene expression, undamaged axons of immature neurons can develop additional axonal terminal arbors or collateral sprouts, as well as redirect axonal growth to denervated targets. Regenerative sprouting of terminal arbors or more distant collaterals may also develop from damaged axons. New or regenerating axons can grow up to several hundreds of micrometers. This new or regenerated axonal growth is also possible because axonal growth inhibitory molecules, present in the adult, have not yet developed to the point that they form a nonpermissive environment for axonal elongation.

ADULT PLASTICITY

Lesion-induced plasticity of adult axonal connections is much more spatially restricted and temporally protracted than in the immature nervous system. Generally new synaptic connections only form by **reactive synaptogenesis,** in which synapses lost as the result of injury are replaced by terminal sprouting from surviving axons in the immediate area (Fig. 26-2). Quantitative studies of reactive synaptogenesis in adult animals have convincingly shown that new synapses formed by surviving afferent terminals are very similar in both number and physiologic efficacy to the lost synaptic inputs. There is a hierarchic specificity in terminal sprouting. Surviving homologous afferents (from the same system) have the highest preference for replacing lost inputs, followed by non-homologous but functionally related surviving afferents (e.g., excitatory surviving afferents replacing lost excitatory afferents), followed by non-homologous, functionally disparate afferents (e.g., inhibitory afferents replacing excitatory afferents). Some synapses can never be replaced as is the case with the patient in the case history at the beginning of this chapter. This patient had CNS trauma that damaged the lateral corticospinal tract including projections to spinal lower motor neurons innervating the intrinsic muscles of the hand. Although there may be partial recovery of some proximal movements, independent, voluntary movements of the fingers will never return.

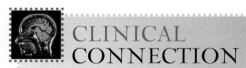

CLINICAL CONNECTION

Two examples illustrate the plasticity of the adult sensory systems. First, after amputation of a digit the cortical area of representation for the lost digit is replaced by sensory inputs expanding from the immediately adjacent representation areas of intact digits, thereby increasing the cortical "sensitivity" for these digits. Cross-modality sensory plasticity occurs in blind patients trained to "read" Braille. Blind patients reportedly have greater tactile discrimination resolution in the fingerpads compared with sighted individuals. In addition, sound localization and speech discrimination are enhanced in blind individuals compared with sighted individuals.

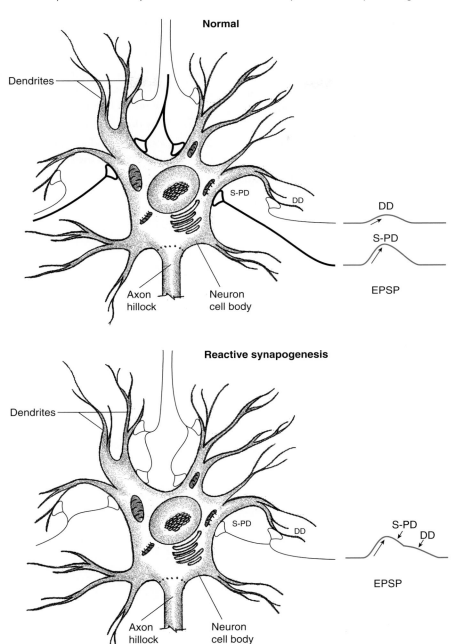

Figure 26-2   Two different afferent pathways are spatially segregated in their terminations on the soma–proximal dendrites (S-PD) or the distal dendrites (DD) of a neuron. Activation of the terminals on S-PD evokes excitatory postsynaptic potentials (EPSPs) with faster rise times (arrow) and greater amplitudes than the EPSPs evoked after activation of terminals on the DD. If the S-PD afferent terminals degenerate, they are replaced by terminal sprouting from the surviving afferents on the DD. Activation of these combined S-PD and DD synapses evokes EPSPs with properties for both their S-PD and DD locations.

Chapter Review Questions

26-1.   What is the causative basis for anterograde axonal (Wallerian) degeneration?

26-2.   What are the characteristic neurohistologic changes in the cell body of an axotomized neuron?

26-3.   What is the critical determinant for a neuron to survive axonal injury?

26-4.   What three factors preclude successful axonal regeneration in the CNS?

26-5.   What is the function of neurotropic molecules synthesized by injury-activated Schwann cells?

26-6.   What type of injury to a peripheral nerve would predictably result in the greatest amount of functional regeneration?

26-7.   Why does a neuroma form?

26-8.   Does lesion-induced plasticity always occur everywhere in the CNS?

Principles for Locating Lesions and Clinical Illustrations

*F*ocal lesions in the central nervous system (CNS) can be localized by the manifestations of long pathway involvement and the segmental distribution of the abnormalities. The most important long pathways in the brainstem and spinal cord are the pyramidal tract, the spinothalamic tract, the dorsal column-medial lemniscus path, and the spinal trigeminal tract. Long pathways in the cerebral hemispheres are the pyramidal and corticobulbar tracts, the somatosensory thalamic radiation, and the visual pathway.

SPINAL CORD

The major long paths in the spinal cord are the pyramidal or lateral corticospinal tract, the spinothalamic tract, and the dorsal column tracts (gracile and cuneate). The level of a spinal cord lesion may be determined by the loss of functions in dermatomes and myotomes.

The key to localizing lesions in the spinal cord is the loss of motor or sensory functions or both below the foramen magnum, i.e., in the area of distribution of the spinal nerves. (Two exceptions are Horner syndrome, which may

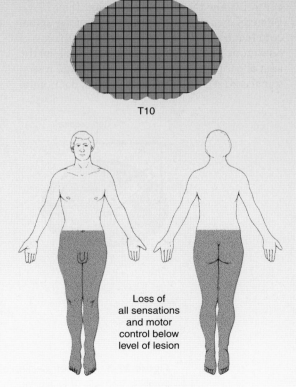

T10

Loss of all sensations and motor control below level of lesion

Figure 27-1 Spinal cord transection.

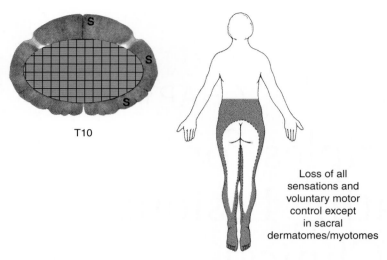

Figure 27-2 Central cord syndrome: sacral sparing. (S = sacral region.)

occur after cervical or upper thoracic spinal cord lesions, and somatosensory losses on the back of the head and scalp, which may occur after lesions in spinal cord segments C2 and C3.) Spinal cord transection results in an immediate and permanent loss of all sensations and voluntary motor control below the level of the lesion (Fig. 27-1). Bilateral damage of the central part of the spinal cord (central cord syndrome) results in the loss of sensations and voluntary motor control in the area of peripheral distribution of the more rostral spinal cord segments below the lesion, but not the

more caudal. This "sacral sparing" phenomenon occurs because of the somatotopic localization in the long ascending and descending pathways, i.e., the more rostral spinal nerves are represented internal to the more caudal (Fig. 27-2). Spinal cord hemisection causes damage to the lateral corticospinal tract and dorsal column, resulting in spastic paralysis and the loss of tactile, vibration, and proprioception senses ipsilaterally, and damage to the spinothalamic tract, resulting in the loss of pain and temperature senses contralaterally (Fig. 27-3). Lesions involving the ventral white

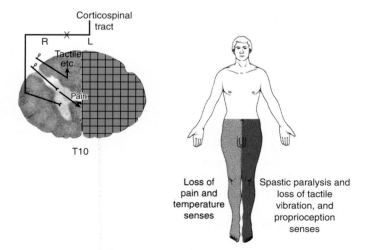

Figure 27-3 Left hemisection of spinal cord at T10. Spastic paralysis and loss of tactile, vibration, and proprioceptive senses on left (L, ipsilateral) side and loss of pain and temperature senses on right (R, contralateral) side.

commissure result in the loss of pain and temperature sensations bilaterally in approximately the same dermatomes as the lesion. This phenomenon usually results from syringomyelia or cavitation of the spinal cord and is called the commissural syndrome (Fig. 27-4).

BRAINSTEM

The major long paths in the brainstem are the pyramidal or corticospinal tract, spinothalamic tract, medial lemniscus, spinal trigeminal tract, and the superior cerebellar peduncle. The level of a brainstem lesion is most readily identified by the cranial nerve involved in the lesion. In general, focal brainstem lesions can be divided into two groups—those located in the medial parts and

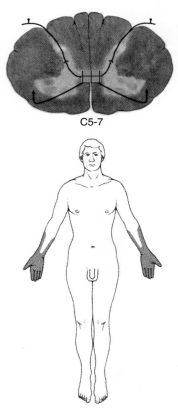

Figure 27-4 Commissural syndrome. Lesion of ventral white commissure results in bilaterally symmetric loss of pain and temperature in dermatomal distribution of spinal cord segments involved.

those located in the lateral parts of the medulla, pons, or midbrain.

MEDIAL BRAINSTEM LESIONS

Lesions located in the medial part of the brainstem involve the pyramidal tract and result in a contralateral spastic hemiplegia. The level of the lesion can be determined by involvement of the hypoglossal, abducens, or oculomotor nerve (Fig. 27-5), all of which emerge close to the pyramidal tract.

LATERAL BRAINSTEM LESIONS

Lesions involving the lateral part of the brainstem usually involve the spinothalamic tract. In the medulla and caudal pons, the spinothalamic and spinal trigeminal tracts are close to each other. When a lesion involves both tracts, pain and temperature sensations are impaired in the face ipsilaterally and the trunk and limbs contralaterally (Fig. 27-6). The level of such a lesion can be determined by involvement of cranial nerves VII, VIII, IX, or X.

Lateral brainstem lesions at more rostral levels involve, in addition to the spinothalamic tract, the motor and principal trigeminal nuclei at midpons (Fig. 27-6), the superior cerebellar peduncle at rostral pons (Fig. 27-7) and caudal midbrain, and the medial lemniscus and trigeminothalamic tracts at rostral midbrain (Fig. 27-8).

CEREBRAL HEMISPHERE

Focal lesions involving the long paths in the cerebral hemisphere are manifested on the contralateral side of the body. The most common site of long pathway involvement in the cerebral hemisphere is the internal capsule, where the pyramidal tract and thalamic somatosensory radiations are adjacent to each other, and the corticobulbar tract is nearby (Fig. 16-5A). Such a lesion results in contralateral spastic hemiplegia, contralateral hemianesthesia, and contralateral lower face weakness (Fig. 27-9), if located in the more dorsal part of the internal capsule. A more ventral capsular lesion may also involve the optic radiation (Fig. 16-5B), resulting in contralateral homonymous hemianopsia in addition to the other three abnormalities.

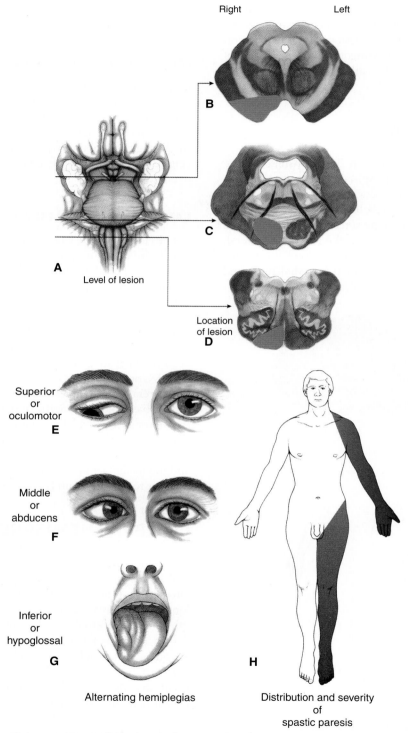

Figure 27-5   Medial brainstem lesions at the levels of cranial nerves (CN) III, VI, and XII. **A.** Level of lesion. **B.** CN III and pyramidal tract lesion. **C.** CN VI and pyramidal tract lesion. **D.** CN XII and pyramidal tract lesion. **E.** Oculomotor palsy. **F.** Abducens palsy. **G.** Hypoglossal palsy. **H.** Spastic weakness, more severe distally in upper and lower limbs.

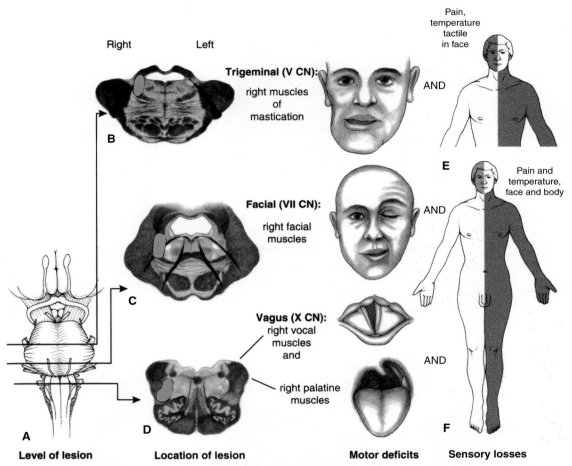

| Level of lesion | Location of lesion | Motor deficits | Sensory losses |

Figure 27-6   Lateral brainstem lesions. **A.** Level of lesion, lesion in lateral tegmentum. **B.** At midpons. **C.** At caudal pons. **D.** At rostral medulla. **E.** All somatosensations in ipsilateral face (principal nucleus and spinal trigeminal tract), pain and temperature in contralateral limbs, trunk, and neck (spinothalamic tract). **F.** Pain and temperature in ipsilateral face (spinal trigeminal tract), and contralateral limbs, trunk, and neck (spinothalamic tract). Dark shading: all sensations. Light shading: pain and temperature only. (CN, cranial nerve.)

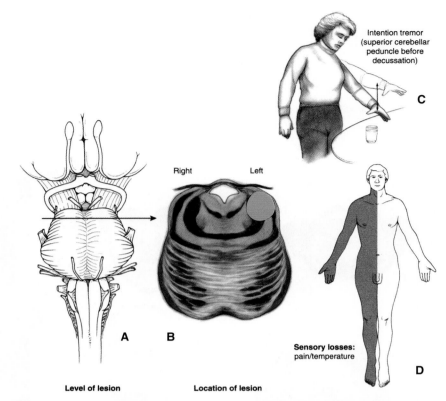

Figure 27-7   Lateral brainstem lesion. **A.** Level of lesion: rostral pons. **B.** Lesion in left lateral tegmentum. **C.** Ipsilateral (left) intention tremor (left superior cerebellar peduncle before decussation). **D.** Contralateral (right) pain and temperature losses (left spinothalamic tract).

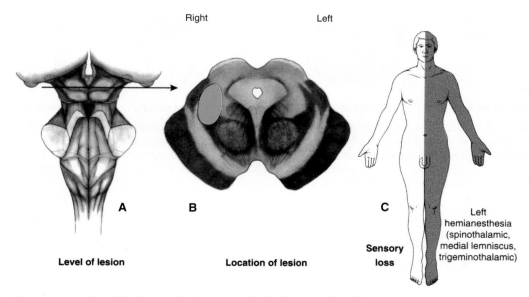

Figure 27-8   Lateral brainstem lesion. **A.** Level of lesion: rostral midbrain. **B.** Lesion in right somatosensory paths. **C.** Contralateral (left) hemisensory loss.

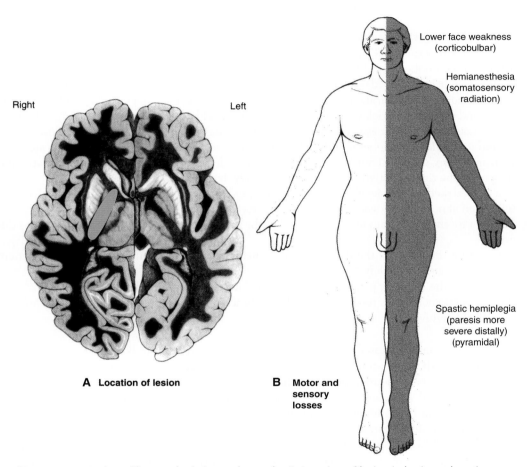

Right

Left

A Location of lesion

Lower face weakness
(corticobulbar)

Hemianesthesia
(somatosensory
radiation)

Spastic hemiplegia
(paresis more
severe distally)
(pyramidal)

**B Motor and
sensory
losses**

Figure 27-9 Lesion of long paths in internal capsule. **A.** Location of lesion in horizontal section. **B.** Motor and sensory losses.

CLINICAL ILLUSTRATIONS

1. An 11-year-old girl complained of pain in the neck and the left shoulder and had a fever of 102° to 103°F. A few days later the left arm, forearm, and hand were paralyzed, the muscles flaccid. Reflexes in the left upper limb were absent. Motor control of other parts of the body was intact. After 4 weeks, the forearm and the hand could be slightly extended by voluntary effort, but no other voluntary movement of these parts could be executed. The paralyzed muscles remained flaccid and showed marked atrophy.
   a. Localize the site of the lesion.
   b. What historical condition was frequently responsible for this clinical picture?

2. A 29-year-old woman, who since the birth of her fourth child 2 years ago had been taking birth control pills, suddenly experienced double vision and weakness in her right upper and lower limbs. Neurologic examination showed right upper and lower limb weakness accompanied by increased resistance to passive stretch, exaggerated tendon reflexes, and an extensor plantar response. In addition, she had a loss of two-point, vibration, and proprioception on the right side in the upper and lower limbs, trunk, and neck and a loss of pinprick sensations on the right side of her face. A corneal reflex on the right could be elicited from either eye. The left side of her face sagged, and she was unable to close the left eye or retract the left side of her mouth. Although her eyes converged for near vision and she could look up and down, she could not look to the left, and her left eye was deviated medially. In attempting to gaze to the right, the right eye abducted normally, but the left eye did not adduct.
   a. In a labeled sketch at the level of the lesion, name and locate precisely the structures involved and tell which abnormality is associated with each structure.
   b. Account for the loss of pain in the right eye but the presence of a corneal reflex on stimulating this eye.
   c. Account for the ability of the right eye to turn medially for near vision but not when the patient attempted to gaze to the left.
   d. Account for the adductor paralysis of the left eye during gaze to the right.
   e. If these phenomena are a result of a vascular occlusion (thrombosis), which major brain artery is most likely involved?

3. A middle-aged woman appeared in the clinic because of difficulties in walking and a sagging of the corner of her mouth. Her history showed that these abnormalities were the latest in a long series of events. About 5 years previously, the woman had a series of dizzy spells and complained of tinnitus in the right ear. Several years later the noise disappeared, and the patient noticed a hearing loss in the same ear. Somewhat later she found it difficult to close her right eye tightly, and the corner of her mouth on the right side began to droop and did not rise when she smiled. Recently, she experienced intermittent painful sensations in the right side of her face, and now it has become numb. Within the past several weeks, she noticed a tendency to sway to the right, and while walking she often staggered and sometimes fell to the right. These recent events have been accompanied by difficulty in swallowing and hoarseness. Neurologic examination also revealed a loss of taste on the right side of her tongue. No corneal reflex could be elicited from the right eye.
   a. Locate the lesion.
   b. Name the structures involved and specify which abnormality is associated with each.
   c. What is the probable etiology of the lesion?

4. The patient is a 45-year-old hypertensive man who suddenly collapsed. He was immediately hospitalized, and it was noted at that time that he had a generalized flaccid paralysis of the right limbs with no response to tendon stimulation. Examination 3 weeks later showed a spastic hemiplegia on the right side of the body. An extensor plantar response was present on the right side, tendon reflexes of the right limbs were exaggerated, and resistance to passive movements was increased. A weakness of

the lower facial muscles on the right was also noted. Pinprick was not sharp and was poorly localized, and a loss of tactile and proprioception senses on the right side of the entire body was evident. In addition, he had a right homonymous hemianopsia.
   a. In a labeled sketch at the level of the lesion, name and locate precisely the structures involved and tell which abnormality is associated with each structure.
   b. Explain the initial flaccid paralysis in the right limbs.
   c. Account for (1) the weakness of the right lower facial muscles and not the upper, and (2) the presence of decreased sensation to pinprick, but the complete absence of tactile and proprioception senses on the right side.
   d. What is a common etiology for this clinical picture?
   e. Describe the pathologic process and common sites of involvement.

5. Locate and describe six neurologic abnormalities you would expect to find in a conscious patient immediately after the right halves of spinal cord segments C8 and T1 are destroyed by a bullet.
   a. How would the abnormalities differ 3 months after the injury?

6. A 56-year-old woman, a heavy cigarette smoker for 35 years, experienced difficulties in walking and in using her right arm, both of which became progressively worse during a period of 4 months. Examination showed an intention tremor and dysmetria in her right upper and lower limbs while she was performing the finger-to-nose and heel-to-shin tests. In addition, she had difficulty with heel-to-toe walking and tended to veer toward the right. She was unable to supinate and pronate her right arm repetitively for even short periods. Although the myotatic reflexes and resistance to passive movements in her right limbs were slightly reduced, neither paralysis nor sensory disturbances were found in these limbs or in any other part of her body. A chest radiograph taken immediately after the physical examination showed a mass in her left lung, and a computed tomography scan of her head showed a CNS mass.
   a. Where would you expect the CNS mass to be located, and what structure or structures would be involved?
   b. Why did the abnormalities occur only when the patient performed a volitional movement?
   c. Define the term "ataxia."
   d. What is the likely etiology?

7. A 63-year-old man has been bothered by the shaking of his hands and generalized stiffness of his body, which have become progressively more severe during the past 3 years. On entering the examining room he moves slowly and deliberately, shuffling his feet, his shoulders and trunk are stooped forward, and his arms are at his sides and not swinging. During the ensuing history and physical examination his face remains masklike with no changes of expression. In both hands, a resting tremor of the pill-rolling type stops only when the patient performs a voluntary movement such as lighting a cigarette or picking up a pencil. Examination reveals the presence of lead-pipe rigidity manifested by a generalized hypertonicity with greatly increased resistance to passive movement. Although the patient moves infrequently, examination reveals no paralysis or sensory disturbances in any part of the body.
   a. Locate the lesion and name the structure or structures involved.
   b. Define the term "dyskinesia."
   c. Which are the positive signs and which are the negative signs manifested by this patient?
   d. Name the likely diagnosis and the rationale for the pharmaceutical and the surgical treatments of this condition.

8. A 28-year-old man was involved in a one-car, high-speed automobile accident. There was no loss of consciousness and no known head injury at the time, and his only complaint thereafter was aching in his neck and left shoulder. He had no other problems until 5 days later when he awoke with dizziness, nausea, vomiting, and an unsteady gait. He was hospitalized 8 hours later.

Neurologic examination revealed a left Horner syndrome. The left gag reflex was absent. Prominent ataxia was noted in the left arm and leg, but strength was normal. Sensation to pinprick was decreased over the left side of the face and over the neck, trunk, and limbs on the right side. The patient could not stand without falling to the left. His upper and lower limb reflexes were symmetric, and the plantar responses were flexor. After 6 days he was discharged from the hospital with a left Horner syndrome, mild left arm and leg dysmetria, and a mildly ataxic gait. All signs and symptoms resolved during the next 4 weeks.

Seven weeks after the injury, he experienced sudden onset of dysphagia, unsteadiness of gait, and left ptosis—all precipitated by lifting a light load. These signs and symptoms lasted about 10 minutes. He was readmitted to the hospital, and angiography revealed partial occlusion of a blood vessel. He was discharged and instructed to refrain from heavy lifting. Eight months later, examination was normal, and he was asymptomatic.

    a. In a labeled sketch at the level of the lesion, name and locate precisely the structures involved and tell which abnormality is associated with each structure.

    b. What blood vessel was partially occluded?

9. A woman, 20 years of age, who had suffered from endocarditis, suddenly fainted and remained unconscious for several hours. On awakening, she was unable to speak although she could say "damn!" repetitively when she was frustrated with being unable to speak. She was able to print words to form sentences with her left hand, but not with her right hand, which was flaccid and paralyzed. Several months later, the loss of speech persisted, and she showed a spastic weakness of the right arm and hand with increased resistance to passive movement and exaggerated tendon reflexes. The lower facial muscles on the right side were paralyzed.

    a. Locate the lesion, name the structures involved, and tell which abnormality is associated with each structure.

    b. If this patient's symptoms are the result of a vascular accident (hemorrhage or thrombosis), which artery is most likely involved?

    c. Define the term "aphasia."

10. A 63-year-old man complained of brief episodes lasting about a minute during which he experienced an unpleasant odor or a feeling of anxiety and fear. Immediately after these episodes, he felt as if he was in a dreamlike state in which he heard and saw things that he had experienced before. He was aware that he was unable to understand what other people were saying to him during these episodes. While experiencing the puzzling episodes, he looked preoccupied, and sometimes his lips and tongue moved as if he had a hair in his mouth. Examination fails to reveal any abnormality except a visual field defect.

    a. Where is the lesion?

    b. What do the episodes represent?

    c. Locate the structures associated with the:

        1. Unpleasant odor

        2. Anxiety and fear

        3. "Déjà vu" phenomenon

        4. Lip and tongue movements

    d. What visual field defect would you expect?

11. A 15-year-old girl became obese and listless during the past year. She also had episodes of high fever without apparent cause and cessation of her menstrual period for several months. She drank copious amounts of water because she was always thirsty, and she urinated excessively. Neurologic examination revealed an obese girl with a visual field defect.

    a. Where is the lesion?

    b. Locate the structures associated with the:

        1. Fever

        2. Obesity

        3. Listlessness

      4. Dysmenorrhea

      5. Thirst and polyuria

  c. What visual field defect would you expect?

12. A professional hockey player complained that his leg felt so tired he could hardly walk, much less play hockey. Neurologic examination showed marked weakness in the left leg and foot accompanied by an extensor plantar response, increased resistance to passive stretch, and exaggerated knee and ankle jerks. Pinprick was not as sharp or well localized below the knee in the left lower limb as compared with the rest of the body. In addition, with his eyes closed, passive flexion and extension of his left leg, foot, and toes were incorrectly described, and the other more discriminative touch senses (tactile localization and two-point sense) in his leg, foot, and toes were also severely impaired.

  a. Give the level and location of the lesion and identify the structures involved in the above abnormalities.

  b. If vascular in nature, what artery would be involved?

13. Robert's college friends noticed that his head tilted to the left. Later Robert noticed a tremor when he attempted a movement, and, when reaching for a glass of soda, he would often knock it over. Disturbed, he went to see a neurologist. On examination, his right eye did not depress fully when adducted. Intention tremor, dysmetria, and dysdiadochokinesia were noted in his right upper and lower limbs. Robert also presented the inability to adduct the left eye when he gazed to the right; but it did adduct when vision was shifted from a far object to a near object.

  a. Locate the level of the lesion and identify the structures for which each abnormality is given.

  b. Why did Robert's head tilt to the left?

  c. What is the likely diagnosis?

14. After sustaining too many blows to the head while playing racquetball, Mary presented with the following abnormalities: She had a left lower homonymous quadrantic anopsia and was unaware of the left side of her body and its surroundings.

  a. In a labeled sketch identify the level and area of the lesion, and name the structures involved and the abnormalities associated with each.

  b. A branch of which blood vessel was most likely damaged?

15. A man came into the city hospital one morning after an evening of excessive drinking. Shortly after a fall in which he struck his head, he complained of inability to use his left eye, and his left upper eyelid drooped. Later, his left eyelid was entirely closed, and, when the eyelid was lifted, the eye was turned down and out. Weakness was noted in the right upper and lower limbs. Examination revealed that muscle tone and reflexes in the right limbs were increased. A Babinski response was detected on the right side. The left pupil was fixed in the dilated position, whereas the right pupil responded normally to increased light intensity in either eye. When the patient smiled, no elevation occurred on the right side of the mouth.

  a. In a labeled sketch at the level of the lesion, name and locate precisely the structures involved and tell which abnormality is associated with each structure.

  b. Explain why the left eye was closed and turned down and out.

  c. Explain why only the right pupil responded to increased light in the left eye.

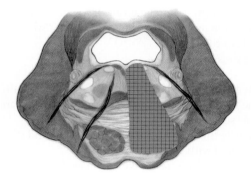

1. a. The extent of the paralysis indicates that the lesion is on the left side and extends from C5 to T1 segments inclusively.
    b. Acute anterior poliomyelitis was an infective disease that resulted in degenerative lesions mainly affecting the alpha motor neurons in the anterior horn of the spinal cord.

2. a. Level: caudal pons

        Structures and Abnormalities: Left corticospinal—weakness in the right upper and lower limbs with increased resistance to passive stretch, exaggerated tendon reflexes, and an extensor plantar response

        Left medial lemniscus: loss of two-point, vibration, and proprioception in the upper and lower limbs, trunk, and neck on the right side

        Left trigeminothalamic tract: loss of pinprick on the right side of the face

        Left ascending root of facial nerve: paralysis of the left facial muscles (upper and lower)

        Left abducens nucleus and nerve: left eye esotropia and paralysis of abduction

        Left paramedian pontine reticular formation (PPRF): paralysis of gaze to the left

    b. Loss of pain in right eye is attributable to left trigeminothalamic tract injury. The corneal reflex involves the spinal trigeminal tract and its nucleus as well as interneurons in the reticular formation that carry impulses to the facial nucleus; the trigeminothalamic tract is not involved in the corneal reflex.

    c. The right eye turns medially during convergence, which does not involve the horizontal gaze center PPRF. It does not turn medially on attempting to gaze to the left because the damaged left PPRF results in paralysis of gaze to the left.

    d. The adductor paralysis of the left eye during gaze to the right is attributable to a lesion of the left medial longitudinal fasciculus (MLF).

    e. Basilar artery

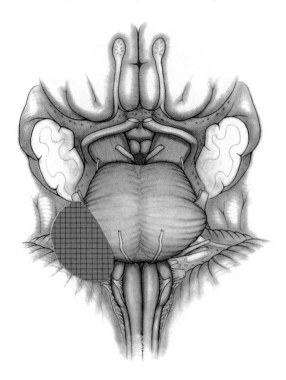

3. a. Location: cerebellar angle
   b. Structures and Abnormalities:
      1. Vestibular nerve (dizziness)
      2. Cochlear nerve (tinnitus → deafness)
      3. Facial nerve (facial paralysis)
      4. Trigeminal nerve (face pain and numbness)
      5. Cerebellum and inferior cerebellar peduncle (ataxia)
      6. Glossopharyngeal and vagus nerve (swallowing—hoarseness)
      7. Facial and glossopharyngeal nerves (taste)
      8. Facial or trigeminal nerve (corneal reflex loss)
   c. Acoustic neurinoma (starting along vestibular nerve just inside internal acoustic meatus—proceeding to cerebellar angle)

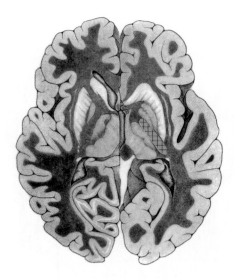

4. a. Level: posterior limb of the internal capsule
Structures and Abnormalities:
1. Left corticospinal tract: right spastic hemiplegia
2. Left corticobulbar tract: right lower facial muscle weakness
3. Left thalamocortical radiation: pinprick not sharp and poorly localized and severe loss of tactile and proprioception senses on the entire right side of the body
4. Left geniculocalcarine tract: right homonymous hemianopsia
b. Initial flaccid paralysis in right limbs attributable to CNS shock phenomenon in right lower motor neurons immediately after sudden release from cortical control
c. The corticobulbar tract influences the upper facial nucleus (for the upper facial muscles) bilaterally but influences the lower facial nucleus only contralaterally. Decreased sensation to pinprick occurs because the pain paths in the brainstem and forebrain are diffuse; hence, only precise localization, intensity, and sharpness of pinprick (the cortical phenomena) are lost with a lesion of the path distal to the thalamus.
d. Hypertensive intracerebral hemorrhage related to longstanding high blood pressure
e. Small vessel disease, especially microaneurysm formation in the distribution of the perforating arteries, most frequently lateral striate.

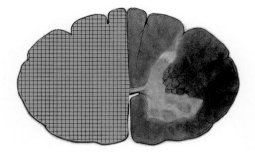

5. Abnormalities and Structures:
  a. Immediately after hemisection:
    1. Flaccid paralysis in the right hand (right anterior horn)
    2. Flaccid paralysis in right lower limb (right lateral corticospinal tract)
    3. Loss of two-point, vibration, and proprioception on the right side from the sole of the foot up the lower limb and trunk to the axilla and medial surface of the upper limb (right gracile and cuneate tracts)
    4. Decreased pain and temperature sensations in the skin on the medial surface of the right upper limb (right tract of Lissauer)
    5. Loss of pain and temperature sensations on the left side from the sole of the foot up the lower limb and trunk to about the second rib (right spinothalamic tract)
    6. Right ptosis, miosis of the right eye, and anhidrosis on the right side of the face: Horner syndrome (right ciliospinal center)
  b. 3 months later:
    1. Paralysis and severe atrophy of the intrinsic muscles in the right hand (lower motor neuron syndrome)
    2. Right lower limb paralysis accompanied by increased resistance to passive stretch, exaggerated myotatic reflexes, clonus, and extensor plantar response (upper motor neuron syndrome)
    3. Would remain the same

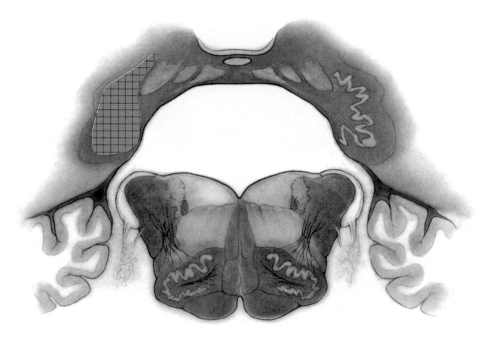

6. a. Level: cerebellum
        Structure: right dentate nucleus
    b. Cerebellar abnormalities are present only when volitional movements are commanded or initiated.
    c. Ataxia is the loss of muscular coordination.
    d. Metastatic carcinoma of lung

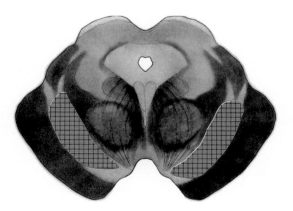

7. a. Level: midbrain
        Structure: substantia nigra (pars compacta)
    b. Dyskinesia is a disorder of movement that occurs spontaneously and is usually associated with basal ganglia disease.
    c. Positive signs: resting tremor, lead-pipe rigidity. Negative signs: slow movements (bradykinesia), shoulders and trunk stooped forward, arms at sides and not swinging, and masklike facial expression
    d. Paralysis agitans (Parkinson disease)—pharmaceutical treatment with levodopa replaces the dopamine in the striatum. Surgical procedures: Transplantation of fetal dopamine-producing tissue (suprarenal medulla) has shown some success. Cryosurgical lesions of the pallidothalamic path in the motor thalamus and of the medial segment of the pallidum have also been used somewhat successfully. The current procedure of choice is deep brain stimulation in which electrodes are implanted in the subthalamic nuclei.

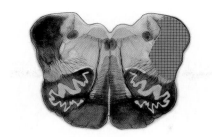

8. a. Level: Rostral medulla
   Structures and Abnormalities:
   Left spinal trigeminal tract: decreased pinprick in left side of face
   Left spinothalamic tract: decreased pinprick in neck, trunk, and limbs on right side
   Left inferior cerebellar peduncle: ataxia and dysmetria in left limbs
   Left vagus nerve rootlets: absence of left gag reflex
   Interruption of fibers in left lateral reticular formation carrying descending input to ciliospinal
      center: left Horner syndrome
   b. Vertebral artery or posterior inferior cerebellar artery (lateral medullary or Wallenberg syndrome)

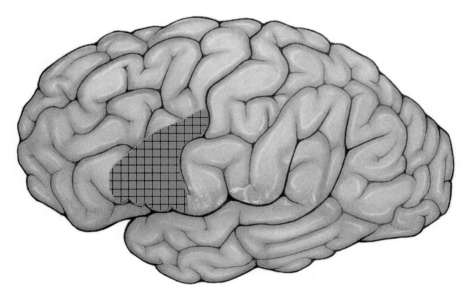

9. a. Level: Cerebral cortex
   Structures and Abnormalities:
   Broca speech area in left inferior frontal gyri: loss of speech (motor aphasia)
   Ventral part of the left precentral gyrus: spastic weakness of right hand and weakness of right lower
      facial muscles
   b. Middle cerebral artery: branches to the inferior frontal and ventral precentral areas
   c. Aphasia is the inability to understand or communicate speech, writing, or signs.

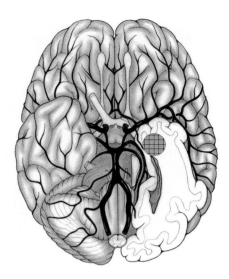

10. a. Level: Temporal lobe—tumor deep to uncus and parahippocampal gyrus
   b. Temporal lobe epilepsy
   c. Structures:
      1. Unpleasant odor—olfactory center at uncus
      2. Anxiety and fear—temporal pole
      3. Déjà vu—amygdala and temporal cortex (memory)
      4. Lips and tongue movements—amygdala
      5. Inattention—hippocampal formation
   d. Contralateral upper homonymous quadrantic anopsia—loop of Meyer

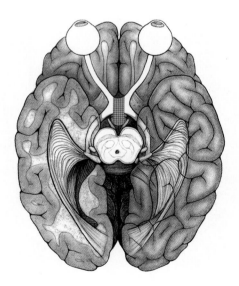

11. a. Level: Hypothalamus (case of craniopharyngioma)
   b. Abnormalities and Structures:
      1. Fever—preoptic area
      2. Obesity—tuberal area (ventromedial nucleus)
      3. Listlessness—posterior hypothalamus
      4. Dysmenorrhea—tuberal area (releasing factors for anterior pituitary)
      5. Thirst and polyuria—supraoptic and paraventricular nuclei (diabetes insipidus)
   c. Visual field defect: bitemporal heteronymous hemianopsia

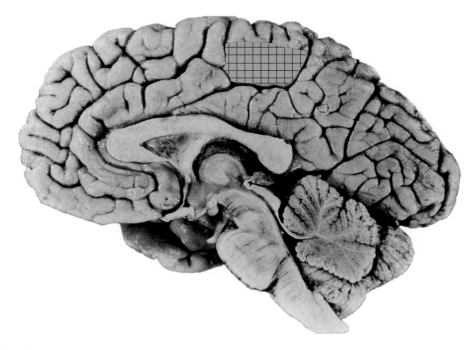

12. a. Level: Cerebral cortex
    Structures and Abnormalities:
    Anterior part of right paracentral lobule: spastic weakness, and so forth in left leg and foot
    Posterior part of right paracentral lobule: somatosensory loss in left leg and foot
  b. Vascular supply: Right anterior cerebral artery

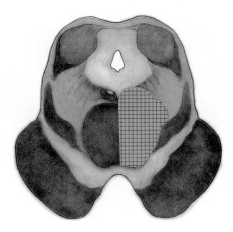

13. a. Level: Inferior colliculus (distal to the decussation of the superior cerebellar peduncle
    Left superior cerebellar peduncle: intention tremor, dysmetria and dysdiadochokinesia in right limbs
    Left trochlear nucleus: right eye, when adducted, has weakness in depression
    Left medial longitudinal fasciculus: left internuclear ophthalmoplegia (left eye does not adduct on
      gaze to right)
  b. With trochlear lesions the affected eye is slightly extorted, and the person compensates by tilting
    the head downward to the opposite side.
  c. Demyelinating process such as multiple sclerosis

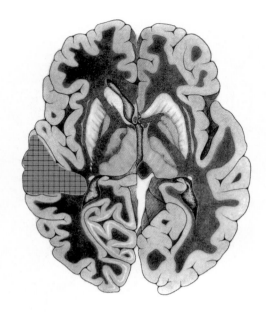

14. a. Level: Parietal lobe
   Structures and Abnormalities:
   Dorsal part of right optic radiation: lower left homonymous quadrantic anopsia
   Right posterior parietal lobe: neglect of left side of body and surroundings
   b. Vascular supply: Middle cerebral artery

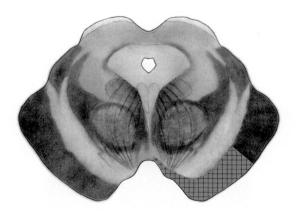

15. a. Level: Superior colliculus
   Structures and Abnormalities:
   Left corticospinal tract: weakness in the right upper and lower limbs with increased muscle tone, reflexes, and a Babinski response
   Left corticobulbar tract: paralysis of the right lower facial muscles
   Left oculomotor nerve: left ptosis, left eye turned down and out, and left pupil dilated
   b. The oculomotor nerve innervates all the eye muscles except the superior oblique and the lateral rectus muscles, which depress and abduct the eye, respectively. With paralysis of the superior levator the eyelid droops severely.
   c. The left optic nerve and right oculomotor nerve are intact, but the left oculomotor nerve (containing the pupilloconstrictor fibers) is not.

Answers to Chapter Questions

CHAPTER 1
Introduction, Organization, and Cellular Components

1-1. The two main classes of cells in the CNS are neurons, the functional units, and neuroglia, the supporting units.

1-2. A synapse is the site of functional contact where impulses pass unidirectionally from one neuron to the other. Most synapses occur between axons and dendrites (axodendritic) or between axons and cell bodies (axosomatic). Histologically, most synapses consist of a terminal enlargement—the bouton—closely apposed to the surface of a dendrite or a neuronal cell body. Ultrastructurally, the bouton contains mitochondria and synaptic vesicles, and its synaptic surface (the presynaptic membrane) is separated from the target's surface (the postsynaptic membrane) by a gap, the synaptic cleft.

1-3. The integrity of axons, some of which may be 3 feet in length, is maintained by elaborate axoplasmic transport systems between the cell bodies, which are the metabolic centers of neurons, and the distant terminals of the axons. Anterograde axonal transport, i.e., movement from the cell body to the terminals, is of two main types: (1) fast transport of membranous organelles and synaptic vesicles or their precursors and (2) slow transport of cytoskeletal materials. Retrograde axonal transport brings worn-out synaptic materials and exogenous substances such as toxins or viruses from the axon terminals back to the cell body.

1-4. The chief differences between astrocytes and oligodendrocytes are as follows: Astrocytes have numerous and voluminous processes that form the CNS packing material, which is metabolically very active. The ends of their processes aid in the formation of the external and internal limiting membranes. They are highly susceptible to CNS insults and form glial scars. Oligodendrocytes have fewer branches and their main functions are to form and maintain the CNS myelin.

1-5. a. Subdural hematoma—between the dura mater and the arachnoid membrane

b. Cerebrospinal fluid—in the subarachnoid space between the arachnoid membrane and the pia mater

c. Epidural hematoma—between the dura and the bony wall of the cranial cavity.

1-6.   (b) Myelin formation and maintenance is a function of oligodendrocytes in the CNS and Schwann cells in the PNS.

1-7.   (d) Retrograde axonal transport is responsible for the movement of substances from the axon terminals to the cell body.

1-8.   (a) Astrocytomas are the most common CNS tumors in both adults and children.

1-9.   (e) Before branching and entering the parenchyma of the brain the cerebral arteries are located in the subarachnoid space. Hence, their leakage results in subarachnoid hemorrhage.

CHAPTER 2
Spinal Cord: Topography and Functional Levels

2-1.   The spinal epidural space contains adipose tissue and blood vessels, the most medically important of which is the internal vertebral venous plexus. This valveless plexus communicates freely with veins of the pelvic, abdominal, thoracic, and cranial cavities and may provide a route for the spread of infections, cancer cells, and so forth from the viscera to the brain.

2-2.   The dural sac contains an enlarged subarachnoid space in which is found chiefly cerebrospinal fluid and the lumbosacral nerve roots that form the cauda equina.

2-3.   Intervertebral dislocations most frequently occur at the articulations between CV5 and CV6, TV12 and LV1, and CV1 and CV2, in order of frequency. The spinal cord-vertebral column relations at each are:

CV1 to CV2 = C2
CV5 to CV6 = C6 or C7
TV12 to LV1 = S1 to S3

2-4.   The spinal cord is not endangered by lumbar puncture in adults below the LV3 level because its caudal extent is usually at the LV1 level, although it may end anywhere between the middle of TV11 and the middle of LV3.

2-5.   The four spinal cord regions can be distinguished in transverse sections on the basis of gray matter size and shape as follows:

	Posterior Horn	Anterior Horn
Sacral	Massive	Massive with lateral extension
Lumbar	Massive	Massive with medial extension
Thoracic	Thin	Thin
Cervical	Thin	Large with lateral extension

2-6.   (d) Unlike all other spinal nerves, the cervical nerves emerge above their respective vertebrae. Because there are only seven cervical vertebrae, the C8 nerve emerges between CV7 and TV1.

2-7.   (e) The cauda equina consists of the lumbosacral dorsal and ventral roots located in the subarachnoid space of the dural sac.

CHAPTER 3
Brainstem: Topography and Functional Levels

3-1.   Ventral surface of (a) Medulla—pyramids, (b) Pons—transverse grooves of basilar part, (c) Midbrain—cerebral peduncles and interpeduncular fossa.

3-2.   Dorsal surface of (a) Closed medulla—gracile and cuneate tubercles, (b) Open medulla—hypoglossal and vagal trigones, (c) Pons—medial eminence and facial colliculus, (d) Midbrain—superior colliculus and inferior colliculus.

3-3.   The brainstem reticular formation is an intermingling of nuclei and nerve fibers in the central core of the brainstem.

3-4.   a. Hypoglossal trigone—open medulla, caudally

        b. Motor trigeminal nucleus—midpons

        c. Superior colliculus—rostral midbrain

        d. Decussation of trochlear nerve—rostral pons

        e. Acoustic tubercle—open medulla, rostrally

        f. Gracile tubercle—closed medulla

        g. Facial colliculus—caudal pons

        h. Inferior colliculus—caudal midbrain

3-5.   (c) The brainstem is located in the posterior cranial fossa, along with the cerebellum. Its anterior surface is related to the clivus, the basal surface of the posterior cranial fossa that slopes downward from the dorsum sellae to the foramen magnum.

3-6.   (b) The superior and inferior foveae are remnants of the embryonic sulcus limitans. Motor structures such as the hypoglossal, vagal, and abducens nuclei are medial, whereas sensory structures such as vestibular and auditory nuclei are lateral to the foveae.

3-7.   (e) The midbrain is divided into a dorsal part, the tectum or roof, and a ventral part, the cerebral peduncle, which from anterior to posterior consists of the cerebral crus, substantia nigra, and tegmentum.

CHAPTER 4
Forebrain: Topography and Functional Levels

4-1.   The 12 cranial nerves attach to the brain and, hence, they travel in the cranial cavity whereas the spinal nerves attach to the spinal cord and travel in the spinal or vertebral canal. Additional differences are that cranial nerves do not have dorsal and ventral roots and their functional components vary, some being purely motor, some purely sensory, and others mixed.

4-2.   Cranial nerves I and II attach to the forebrain, III to the midbrain, and all the others attach to the hindbrain. Note that CN IV originates in the midbrain but emerges from the pons.

4-3.   In the forebrain are the two lateral ventricles, one in each of the cerebral hemispheres, and the third ventricle in the diencephalon. In the hindbrain is the fourth ventricle and in the midbrain is the cerebral aqueduct, which connects the third and fourth ventricles.

4-4.   The terms "anterior or ventral," meaning toward the front, and "posterior or dorsal," meaning toward the back, are synonymous in all parts of the CNS except the forebrain. Because the axis of the forebrain is oriented almost perpendicular to the rest of the CNS, in the forebrain the term "ventral" is synonymous with infe-

rior, meaning toward the base of the skull; "dorsal" is synonymous with superior, meaning toward the top of the skull.

4-5.   (b) The internal medullary lamina (IML) separates the thalamus into anterior, medial, and lateral subdivisions. Within these subdivisions the anterior, medial, ventral, and lateral nuclei lie adjacent to the IML, whereas the metathalamic, midline, and reticular nuclei do not.

4-6.   (e) From anterior to posterior the hypothalamus consists of the chiasmatic, infundibular, tuberal, and mamillary regions or levels.

4-7.   (e) The lateral fissure (of Sylvius) is the deepest and most uniform and prominent landmark on the lateral surface of the cerebral hemisphere. Dorsal to it are the frontal lobe and the anterior part of the parietal lobe; ventral to it is the temporal lobe.

4-8.   (b) The paracentral lobule, so named because it contains the most dorsal part of the central sulcus, includes the continuations of the precentral and postcentral gyri onto the medial surface of the cerebral hemisphere. Hence, it includes parts of the frontal and parietal lobes.

CHAPTER 5
Lower Motor Neurons: Flaccid Paralysis

5-1.   A motor unit is an alpha motor neuron, its axon, and all the muscle fibers it innervates. Those motor units involved in coarse movements comprise as many as 2,000 muscle fibers, whereas those involved in delicate movements may include as few as a dozen or so muscle fibers.

5-2.   Spinal lower motor neuron lesions result in paralysis because commands from the CNS can no longer reach extrafusal muscle fibers, decreased muscle tone because of impaired lower motor neuron activity, loss of motor reflexes because lower motor neurons form their efferent limbs, and severe atrophy as a result of the degeneration of denervated muscle fibers. The hallmark of the lower motor neuron syndrome is flaccid paralysis and severe atrophy.

5-3. Type I muscle fibers are activated when a sustained muscle contraction is required.

5-4. Type II muscle fibers contract faster and with greater force than type I muscle fibers.

5-5. A motor unit is composed of only a single muscle fiber type.

5-6. The membrane properties of smaller lower motor neurons make them more excitable than larger lower motor neurons. Motor neurons are recruited by size, smallest first and largest last.

5-7. Amyotrophic lateral sclerosis or Lou Gehrig disease is a lower motor neuron disorder characterized by weakness, muscle atrophy, and fasciculations.

5-8. Renshaw cells are excited by collaterals of lower motor neuron axons and, in turn, inhibit adjacent lower motor neurons.

5-9. Reciprocal inhibition allows a movement performed by agonist muscles to occur while the lower motor neurons innervating antagonist muscles are inhibited.

5-10. a. Ambiguus nucleus: Hoarse and weak voice as a result of paralysis of the ipsilateral vocal muscles, sagging of the ipsilateral palatal arch, and contralateral deviation of the uvula could be expected with the lesion at this level, which is the vagal part of the nucleus.

   b. Oculomotor nucleus: Ipsilateral ptosis and ophthalmoplegia with the eye turned down and out; mydriasis as a result of interruption of visceral pupilloconstrictor components.

   c. Facial nucleus: Paralysis of ipsilateral muscles of facial expression; inability to close eye tightly or retract corner of mouth.

   d. Motor trigeminal nucleus: Paralysis and atrophy of ipsilateral muscles of mastication; on opening the mouth, the jaw deviates toward ipsilateral side.

CHAPTER 6
The Pyramidal System: Spastic Paralysis

6-1. The pyramidal tract is highly susceptible to injury because it extends without interruption from the cerebral cortex to the caudal end of the spinal cord. Thus, it is subject to injury by trauma, cerebrovascular disease, neoplasms, and so forth that occur at any level of the brain and spinal cord.

6-2. A lower motor neuron lesion affecting the facial muscles is caused by an injury of the facial nucleus or nerve and results in paralysis of all ipsilateral facial muscles. An upper motor neuron lesion affecting the facial muscles is caused by injury of the corticobulbar neurons or their axons and results in paralysis or weakness of the contralateral lower facial muscles only. The upper facial muscles are influenced by both the ipsilateral and contralateral corticobulbar tracts; hence, the upper facial muscles will not be affected by a unilateral corticobulbar tract lesion.

6-3. Rapid, fractionated movements of the fingers are commanded by monosynaptic corticomotoneuronal connections.

6-4. (e) The premotor cortex, primary and secondary somatosensory areas, and the motor thalamus activate upper motor neurons in MI.

6-5. Neuronal activity in the supplementary motor cortex precedes activity in upper motor neurons in MI.

6-6. Cutting the dorsal roots (dorsal rhizotomy) or chronic intrathecal administration of baclofen is used therapeutically for treating severe cases of spasticity.

6-7. a. 1. Corticospinal tract: Contralateral spastic hemiplegia accompanied by exaggerated myotatic reflexes, increased resistance to passive stretch, and an extensor plantar response
   2. Corticobulbar tract: Contralateral lower facial muscle paralysis

   b. 1. Corticospinal tract: (see a. 1.)
   2. Hypoglossal nerve: Paralysis, atrophy, and deviation of protruded tongue to ipsilateral side

   c. 1. Corticospinal tract: (see a. 1.)
   2. Abducens nerve: Medial deviation (esotropia) and abductor paralysis of ipsilateral eye

d. 1. Corticospinal tract: (see a. 1.)
   2. Corticobulbar tract: (see a. 2.)
   3. Oculomotor nerve: Ipsilateral ptosis and ophthalmoplegia with eye turned down and out (mydriasis also, owing to visceromotor fibers in CN III)

CHAPTER 7
Spinal Motor Organization and Brainstem Supraspinal Paths: Postcapsular Lesion Recovery and Decerebrate Posturing

7-1. Spinal lower motor neurons are arranged from medial to lateral in the anterior horn. The most medial supply the most proximal muscles, and the most lateral, the most distal muscles. The brainstem supraspinal paths have the strongest influence on the closest lower motor neurons. The ventromedial paths, i.e., medial vestibulospinal and reticulospinal, descend in the anterior funiculus near the more medial lower motor neurons and have their greatest influence on the axial muscles. The lateral supraspinal paths, the lateral vestibulospinal and reticulospinal and the rubrospinal, descend in the lateral funiculus and have their greatest influence on the proximal and distal limb muscles.

7-2. The contralateral limb paralysis resulting from a lesion of the pyramidal tract by capsular stroke is, in most cases, gradually overcome initially and quite completely by neck and trunk movements, which receive strong input from the ventromedial descending paths. From proximal to distal, limb movements receive stronger to weaker input from the lateral descending paths. Hence, from proximal to distal, limb movements recover, but more slowly and less completely. Therefore, the recovery of function after capsular stroke is thought to occur because of the actions of the brainstem ventromedial and lateral supraspinal paths. Fine movements of the most distal muscles are controlled solely by the pyramidal tract through numerous monosynaptic connections with the appropriate lower motor neurons. Hence, rapid and

independent finger movements are permanently lost.

7-3. a. Decorticate posturing occurs with brainstem impairment rostral to the red nucleus, that is, in the forebrain.

b. Decerebrate posturing occurs with brainstem impairment anywhere between the forebrain-midbrain junction and the rostral extent of the vestibular nuclei, that is, in the midbrain or rostral pons.

CHAPTER 8
The Basal Ganglia: Dyskinesia

8-1. Anatomically, the corpus striatum is composed of the caudate and lentiform nuclei, the latter being further subdivided into a lateral segment, the putamen, and two medial segments, the globus pallidus. Functionally, the corpus striatum is divided into the striatum, consisting of the caudate nucleus and putamen, and the pallidum, which is the globus pallidus.

8-2. Medium spiny neurons, the principal cell type in the striatum, have either dopaminergic D1 receptors or D2 receptors. Through these receptors dopamine is selectively excitatory or inhibitory on striatal neurons.

8-3. The chief input to the basal ganglia is directed to the striatum and is composed largely of the massive and highly topographically organized corticostriate projections from all parts of the neocortex. The putamen, which is closely associated with limb movements, receives projections from the motor, premotor, and somatosensory cortical areas.

8-4. Activation of the direct pathway is responsible for decreased inhibition, referred to as disinhibition, allowing thalamic ventral anterior neurons to fire, thereby enabling the desired movement to occur.

8-5. Activation of the indirect pathway is largely responsible for the inhibition of thalamic ventral anterior neurons involved with competing or undesired movements.

8-6. Ventral anterior thalamocortical projections to premotor and supplementary motor areas indirectly regulate MI upper motor neurons.

8-7.   (a) Lead-pipe rigidity is characterized by the co-contraction of agonist and antagonist muscles, resulting in bidirectional increased resistance to passive stretch.

8-8.   The cardinal manifestations of basal ganglia diseases are disorders of movement and alterations in muscle tone. The disorders of movement, or dyskinesia, take the form of tremors, athetosis, chorea, or ballismus. They are more prevalent while the patient is "at rest," i.e., not intending to perform a movement. Dyskinesia can be neither prevented nor interrupted. The alteration in muscle tone in basal ganglia diseases usually takes the form of hypertonicity.

8-9.   The basal ganglia influence voluntary movements through the pyramidal system.

8-10.   a. Structure—Bilateral compact parts of substantia nigra

        Abnormality—Parkinson disease: Mask-like facial expression, pill-rolling tremor, bradykinesia, lead-pipe rigidity, and impairment of postural adjustments

        b. Structures—Bilateral striatal degeneration (caudate nucleus and putamen)

        Abnormality—Huntington chorea: Head jerking, lip and tongue smacking, gesticulations of distal parts of limbs

        c. Structures—Subthalamic nucleus

        Abnormality—Contralateral hemiballismus: Violent flinging of upper and lower limbs

CHAPTER 9
The Cerebellum: Ataxia

9-1.   The inferior cerebellar peduncle emanates from the medulla and its more lateral part, the restiform body, and contains chiefly the olivocerebellar, dorsal spinocerebellar, and cuneocerebellar tracts. Its more medial part, the juxtarestiform body, comprises the incoming vestibulocerebellar and the outgoing cerebellovestibular connections. The middle cerebellar peduncle is largest and is made up of the pontocerebellar projections. The superior cerebellar peduncle is composed chiefly of the cerebellar output to the thalamus, although it also contains some output to the red nucleus.

9-2.   Climbing fiber activation evokes a very powerful and excitatory complex spike in Purkinje cells.

9-3.   (e) Granule cells are the only excitatory neurons in the cerebellar cortex.

9-4.   Long-term synaptic depression refers to the decreased postsynaptic responsiveness in some Purkinje cells to those parallel fibers activated temporally coincident with complex spikes activated when acquiring a new motor skill.

9-5.   The cerebellar nuclei are, from medial to lateral, the fastigial, the interposed (composed of the globus and emboliform nuclei), and the dentate. Each receives an excitatory input from collaterals of the climbing and mossy fibers and an inhibitory input from the Purkinje neurons.

9-6.   The three sagittal zones of the cerebellum are, from medial to lateral, vermis, paravermal or intermediate, and lateral. Purkinje neurons in the vermis project to the fastigial nucleus, whereas those in the paravermal or intermediate zone project to the interposed nucleus, and those in the lateral cerebellum project to the dentate nucleus.

9-7.   The flocculonodular syndrome is characterized by truncal ataxia, the anterior lobe syndrome by gait ataxia, and the posterior lobe syndrome by a generalized ataxia that includes intention tremor, dysmetria, dysdiadochokinesia and, if bilateral, explosive speech.

9-8.   (a) The lateral hemisphere and dentate nuclei are involved with the planning of voluntary movements, and accordingly there is an increase in unitary activity in these structures before activity in the primary motor cortex.

9-9.   Delayed activation of antagonist muscles to slow the movements started by the agonist muscles is characteristic in past-pointing.

9-10.   The anterior lobe cortex compares information about an intended movement transmitted by collaterals of corticospinal axons via pontocerebellar projections, and information about the movement as it is occurring transmitted by spinocerebellar projections.

9-11.   A midline medulloblastoma will result in truncal ataxia. If the patient is provided with postural support, such as that provided by lying in bed, movements involving the distal parts of the limbs will be relatively normal.

9-12. A lesion of the inferior cerebellar peduncle damages the dorsal spinocerebellar and cuneocerebellar tracts and results in ipsilateral lower and upper limb ataxia. A lesion of the red nucleus damages the fibers of the crossed superior cerebellar peduncle and results in a contralateral posterior lobe syndrome.

9-13. a. Anterior cerebellar lobe (lower limb area): Gait ataxia

   b. Superior cerebellar peduncle (before decussation): Posterior lobe syndrome; ipsilaterally—intention tremor, dysmetria, dysdiadochokinesia, and so forth

   c. Flocculonodular lobe: Truncal ataxia

CHAPTER 10
The Oculomotor System: Gaze Disorders

10-1. Right oculomotor nerve

10-2. Right abducens nerve

10-3. Internuclear ophthalmoplegia resulting from lesion of the right medial longitudinal fasciculus in the rostral pons or in the midbrain

10-4. If transient—left frontal eye field. If permanent—right horizontal gaze center in paramedian pontine reticular formation.

CHAPTER 11
The Somatosensory System: Anesthesia and Analgesia

11-1. The three tactile receptors are Meissner corpuscles, Merkel discs, and hair follicle receptors. Merkel disc receptors have the smallest receptive fields of all mechanoreceptors and accordingly signal the most discrete tactile stimulation.

11-2. Stimulus intensity is signaled by the frequency and number of action potentials transmitted by the primary afferent axon.

11-3. A receptive field defines the spatial cutaneous area from which a specific type of stimulus will activate a receptor. Cutaneous receptive fields are smallest in areas of greatest tactile sensitivity (fingertips) and largest in areas of poor tactile localization (back).

11-4. Mechanical distortion stretches the receptor membrane, resulting in the opening of ionic channels leading to the receptor's depolarization and generation of an action potential in the primary afferent axon.

11-5. Sensory adaptation is a decline in receptor sensitivity with a constant stimulus intensity for a relatively long duration.

11-6. Surround inhibition serves to maintain the "sharpness" of tactile information processing in brainstem and thalamic relay nuclei. It is the physiologic basis for two-point discrimination.

11-7. The fast pain path synapses in the lateral thalamus, which projects to the SI cortex where the precise localization, sharpness, and intensity of pinprick are perceived. The slow pain path synapses in the medial thalamus, which projects to the limbic area of the cerebral cortex where emotional or affective feelings are perceived.

11-8. TENS is based on the selective stimulation of large cutaneous touch fibers that activate spinal interneurons, which inhibit secondary slow pain neurons, thereby resulting in the relief of chronic pain.

11-9. a. Cutaneous touch and pain sensations in dermatome L5 (first four toes and the dorsum of the foot)

   b. Tactile, vibration, and proprioception senses below the umbilicus on the left side and pain and temperature sensations below the inguinal ligament on the right side

   c. Pain and temperature sensations bilaterally at the level of the nipples

   d. Pain and temperature sensations in the face on the left side and pinprick and temperature in the occiput, neck, trunk, and limbs on the right side

   e. Tactile and proprioception senses in the occiput, neck, trunk, and limbs on the left side and pinprick and temperature sensations in the face on the left side

f. Tactile, proprioception, pinprick, and temperature senses on the entire right side

g. Loss of tactile and proprioception senses and some diminution of pinprick and temperature sensations and their precise localization, all in the left lower limb. Only precise localization and fine tactile discrimination depend on an intact primary somatosensory cortex for recognition.

CHAPTER 12
The Auditory System: Deafness

12-1. Bending of the stereocilia toward the scala vestibuli results in the influx of potassium from the endolymph in the cochlear duct, resulting in depolarization of the hair cells and the activation of primary auditory afferent axons.

12-2. The tone and loudness of sound are primarily signaled by inner hair cell receptors.

12-3. The bilateral representation of sound in the auditory system occurs because of the bilateral connections of (1) the superior olivary and trapezoid nuclei, (2) the nuclei of the lateral lemniscus, and (3) the inferior colliculi. Hence, a unilateral lesion in the auditory path anywhere from the level of the superior olivary nuclei to the cerebral cortex results in virtually no loss of hearing in either ear.

12-4. Complete ipsilateral deafness occurs after unilateral destruction of the spiral organ, the spiral ganglion, the cochlear nerve, or the dorsal and ventral cochlear nuclei.

12-5. An enlarging acoustic neurinoma on the vestibular nerve causes impairment of

a. The cochlear and facial nerves in the internal acoustic meatus

b. The trigeminal, glossopharyngeal, and perhaps vagus and abducens nerves in and near the cerebellar angle

12-6. Conduction deafness occurs as a result of external or middle ear diseases and injuries, which interfere with the conduction of sound waves or with the vibrations of the tympanic membrane or middle ear ossicles. Nerve deafness results from diseases and injuries of the spiral organ or the cochlear nerve. Conduction deafness is incomplete because sound waves are still transmitted through the cranial bones. In the event of total destruction of the spiral organ or cochlear nerve, the resulting "nerve deafness" is complete.

CHAPTER 13
The Vestibular System: Vertigo and Nystagmus

13-1. Impulses from the maculae of the utricles and saccules pass via the vestibular ganglion and nerve to the vestibular nuclei. From the left lateral vestibular nucleus, impulses descend via the left lateral vestibulospinal tract to the lower motor neurons that facilitate the extensor muscles of the left limbs.

13-2. a. The otolithic membranes in the maculae of the utricle and saccule shift on tilting the head or on linear acceleration, thereby initiating the vestibulospinal reflexes associated with equilibrium.

b. The cupulae of the ampullary crests in the semicircular ducts shift on rotation of the head, thereby initiating the vestibulo-ocular reflexes associated with visual fixation, that is, keeping the eyes on a target when the head is in motion.

13-3. The anatomic basis for the slow phase of rotary and caloric nystagmus is the vestibulo-ocular reflex.

13-4. a. In a conscious patient with a normal VOR, cold water irrigation of the right external auditory meatus will result in a left nystagmus, that is, the fast phase will be opposite to the irrigated side (COWS).

b. In a comatose patient with a normal VOR, cold water irrigation of the right external auditory meatus will result in turning of the eyes to the same side as long as the irrigation is continued. This phenomenon is the same as the slow phase of nystagmus induced by the

VOR. There is no fast phase in the comatose state.

13-5.   The vestibulo-ocular reflex is interrupted in the central brainstem somewhere between the levels of the vestibular and oculomotor nuclei (midpons to rostral midbrain).

CHAPTER 14
The Visual System: Anopsia

14-1.   Glaucoma results from increased intraocular pressure, which causes impaired vision as a result of retinal and optic nerve damage. Cataract is opacification of the lens, which causes impaired vision by interfering with the light rays passing through it.

14-2.   Detachment of the retina occurs between the pigment cells (layer 1) and the photoreceptor cells (layer 2). The detached part ceases to function because the rods and cones are metabolically dependent on the pigment cells.

14-3.   Retinal layers 4, 6, and 8 contain the cell bodies of the photoreceptors, bipolar cells, and ganglion cells, respectively.

14-4.   Night blindness is associated with deficiency of vitamin A, which aids in the restoration of the photopigment rhodopsin in the rods.

14-5.   Color blindness is associated with the absence of the red-, green-, or blue-sensitive photopigments in the cones.

14-6.   The fovea centralis is the area for most acute vision, and here most of the inner layers of the retina are pushed aside so the light rays can reach the cones of the foveola with as little interference as possible. Thus, only layers 1, 2, 3, 4, and 10 are found at the fovea. The optic disc is the area where the ganglion cell axons gather together and emerge from the eye as the optic nerve. It possesses only layers 9 and 10 and is the blind spot because of the absence of photoreceptors.

14-7.   As a component of the PNS, the optic nerve is unique because histologically it is similar to a CNS structure. Because it develops as an evagination of the diencephalon, the retina and its connection to the brain, the optic nerve, possess CNS morphologic characteristics. Histologically, the optic nerve resembles a spinal cord or brainstem tract in that its axons are supported by glial cells, and in the absence of neurolemma cells optic nerve axons do not regenerate if injured. Moreover, like the brain and spinal cord, the optic nerve is enveloped by the meninges, an arrangement that becomes medically important in the case of increased intracranial pressure, which exerts force on the optic nerve through the cerebrospinal fluid in the subarachnoid space surrounding it. Thus, increased intracranial pressure may be the cause of an edematous swelling of the optic disc, a phenomenon referred to as disc edema, papilledema, or choked disc.

14-8.   A photon of light hitting the retina triggers a biochemical change in the visual pigments rhodopsin and iodopsin, whereas in the somatosensory system a mechanical stimulus alters the receptor membrane potential as the result of changes in ionic conductance.

14-9.   a. Blindness in left eye

b. Bitemporal hemianopsia

c. Left homonymous hemianopsia

d. Right homonymous superior quadrantic anopsia

e. Left homonymous hemianopsia

14-10.   Retinal ganglion cells and lateral geniculate neurons respond to focused spots of light with on-center or off-center response properties. Neurons in the primary visual cortex transform this input to lines or bars of different orientations.

14-11.   The conscious perception of shape, color, and movement is interpreted in cortical areas away from the primary visual cortex. The shape and color recognition of an object occurs in the inferior temporal cortex, whereas movement is interpreted in the posterior parietal cortex.

14-12.   The direct light reflex involves the ipsilateral optic and oculomotor nerves, whereas the consensual light reflex involves the ipsilateral optic nerve and the contralateral oculomotor nerve. Central connections are made in the light reflex center in the pretectal nuclei, which connects with the ipsilateral and contralateral Edinger-Westphal nuclei; hence, the rostral midbrain must be intact for these reflex responses to occur.

14-13. CNS and PNS structures whose damage interrupts the pupillary dilation path are:

CNS   lateral reticular formation of medulla
lateral funiculus of cervical spinal cord
ciliospinal center at C8 and T1
intramedullary ventral rootlets at T1 and T2

PNS   ventral roots of T1 and T2
T1 and T2 spinal nerves
white communicating rami of T1 and T2
cervical sympathetic trunk
superior cervical ganglion
internal carotid plexus

14-14. Accommodation is the phenomenon whereby images remain in focus as the gaze shifts from far to near objects. It includes (1) contraction of the ciliary muscles, which allows the lens to bulge; (2) constriction of the pupil; and (3) convergence of the eyes. The center for accommodation is thought to be located in the region of the pretectum and superior colliculus. Its input comes from the visual cortex, and its output passes to the Edinger-Westphal and oculomotor nuclei. Both of these give rise to fibers in the oculomotor nerve: those from the Edinger-Westphal nucleus are preganglionic parasympathetic axons that synapse in the ciliary ganglion from whence postganglionic fibers pass via the short ciliary nerves to the ciliary and pupilloconstrictor muscles; those from the oculomotor nuclei pass directly to the medial rectus muscle of each eye.

CHAPTER 15
The Gustatory and Olfactory Systems: Ageusia and Anosmia

15-1.   Three cranial nerves contain taste fibers: the facial, the glossopharyngeal, and the vagus. The taste fibers in the facial nerve supply the anterior two-thirds of the tongue and have their cell bodies located in the geniculate ganglion. The glossopharyngeal nerve taste fibers are distributed to the posterior third of the tongue and their cell bodies are in the petrosal ganglion, whereas the vagal nerve taste fibers are distributed to the epiglottic and palatal regions and their cell bodies are in the nodose ganglion. The central branches of all the primary gustatory neurons enter the solitary tract and are distributed to the rostral part of the solitary nucleus sometimes called the gustatory nucleus.

15-2.   The primary gustatory area is located in the parietal operculum and the adjacent part of the insula.

15-3.   The olfactory membrane is 1 square inch of epithelium on the superior nasal concha and the adjoining nasal septum. It contains the bipolar olfactory neurons whose peripheral processes (dendrites) extend to the surface and possess chemosensitive cilia that are bathed in mucus. The central processes of these primary olfactory neurons form the axons of the olfactory nerves.

15-4.   The primary olfactory area is located in the region of the uncus. Unlike the other cortical sensory areas, it receives only ipsilateral olfactory impulses.

CHAPTER 16
The Cerebral Cortex: Aphasia, Agnosia, and Apraxia

16-1.   The neocortex is composed of six layers. Layer IV is abundant in granule cells and is the chief recipient of the afferent projection fibers. The infragranular layers are efferent in nature and give rise to the massive efferent projection fibers. The efferent projection fibers arise chiefly from the large pyramidal neurons in layer V and to a lesser extent from the fusiform neurons in layer VI. The supragranular layers are for association. Layer II is rich in granule cells and receives input from other cortical areas. Layer III contains numerous pyramidal neurons, which give rise to association and commissural fibers. Layer I provides for association between adjacent cortical areas.

16-2. The planning of a complex movement occurs in the supplementary motor cortex in the medial surface of the superior frontal gyrus. Focal lesions of the supplementary motor area result in motor apraxia, the inability to perform complex movements on command in the absence of any paralysis.

16-3. a. Right paracentral lobule

b. Frontal eye field chiefly in the posterior part of the left middle frontal gyrus

c. Right primary visual cortex in the parts of the cuneus and lingual gyrus along the calcarine fissure

d. Dorsal part of the primary motor area in the left precentral gyrus

e. Wernicke speech area in the posterior part of the left superior temporal gyrus

f. Right posterior parietal lobe

16-4. A vascular accident involving the left inferior frontal and precentral gyri and underlying white matter results in a sudden loss of speech (Broca aphasia), weakness in the right lower facial muscles (corticobulbar neurons in ventral part of precentral gyrus), and weakness in the right hand (corticospinal neurons in intermediate part of precentral gyrus).

16-5. The smallest lesion resulting in left spastic hemiplegia, lower facial weakness, hemianesthesia, and homonymous hemianopsia occurs in the posterior limb of the right internal capsule where the pyramidal tract, corticobulbar tract, thalamocortical somatosensory radiation, and optic radiation are located.

CHAPTER 17
The Limbic System: Anterograde Amnesia and Inappropriate Social Behavior

17-1. The limbic lobe borders the corpus callosum and rostral brainstem and is composed of the cingulate gyrus and its anterior extension, the septal area, and the parahippocampal gyrus. The limbic system consists of the limbic lobe and the various structures related to it and connected with it that are associated with the consolidation of memory, behavior, and emotions.

17-2. The two key functional centers of the limbic system are the amygdala and hippocampus, both of which are located in the medial part of the temporal lobe. The amygdala is deep to and continuous with the uncus, whereas the hippocampus is deep to and continuous with the posterior part of the parahippocampal gyrus.

17-3. The Papez circuit begins in the hippocampus and passes via the fornix to the mamillary body, from whence the mamillothalamic tract travels to the anterior thalamic nucleus. This nucleus then sends impulses to the cingulate gyrus, which projects via the cingulum to the entorhinal part of the parahippocampal gyrus; this then completes the circuit by connecting with the hippocampus. Although the Papez circuit was initially thought to be concerned with emotions, it is now thought to play a role in memory and learning.

17-4. Bilateral lesions of the hippocampi (or posterior parts of the parahippocampal gyri) result in profound impairment of the ability to recall recent events and to form new memories. Bilateral lesions of the amygdalae result in behavioral alterations usually described as apathy or docility and a profound loss of fear.

17-5. Alzheimer disease: hippocampus or entorhinal area—recent memory; cholinergic neurons of basal nucleus of Meynert—disorientation and long-term memory loss.

Klüver-Bucy syndrome: amygdalae

Korsakoff psychosis: medial parts of medial dorsal thalamic nuclei

17-6. The limbic loop of the basal ganglia includes the ventral striatum or accumbens nucleus and its projections to the ventral pallidum, which sends impulses to the medial dorsal thalamic nucleus that connects with the prefrontal cortex which, in turn, projects to the ventral striatum, thus completing the loop. The limbic loop is associated with behavior and the accumbens nucleus with pleasure or reward.

CHAPTER 18
The Hypothalamus: Vegetative and Endocrine Imbalance

18-1.   The hypothalamus is divided, from anterior to posterior, into chiasmatic, tuberal, and mamillary regions.

18-2.   The neural hypothalamic output passes chiefly to the anterior thalamic nucleus, to the medial dorsal thalamic nucleus, and to brainstem and spinal motor and autonomic centers.

18-3.   The hypophysial portal system is a vascular connection between the tuberal region of the hypothalamus and the anterior pituitary. Hypothalamic regulatory hormones, called excitatory and inhibitory releasing factors, produced chiefly in the arcuate and paraventricular nuclei, are secreted into the hypothalamic capillaries and transported through this portal system to target secretory cells in the anterior pituitary, thus allowing for the widespread hypothalamic influence on endocrine activity.

18-4.   a. Heat loss center in the anterior and preoptic nuclei, heat gain center in the posterior nucleus

   b. Parasympathomimetic activity in anterior and preoptic parts

   c. Sympathomimetic activity in posterior part

   d. Hypothalamic regulatory hormones in tuberal part

   e. Water balance in anterior part

   f. Sleep–wake cycle in anterior part

   g. Emotion in ventromedial and posterior nuclei

CHAPTER 19
The Autonomic Nervous System: Visceral Abnormalities

19-1.   The somatic efferent system is under voluntary control and comprises the alpha motor neurons and their axons, which directly innervate skeletal muscle. The autonomic or general visceral efferent system is involuntary and is composed of two efferent neurons: a preganglionic neuron, located in the brainstem or spinal cord, whose axon synapses in a ganglion; and a postganglionic neuron, located in an autonomic ganglion, whose axon innervates smooth muscle, cardiac muscle, or glandular tissue.

19-2.   The cranial parasympathetic system consists of the following:

   a. Preganglionic neurons in the Edinger-Westphal nucleus whose axons are in the oculomotor nerve;

   b. Preganglionic neurons in the superior salivatory nucleus whose axons travel in the facial nerve;

   c. Preganglionic neurons in the inferior salivatory nucleus whose axons are in the glossopharyngeal nerve;

   d. Preganglionic neurons in the dorsal vagal nucleus and near the nucleus ambiguus whose axons travel in the vagus nerve.

19-3.   The preganglionic sacral parasympathetics arise from neurons in and near the intermediolateral nucleus of S2, S3, and S4.

19-4.   All preganglionic sympathetic fibers arise from the sympathetic nucleus, which extends from about C7 or C8 to L2 or L3. This nucleus comprises an intermediolateral part in the lateral horn, an intermediomedial part in the medial part of lamina VII, an intercalated part that bridges the previous two, and neurons scattered in the lateral funiculus near the lateral horn.

19-5.   Autonomic afferent fibers are very abundant in the glossopharyngeal and vagus nerves. The glossopharyngeal nerve distributes them chiefly to the oral cavity, the pharynx, and the carotid body and sinus. Through the vagus nerve, autonomic afferents are distributed to the thoracic and abdominal viscera. The autonomic afferents in these nerves synapse in the solitary nucleus and are distributed to visceral and somatic nuclei subserving cardiovascular, respiratory, and gastrointestinal reflexes.

19-6.   As a general rule, pain fibers from the thoracic, abdominal, and pelvic viscera reach the spinal cord via the sympathetic nerves and trunks and the T1 to L2 spinal nerves and their dorsal roots. Exceptions to this are the sigmoid colon and rectum, the neck of the bladder, the prostate gland, and the cervix of the uterus, from which pain fibers reach the spinal cord via the pelvic nerves and the S2, S3, and S4 spinal nerves and their dorsal roots.

19-7.   Referred pain is the phenomenon in which pain is localized in a part of the body remote from its source. The basis for the referral is the convergence within the spinal cord of visceral impulses onto somatic neurons, thereby eliciting spinothalamic tract activity that is erroneously interpreted by the cerebral cortex as having originated in cutaneous sites. Thus, referred pain is always located in the somatic area supplied by the spinal cord segments common to both the visceral afferent and the somatic afferent input.

19-8.   Cardiac pain fibers travel centrally in the cardiac nerves to the sympathetic trunk. They then descend in the trunk and travel via the white communicating rami to the spinal nerves and their dorsal roots (where their cell bodies are located) and into the spinal cord. The chief central connections are made at T2 through T4; hence, the retrosternal location of cardiac pain. As the intensity of the pain increases, the T1 and T2 segments become involved and the pain then radiates to the inner aspect of the left arm.

19-9.   Parasympathetic stimulation results in decreased heart rate (bradycardia), emptying of the urinary bladder, and erection of the clitoris or penis. Sympathetic stimulation results in increased heart rate (tachycardia), relaxation of the bladder and contraction of the internal urethral sphincter, and vaginal contractions or ejaculation.

CHAPTER 20
Reticular Formation: Modulation and Activation

20-1.   The chief cranial nerve inputs to the reticular formation are the trigeminal and vestibulocochlear nerves. The reticular formation input from the trigeminal is chiefly pain, whereas the vestibulocochlear is equilibrium and hearing. The spinal input comes from the anterolateral quadrants whose ascending components are associated chiefly with nociception. The forebrain input comes mainly from the hypothalamus and the cerebral cortex.

20-2.   The reticular formation integrates cranial nerve output associated with ocular movements, mastication, facial expression, lacrimation, salivation, deglutition, phonation, and tongue movements. Its spinal projections modulate pain and influence the activity of voluntary muscles and the sympathetic and sacral parasympathetic systems. Its ascending projections to the forebrain influence the thalamus, hypothalamus, limbic centers, and the cerebral cortex.

20-3.   Neuronal degeneration in cholinergic basal forebrain nuclei, especially the basal nucleus of Meynert, is associated with impaired cognitive functions in Alzheimer disease.

20-4.   The center associated with pleasure or reward is the accumbens nucleus, which receives a strong dopaminergic projection from the ventral tegmental area in the midbrain. Psychostimulants increase dopamine activity in the accumbens nucleus.

20-5.   The respiratory center, located bilaterally in the ventrolateral part of the reticular formation at and slightly rostral to the obex, controls inspiration via descending projections to the phrenic nuclei that supply the diaphragm and the intercostal nuclei that supply the intercostal muscles. Bilateral lesions of the medulla at or slightly rostral to the obex will damage the respiratory center, and bilateral lesions at the levels between the obex and the C3 spinal cord segment will interrupt the inspiratory pathway and result in respiratory arrest.

20-6.   Neurons in the anterior hypothalamic nucleus and preoptic area are considered to form the sleep center and, when impaired, insomnia results. Neurons in the posterior hypothalamic nucleus are associated with arousal and, when impaired, hypersomnia results.

20-7. Neurons located bilaterally in the dorso-lateral pontine reticular formation near the locus ceruleus are associated with REM sleep. Bilateral lesions of these neurons result in the loss of REM sleep.

20-8. Impaired consciousness in a patient with head trauma accompanied by oculomotor nerve signs is suggestive of damage to the paramedian midbrain reticular formation through which the ascending reticular activating system travels. Irreparable damage to the ARAS at this level results in irreversible coma.

CHAPTER 21
Summary of the Cranial Nerves: Components and Abnormalities

21-1. a. The vagus nerve supplies the muscles of the vocal cords and soft palate. A left vagal palsy results in a weak, hoarse voice and sagging of the left soft palate.

b. The trochlear nerve supplies the superior oblique muscle. A right trochlear palsy results in impaired depression of the adducted right eye. If this abnormality were caused by a nuclear lesion, it would be on the left side because the trochlear nerve is crossed.

c. The hypoglossal nerve supplies the intrinsic muscles of the tongue. A left hypoglossal palsy results in paralysis of the left genioglossus muscle, thereby allowing the intact right genioglossus to deviate the protruded tongue toward the side of the lesion.

d. The right trigeminal nerve with its ophthalmic, maxillary, and mandibular divisions carries somatosensations from the right side of the face (except the angle of the mandible), and its damage results in right facial hemianesthesia.

e. The left vestibular nerve carries the afferent limb of the vestibulo-ocular reflex (VOR), normally induced by movements of the cupula of the ampullary crest in the horizontal semicircular duct as a result of convection currents caused by cold or warm water irrigation of the left external auditory meatus. Damage to the left vestibular nerve interrupts the afferent limb of the VOR, resulting in the absence of the slow and fast phases of nystagmus. The VOR is responsible for the slow phase, without which there is no fast phase.

f. The right abducens nerve supplies the right lateral rectus muscle whose paralysis results in the absence of abduction in the right eye accompanied by esotropia caused by the pull of the normal medial rectus muscle.

g. The left glossopharyngeal nerve carries gustatory impulses from taste buds in the posterior third of the left side of the tongue and, when damaged, ageusia occurs in this area.

21-2. a. Corneal reflex:
afferent limb—trigeminal nerve
interneurons—spinal trigeminal nucleus
efferent limb—facial nerve

b. Light reflex:
afferent limb—optic nerve
interneurons—pretectal nuclei
efferent limb—oculomotor nerves (to ciliary ganglia)

c. Gag reflex:
afferent limb—glossopharyngeal nerve
interneurons—solitary nucleus
efferent limb—vagus nerve

d. Oculocardiac reflex:
afferent limb—trigeminal nerve
interneurons—spinal trigeminal nucleus
efferent limb—vagus nerve

e. Lacrimation/salivation reflex:
afferent limb—trigeminal nerve
interneurons—spinal trigeminal nucleus
afferent limb—facial nerve (to pterygopalatine and submandibular ganglia)

f. Masseter reflex or jaw jerk:
afferent limb—trigeminal nerve fibers from mesencephalic nucleus
interneuron—none: monosynaptic stretch reflex
efferent limb—trigeminal nerve

g. Vomiting reflex:
afferent limb—vagus nerve
interneurons—solitary nucleus
efferent limb—vagus nerve (plus spinal
nerves to diaphragm and abdominal
muscles)

CHAPTER 22
The Blood Supply of the Central Nervous System: Stroke

22-1. The chief morphologic features of cerebral arteries are a thin intima with many elastic fibers and a prominent internal elastic membrane, a thin media that is frequently absent where the vessels branch, and a thin adventitia with no external elastic membrane. Thus, as compared with extracranial arteries, the cerebral arteries are extremely thin and their structure is conducive to the formation of aneurysms.

22-2. The anatomic substrate of the blood–brain barrier is the nonfenestrated capillary endothelium with its tight junctions.

22-3. The arterial circle of Willis is an anastomosis between the anterior and posterior cerebral circulations, which is found on the ventral surface of the brain surrounding the hypothalamus and interpeduncular fossa. It is formed by the right and left internal carotid arteries laterally and the basilar artery and its right and left posterior cerebral branches posteriorly. The circle is completed posterolaterally by the posterior communicating branches of the internal carotid arteries, which anastomose with the posterior cerebral arteries, anterolaterally by the anterior cerebral branches of the internal carotids, and anteriorly by the anterior communicating arteries that connect the right and left anterior cerebral arteries. The circle is rarely symmetric; in most cases, one of the communicating arteries or a posterior cerebral artery is atrophic. Functionally, the circle serves as a potential vascular shunt.

22-4. The spinal cord is supplied by a single large anterior spinal artery and paired small posterior spinal arteries. These vessels are sup-
plemented along the length of the spinal cord by the radicular branches of the vertebral, ascending cervical, intercostal, and lumbar arteries.

22-5. a. Middle cerebral
b. Anterior cerebral
c. Posterior cerebral
d. Dorsal part by lateral striate branches of middle cerebral and ventral part by anterior choroidal
e. Vertebral or posterior inferior cerebellar
f. Anterior spinal

CHAPTER 23
The Cerebrospinal Fluid System: Hydrocephalus

23-1. CSF functions as protection for the brain and spinal cord against surface contact pressure and sudden motion, as support for cerebral vessels and cranial nerves, and as sustenance for the neuronal internal milieu.

23-2. The lateral ventricle is composed of (1) an anterior or frontal horn that is anterior to the interventricular foramen, (2) a body located beneath the trunk of the corpus callosum, (3) a posterior or occipital horn whose size is highly variable, and (4) an inferior or temporal horn that ends about 3 cm behind the temporal pole. The largest part of the lateral ventricle is at the atrium, a triangular space at the confluence of the body and the occipital and inferior horns. It is located beneath the splenium of the corpus callosum and contains the glomus, a large tuft of choroid plexus.

23-3. CSF is secreted by the choroid plexuses into the lateral, third, and fourth ventricles. It flows from the lateral ventricles into the third ventricle through the paired interventricular foramina (of Monro) and from the third to the fourth ventricle through the cerebral aqueduct. It flows out of the ventricular system through three openings in the fourth ventricle: a median aperture (foramen of Magendie) and paired lateral apertures (foramina of Luschka). It enters the subarachnoid space and then flows around the ventral and dorsal surfaces of the brainstem and over the cerebellum. It eventually passes along the convexity of the cerebral hemispheres toward the superior sagittal sinus into which it is absorbed through the pressure-dependent arachnoid villi and their one-way valves.

23-4. Noncommunicating or obstructive hydrocephalus refers to the blockage of CSF flow anywhere within the ventricular system whereby flow is obstructed from one ventricle to another or from the ventricular system into the subarachnoid space. Communicating hydrocephalus refers to any disruption to the flow of CSF through the subarachnoid space and cisterns or across the arachnoid villi.

CHAPTER 24
Development of the Nervous System: Congenital Anomalies

24-1. The CNS develops from specialized surface ectoderm along the midline of the gastrula.

24-2. The neural crest gives rise to (1) neurons in cranial sensory, spinal sensory, and autonomic ganglia, (2) supporting cells in ganglia and peripheral nerves, and (3) the meninges surrounding the brain and spinal cord.

24-3. Anencephaly results from failure of the anterior neuropore to close, resulting in the malformed rostral end of the brain being exposed. This condition is always fatal.

24-4. The notochord induces by diffusible trophic signals the formation of the neural plate, the neural folds, and the neural tube.

24-5. Radial glia extend processes from the ventricular lumen to the surface of the incipient brain to physically guide migrating neurons toward their target destinations.

24-6. Neurons survive developmental apoptosis because they successfully compete for a limited amount of trophic signal in their targets.

24-7. In the developing cerebellar cortex early outward migration of Purkinje, basket, stellate, and Golgi neurons is followed by the inward migration of granule cells from

the surface of the cortex. In the cerebral cortex all neurons migrate outward from the ventricular germinal epithelium. There is a stratification of neurons in the cerebral cortex based on their age: earlier generated neurons form the deeper layer of the cortex, whereas later generated neurons form progressively more superficial layers of the cortex.

24-8. Lissencephalous occurs when neurogenesis or abnormal neuronal migration fails to form cortical gyri.

CHAPTER 25
Aging of the Nervous System: Dementia

25-1 Neurofibrillary tangles and amyloid plaques are the hallmark pathologic changes in the brains of Alzheimer patients.

25-2. Alzheimer disease is the leading cause of senile dementia.

25-3. Magnetic resonance images of an atrophied brain show widening of the sulci and shrinkage of the gyri as a result of neuronal degeneration and dendritic atrophy in selected areas of the cortex.

25-4. Most neuropathologic changes in the aging cerebral cortex occur in the prefrontal and posterior parietal areas and in the temporal lobe.

CHAPTER 26
Recovery of Function of the Nervous System: Plasticity and Regeneration

26-1. Interruption of anterograde axoplasmic transport is the basis for Wallerian degeneration distal to the site of injury.

26-2. Chromatolysis, an eccentrically located nucleus, swelling of the cell body, and enlargement of the nucleolus occur in axotomized neurons.

26-3. The relative amount of axoplasm lost as the result of injury is the critical determinant for a neuron to survive axonal injury.

Neurons with numerous collateral branches proximal to the injury site or injury located at a distance from the cell body increase the survivability of axotomized neurons.

26-4. The formation of an astrocytic glial scar at the site of injury, the presence of Nogo receptor–recognized proteins in the myelin of oligodendroglia, and a cavity formed at many injury sites collectively block the regrowth of damaged CNS axons.

26-5. Neurotropic molecules serve as chemo-attractants for regenerating axons in the PNS. The effect of the chemoattractants is concentration dependent and determined by the distance the molecules can diffuse from the distal nerve stump to the site of injury.

26-6. A crushing-type injury that does not disrupt the Schwann cell neurolemmal tubes and the basal lamina will result in greater functional recovery than physical separation of the nerve into distal and proximal nerve stumps.

26-7. A neuroma forms by physically blocking regenerating peripheral axons from growing distally past the site of injury. This can result in the formation of abnormal axonal endings that are activated by non-physiologic stimuli such as mechanical distortions.

26-8. Lesion-induced plasticity is age and systems dependent. Damage to the visual pathway from the retina to the visual cortex always results in permanent blindness.

Glossary

Ia nerve fiber axons of dorsal root ganglion cells that supply muscle spindles and excite alpha motor neurons; form afferent limb of myotatic reflex.

Ib nerve fiber axons of dorsal root ganglion cells that supply tendon organs and inhibit alpha motor neurons via spinal interneurons; form afferent limb of inverse myotatic reflex and clasp-knife response.

accommodation center neurons in the tectum of the rostral midbrain that receive input directly from the occipital cortex and integrate the actions of the ciliary muscles, iris muscles, and medial rectus muscles to maintain a focused image on the retina during near or far vision.

accumbens nucleus ventral, medial, and dorsal expansion of the striatum where the head of the caudate nucleus meets the putamen, adjacent to the base of the septum pellucidum at the levels of the basal forebrain and the septal region; syn. ventral striatum.

acoustic neurinoma benign tumor arising from Schwann cells of the VIII cranial nerve (CN). As the tumor grows within the internal acoustic meatus, it progressively affects the cochlear, vestibular, and facial nerves; with further enlargement it invades the cerebellopontine angle affecting the cerebellum and eventually the V, IX, X, and XI CN; syn. acoustic neuroma, neurilemoma or Schwannoma; cerebellopontine angle tumor.

acute sympathetic shock syndrome characterized by bradycardia, hypotension, and bilateral Horner syndrome; occurs in acute bilateral cervical spinal cord injuries as a result of the interruption of the descending impulses to the sympathetic nuclei.

afferent conducting impulses toward.

agnosia inability to recognize sensory stimuli.

agraphesthesia inability to recognize figures written on the skin.

agraphia loss of ability to write.

akinesia loss of ability to initiate and execute voluntary movement.

alar plate that part of the neural tube dorsal to the sulcus limitans that develops into sensory structures.

alexia word blindness; loss of ability to interpret written words.

alpha motor neuron neuron located in anterior horn of spinal cord and in certain brainstem nuclei whose axon passes directly to extrafusal fibers of voluntary muscle; syn. lower motor neuron, α-motor neuron.

alternating hemiplegia combined upper and lower motor neuron brainstem lesion affecting pyramidal tract, which results in contralateral spastic hemiplegia, and affecting oculomotor, abducens, or hypoglossal nerve rootlets, which results in ipsilateral palsies in the respective nerves.

Alzheimer disease presenile dementia in which large numbers of neurofibrillary tangles and neuritic (senile) plaques occur in the cortex. This disease is associated with neuronal degeneration in the hippocampus and parahippocampal gyrus and decreased cortical levels of choline acetyl transferase owing to degeneration of neurons in such basal forebrain structures as the basal nucleus of Meynert and the diagonal band nuclei.

amacrine cell local circuit neuron in the internal nuclear layer of the retina that influences synaptic

359

transmission between the bipolar and the ganglion cells.

ampulla (L., a jug) swelling at end of each semicircular duct which contains the ampullary crest.

ampullary crest (L., crista = crest + ampulla = a jug) sensory organ of kinetic equilibrium occurring as an elevation on the inner aspect of the membranous ampulla of each semicircular duct.

amygdala (G., almond) collection of nuclei within and deep to the uncus of the temporal lobe, forming an important behavior and emotions center of the limbic system; syn. amygdaloid nucleus.

amyloid precursor protein inserted into the membrane of neurons; the external component is cleaved to form amyloid senile plaques in Alzheimer disease.

amyloid senile plaques intracellular and extracellular proteins that are pathologic to surrounding neurons.

amyotrophic lateral sclerosis disease involving coincident degeneration of brainstem and spinal cord lower motor neurons and the corticospinal tracts; syn. Lou Gehrig disease.

analgesia (G., insensibility) relief of pain without loss of consciousness.

anencephaly a congenital absence of the brain caused by the lack of closure of the anterior neuropore of the developing neural tube; always fatal.

anesthesia loss of sensation as a result of pharmacologic depression of nerve function or of neurologic disease.

aneurysm dilation in the wall of a blood vessel.

anhidrosis (G., an = without + hidros = sweat) absence of sweating.

annulospiral stretch receptor afferent nerve ending, located at central portion of a muscle spindle, that responds to muscle stretch.

anomia (G., a + onoma = name) inability to recall names of objects or persons.

anopsia (G., an + opsis = sight) nonuse of vision in one eye.

anosmia (G., an + osmesis = sense of smell) absence of sense of smell.

ansa (L., loop, handle) any anatomic structure in the form of a loop or an arc.

ansa lenticularis outflow tract of the medial pallidum that loops in front of the posterior limb of the internal capsule and enters the prerubral field.

anterior commissure complex fiber system crossing midline in lamina terminalis; interconnects middle and inferior temporal gyri and olfactory bulbs.

anterior limb of internal capsule that part of the internal capsule between the head of the caudate nucleus medially and the lentiform nucleus laterally.

anterior lobe syndrome cerebellar disorder characterized by loss of coordination initially in the lower limbs (gait ataxia), frequently as a result of Purkinje cell degeneration caused by chronic nutritional deficiency frequently associated with alcoholism.

anterior perforated substance region behind orbital surface of frontal lobe and medial and lateral olfactory striae, through which numerous small arteries reach internal structures.

anterograde axonal transport passage from the cell body; two rates occur: (1) fast transport, 400 mm/day; requires neurotubules; membranous organelles, synaptic vesicles, and their precursors are carried this way; (2) slow transport, 1 to 2 mm/day; carries entire cytoskeleton and nonpackaged macromolecules.

anterolateral cordotomy surgical sectioning of anterolateral quadrant of spinal cord for relief of chronic pain.

anterolateral quadrant area of spinal white matter between attachment of denticulate ligaments and emergence of anterior roots; the spinothalamic tract is located here.

antidiuretic hormone (ADH) hormone produced by neurosecretory cells in the supraoptic and paraventricular nuclei of the hypothalamus that stimulates water reabsorption from kidney.

aperture (L., apertura = to open) an opening.

aphasia (G., a + phasis = speech) inability to understand or communicate speech, writing, or signs.

apneustic breathing prolonged inspiration alternating with prolonged expiration; results from damage to dorsolateral tegmentum in the rostral pons.

apraxia (G., a + pratto = to do) inability to carry out a voluntary movement in the absence of paralysis, sensory loss, and ataxia.

aqueous humor fluid of anterior and posterior chambers of the eye; it is secreted by the ciliary body and absorbed through the trabecular spaces at the iridocorneal angle; an increase in its volume is associated with glaucoma.

arachnoid (G., spider) middle of three membranes covering the central nervous system (CNS).

arachnoid granulations groups of arachnoid villi, found predominantly in lacunae of the superior sagittal sinus, through which cerebrospinal fluid (CSF) is absorbed into the venous system; syn. arachnoid villi.

archicerebellum (G., archi = beginning) oldest part of cerebellum; the flocculonodular lobe or vestibulocerebellum located inferiorly, anterior to the posterolateral fissure.

arcuate fasciculus large association bundle connecting the inferior and middle frontal gyri with the superior temporal gyrus; sometimes also considered to include the superior longitudinal fasciculus.

arcuate fibers short association fibers that lie immediately beneath the cortex adjacent to a cerebral sulcus and connect adjacent gyri; syn. U-fibers.

area postrema paired circumventricular organs in the floor of the fourth ventricle near the obex; considered the vomiting center.

Argyll Robertson pupil small pupil that does not react to light but does constrict on accommodation.

ascending reticular activating system (ARAS) components of the brainstem reticular formation that project to parts of the thalamus and subthalamus and pace the activity of the cerebral cortex; if interrupted at the midbrain, coma results; associated with the sleep-wake cycle; sleep centers in the pons, medulla, and hypothalamus project to the ARAS to turn it off to induce sleep; syn. reticular activating system.

astereognosis (G., a + stereos = solid + gnosis = knowledge) inability to identify an object by touch; syn. tactile amnesia.

astrocyte (G., astron = star) star-shaped neuroglial cell with cytoplasmic processes whose terminal expansions or "end-feet" ensheathe blood vessels and the surfaces of the brain and spinal cord.

ataxia (G., a + taxis = order) loss of muscular coordination.

ataxic breathing characterized by irregular and uneven depths of breathing; results from impairment of dorsomedial reticular formation in caudal pons or rostral medulla.

athetosis (G., athetos = without position or place) disorder of movement involving slow writhing movements of the limbs, particularly the fingers and hands; associated with basal ganglia disorders.

auditory ossicles the small bones of the middle ear; malleus, incus, and stapes; they are articulated to form a chain for the transmission of sound-induced vibrations from the tympanic membrane to the oval window.

auditory radiation fibers carrying auditory impulses from the medial geniculate nucleus via the sublenticular part of the internal capsule to the transverse temporal gyri of Heschl.

automatic reflex bladder incontinence and retention; occurs after spinal cord lesions above sacral levels.

autonomic plexus ganglion sympathetic neurons located in plexuses along abdominal aorta and its branches; syn. prevertebral or collateral ganglion.

axon nerve cell process conducting impulses away from cell body.

axon hillock the part of a nerve cell body at the origin of the axon that is characterized by the absence of Nissl substance.

axon reaction response of the neuron to axotomy that includes swelling of the soma, movement of the nucleus to an eccentric location, chromatolysis, enlargement of the nucleolus, and disengagement of presynaptic boutons.

axotomy functional or physical separation of an axon into distal and proximal parts.

Babinski response abnormal upward extension (dorsiflexion) of great toe in response to stroking outer border of the sole; usually indicates pyramidal tract damage; syn. extensor plantar reflex or response.

ballismus (G., ballismos = a jumping about) violent jerking or flinging movements of proximal parts of limbs and shoulders and pelvic girdle musculature; associated with lesions of the subthalamic nucleus.

basal ganglia nuclear masses in the cerebral hemisphere, diencephalon, and midbrain that influence voluntary movements; include corpus striatum, subthalamic nucleus, and substantia nigra.

basal nucleus (of Meynert) extensive group of neurons located in the substantia innominata of the anterior perforated substance; major source of cholinergic projections to neocortex and implicated in Alzheimer disease.

basal plate that part of the neural tube ventral to the sulcus limitans that develops into motor structures.

basilar membrane membrane supporting the organ of Corti; stretches between the osseous spiral lamina and spiral ligament; syn. membranous spiral lamina.

basket cell inhibitory neuron found deep in molecular layer of cerebellar cortex, whose axon forms a basketlike ramification around the base of a Purkinje cell body.

Bell palsy weakness of upper and lower facial muscles and inability to close the eye completely; usually caused by inflammation of facial nerve in the facial canal.

bitemporal hemianopsia loss of temporal vision in both eyes; results from median lesion of optic chiasm.

blind spot area in the retina at the origin of the optic (II) nerve in which there are no photoreceptor cells.

blood-brain barrier permeability control system governing the passage of substances between capillaries and the CNS parenchyma; related to tight junctions between endothelial cells.

bone conduction sound vibrations conducted to the internal ear by the temporal bone.

bony labyrinth series of cavities within the petrous portion of the temporal bone forming the vestibule, cochlea, and semicircular canals of the inner ear; syn. osseous labyrinth.

brachium (L., arm) a large bundle of nerve fibers connecting one structure with another.

brachium of the inferior colliculus prominent bundle on lateral surface of rostral midbrain containing fibers passing from the inferior colliculus to the medial geniculate nucleus; landmark for neurosurgical transection of spinothalamic tract for relief of intractable pain.

brachium of the superior colliculus fibers arising mainly from the optic tract and passing between the medial geniculate nucleus and the pulvinar to enter the superior colliculus and pretectal area.

bradycardia slowness of the heart beat, usually defined as a rate under 60 beats per minute.

bradykinesia (G., brady = slow + kinesis = movement) extreme slowness in purposeful movements, frequently associated with basal ganglia disease.

brain atrophy occurs as the result of shrinkage of cortical gyri owing to neuronal death or dendritic wasting and the increase in the width of the separating sulci.

Broca area opercular and triangular parts of inferior frontal gyrus in dominant hemisphere; associated with motor programs for production of words; nonfluent (motor or expressive) aphasia is attributed to its injury.

Brodmann numerical areas numeric subdivisions of the cerebral cortex, originally based on cytoarchitectural characteristics but now related to functions.

Brown-Séquard syndrome hemisection of the spinal cord; causes ipsilateral spastic paralysis and loss of tactile, vibration, and proprioception and contralateral loss of pain and temperature sensations below the level of the lesion.

calcar avis that part of the medial wall of the posterior horn of the lateral ventricle which lies deep to the calcarine fissure.

canal of Schlemm canal that drains aqueous humor; found encircling cornea at corneoscleral junction; syn. sinus venosus sclerae.

capsular cell supporting cells surrounding the cell bodies of dorsal root and autonomic ganglion cells.

carotid plexuses postganglionic sympathetic fibers traveling along carotid arteries to smooth muscle and glands of head.

carotid siphon hairpin bend formed by internal carotid artery within the petrous canal and cavernous sinus.

cataract a loss of transparency of the lens of the eye, or of its capsule.

cauda equina (L., cauda = tail + equus = horse) roots of lumbar and sacral nerves as they travel in the vertebral canal below the spinal cord to their respective lumbar intervertebral or sacral foramina.

caudal a position more toward the tail or more inferior.

central neurogenic hyperventilation sustained, rapid, deep hyperpnea; results from impairment of deep periaqueductal gray and paramedian reticular formation in midbrain or isthmus of pons.

cephalic flexure fold where the prosencephalon of the developing neural tube bends ventrally just anterior to the mesencephalon.

cerebellar angle area on ventrolateral surface of brainstem where cerebellum, pons, and medulla meet; VII, VIII, and IX CN attach at this point.

cerebellar peduncle fiber bundles connecting the cerebellum to the brainstem.

cerebral aqueduct midbrain channel connecting third and fourth ventricles; syn. aqueduct of Sylvius, iter.

cerebral arterial circle arterial ring found on base of brain and formed by branches of the internal carotid and basilar arteries; connects the anterior and posterior circulations; syn. circle of Willis.

cerebral crus ventral part of cerebral peduncle of midbrain; contains corticospinal and corticobulbar fibers in its middle part and corticopontine in its medial and lateral parts.

cerebral edema brain swelling caused by increased uptake of water in the neuropil and white matter.

cerebral ischemia decreased blood supply in the brain.

cerebral palsy neurologic disorder generally diagnosed in infants to 3-year-old children that affects muscle contractions and coordination of movements. Movements are generally ataxic, and increased muscle tone (spasticity) and exaggerated reflexes are present. There is not a common cause for cerebral palsy. In utero hypoxia, asphyxia during the birthing process, and postnatal infections or head injuries can result in cerebral palsy. There is no cure for this disorder.

cerebral peduncle ventral part of midbrain that connects the forebrain to the hindbrain and consists of the cerebral crus, substantia nigra, and tegmentum.

cerebrocerebellum posterior lobe of the cerebellum having strong connections with the cerebrum; syn. neocerebellum.

cerebrospinal fluid (CSF) clear, colorless liquid secreted by the choroid plexuses and found in the ventricular system and subarachnoid space; total volume is approximately 150 mL; rate of formation is approximately 500 mL/day.

Charcot-Marie-Tooth disease one of the most common inherited neurologic disorders affecting peripheral nerves. This neuropathy affects both motor and sensory nerves, resulting in abnormalities initially in the distal part of the lower limb and later in the distal part of the upper limb. Motor abnormalities include weakness and muscle atrophy.

Cheyne-Stokes respiration characterized by alternating hyperpnea and apnea; results from bilateral dysfunction of structures deep in the cerebral hemispheres or diencephalon.

chiasm (G., chiasma = two crossing lines) the crossing of optic nerve fibers beneath the anterior part of the hypothalamus.

chorea (G., dance) jerky, spasmodic involuntary movements of limbs or facial muscles; associated with lesions of the caudate nucleus and putamen.

choroid (G., skin-like) the vascular tunic of the eye located between the sclera and retina.

choroid plexus epithelium and blood vessels of the lateral, third, and fourth ventricles; secretes CSF.

chromatolysis (G., chroma = color + lysis = dissolution) the dissolution of Nissl substance in response to damage of a neuron or its axon.

ciliary (L.) resembling an eyelid or eyelash.

ciliary body thickening of the uvea of the eye; suspends the lens and contains smooth muscles that pull forward in accommodation; also secretes aqueous humor.

ciliospinal center neurons in the upper one or two thoracic segments giving rise to sympathetic preganglionic fibers that convey impulses to the superior cervical ganglion from whence postganglionic sympathetic fibers elicit pupillary dilation.

ciliospinal reflex dilation of pupils in response to pain, usually elicited by stroking the side of the head or neck; dependent on intact path that includes descending central autonomic path, ciliospinal center neurons, and their preganglionic sympathetic fibers, which ascend in the cervical sympathetic trunk, and includes superior cervical ganglion cells whose postganglionic fibers reach the dilator muscle of the iris.

cingulum (L., girdle) a large association bundle passing longitudinally in the white matter of the cingulate gyrus; connects frontal, parietal, and occipital lobes with parahippocampal gyrus and adjacent temporal cortex.

circadian rhythm biologic activity (such as sleep) that occurs in approximately 24-hour periods or cycles; the "clock" resides in the suprachiasmatic nucleus of the hypothalamus.

circle of Willis see *cerebral arterial circle*.

circumventricular organs highly vascularized areas with fenestrated capillaries; found chiefly in the diencephalon and lacking the blood-brain barrier.

clasp-knife response sudden relaxation or decrease in resistance to passive stretch of a limb after initial increased resistance; involves Golgi tendon organ (Ib) activity and is seen in pyramidal tract damage.

claustrum (L., barrier) a thin sheet of gray matter deep to the insula and between external and extreme capsules; has reciprocal connections with neocortex.

climbing fibers axons arising from the contralateral inferior olivary nucleus and carrying excitatory impulses to the Purkinje neurons of the cerebellar cortex; collaterals also excite cerebellar nuclei.

clonus series of alternating contractions and relaxations of flexors and extensors produced by passive stretch of a limb; seen in pyramidal tract damage.

cluster breathing characterized by several rapid deep breaths alternating with periods of apnea; results from damage at midpontine levels.

cochlea (L., snail shell) spiral part of internal ear concerned with audition; located in anterior part of labyrinth in petrous part of temporal bone.

cogwheel rigidity type of rigidity in which passive movements exhibit intermittent resistance as if cogwheels were moving on one another; a manifestation of tremor superimposed on rigidity, frequently seen in parkinsonism.

colliculus (L.) a mound or small elevation.

commissural syndrome loss of pain and temperature bilaterally caused by lesion of ventral white commissure of spinal cord.

commissure (L., a joining together) a bundle of nerve fibers joining corresponding parts of both sides with each other.

communicating hydrocephalus disruption of CSF flow outside the ventricular system, usually in the cisterns, subarachnoid space, or arachnoid villi.

conduction aphasia associative aphasia; a form of aphasia in which the patient can speak and write in a way, but skips or repeats words or substitutes; associated with lesions in arcuate fasciculus.

conduction deafness incomplete deafness caused by interference with passage of sound waves through the external ear or sound-induced vibrations through the middle ear.

cone photoreceptor of retina concerned with color perception and visual acuity.

conjugate eye movements movements of both eyes together.

consensual light reflex pupillary constriction of one eye in response to light reaching the retina of the other eye; dependent on intact optic nerve ipsilaterally and oculomotor nerve contralaterally.

contralateral (L., contra = opposite + lotus = side) related to the opposite side.

cornea the anterior, transparent part of the external layer of the eye.

corneal reflex closure of the eye on stimulation of the cornea; dependent on afferent impulses in ophthalmic division of trigeminal nerve and spinal trigeminal tract and efferent impulses through facial nucleus and nerve.

corona radiata (L., corona = crown) fibers fanning out from the internal capsule to the cortex.

corpora quadrigemina (L., corpora = body + quadri = four + geminus = twin) the two superior colliculi and the two inferior colliculi.

corpus callosum the major commissure connecting the cerebral hemispheres.

corpus striatum caudate and lentiform nuclei.

cortical columns columns of neurons in cerebral cortex oriented perpendicular to six layers of cortex; make up the vertical functional units of the cortex.

corticofugal fibers axons carrying impulses away from the cortex.

corticopetal fibers axons carrying impulses toward the cortex.

cough reflex coughing response elicited by irritation of larynx or tracheobronchial tree; dependent on intact afferent fibers in vagus nerve.

crossed extension reflex automatic response coupled with the flexor reflex that results in the contraction of extensor muscles contralateral to flexor muscles reflexively activated because of an ipsilateral painful stimulus.

cuneus (L., wedge) wedge-shaped part of occipital lobe on medial surface between calcarine and parieto-occipital fissures.

cupula of ampullary crest (L., dome-shaped cup; cupa = a tub) the gelatinous substance lying over the hair cells of the ampullary crest.

cyton the cell body of a neuron; syn. soma.

decerebrate posturing describes one whose brain has been impaired between the vestibular nuclei and the red nucleus, that is, in the midbrain or rostral pons; characterized by extension of upper and lower limbs.

decibel unit of measurement expressing the relative loudness of a sound on a logarithmic scale.

decorticate posturing describes one whose brain has been impaired above the red nucleus, that is, in the forebrain; characterized by extension of lower limbs and flexion of upper limbs.

decussation a crossing of nerve tracts.

deglutition the act of swallowing.

dementia temporally progressive impairment of higher mental function and memory. Dementia can be irreversible or reversible depending on the underlying cause.

dendrite (G., dendron = tree) a branching neuronal protoplasmic process carrying impulses to the cell body.

dendritic spine cytoplasmic bud on surface of a dendrite for synaptic contact; syn. gemmule.

dentate nucleus most lateral of the cerebellar nuclei; receives Purkinje cell axons from lateral part of hemisphere.

denticulate ligament fibrous sheath attached medially to the pia at the lateral surface of the spinal cord, midway between the dorsal and ventral roots; anchors the spinal cord to the dura mater by its lateral serrated part consisting of 21 toothlike processes.

dermatome (G., derma = skin + tome = a cutting) an area of skin supplied by one spinal nerve and its ganglion.

dermatomyositis a progressive decrease in muscle strength coupled with the appearance of a purplish-red skin rash.

detrusor muscle muscle in the wall of the urinary bladder.

diabetes insipidus condition caused by hyposecretion of ADH and characterized by thirst and the excretion of large amounts of urine.

diaphragma sellae dural fold covering the pituitary gland; extends across sella turcica.

dichromatic vision abnormal perception of only two of the three primary colors.

diencephalon (G., dia = through + enkephalos = brain) that part of the forebrain consisting of the thalamus, subthalamus, hypothalamus, and epithalamus; syn. through-brain.

diffuse modulating systems groups of neurons chiefly in the brainstem and associated with neurotransmitters that are distributed diffusely in the CNS via axons with innumerable branches; function to regulate the excitability of vast numbers of neurons.

diplopia double vision.

direct light reflex pupillary constriction in one eye in response to increased light reaching the retina of the same eye; dependent on intact ipsilateral optic and oculomotor nerves.

disc edema edema of the optic disc; may be caused by elevated intracranial pressure; syn. papilledema, choked disc.

doll's eye movements turning of the eyes in the direction opposite to that of rotation of the head; signifies intact vestibulo-ocular reflex in comatose patient; syn. oculocephalic reflex.

dominant hemisphere the hemisphere responsible for speech, usually the left.

dorsal rhizotomy section of the dorsal roots of spinal nerves for the relief of pain or spasticity.

dorsal root entry zone (DREZ) area in spinal cord where the dorsal roots attach, just external to dorsal horn; DREZ lesions are surgical procedures to abolish chronic deafferentation pain.

dorsal root ganglion groups of unipolar afferent neurons in the dorsal root of each spinal nerve; syn. spinal ganglion.

dorsolateral fasciculus spinal cord tract located between the posterior horn and the posterolateral sulcus; composed of short ascending and descending branches of dorsal root fibers carrying pain and temperature impulses and axons of substantia gelatinosa neurons; syn. tract of Lissauer.

Down syndrome mongolism; trisomy 21 syndrome; a syndrome of mental retardation associated with a variable constellation of abnormalities caused by representation of at least a critical portion of chromosome 21 three times instead of twice in some or all cells.

dura mater (L., dura = hard + mater = mother) the thick outer layer of the meninges.

dural sac continuation of dura mater from LV2 to SV2 containing CSF and the cauda equina.

dural sinus valveless, venous channel found in dural attachments and folds.

dys a prefix denoting disordered, difficult, bad, painful, and so forth.

dysdiadochokinesia (G., dys + diadochos = succeeding + kinesis = movement) a cerebellar disorder manifested by difficulty in rapidly alternating diametrically opposite movements, e.g., pronation and supination.

dyskinesia (G., dys + kinesis) disorder of voluntary movement frequently associated with basal ganglia disease.

dyslexia (G., dys + lexis = word, speech) a disturbance of the ability to read caused by a central lesion.

dysmetria (G., dys + metron = measure) a cerebellar disorder manifested by difficulty in controlling the range and force of movement.

dysphagia (G., dys + phagein = to eat) difficulty in swallowing.

dysphasia (G., dys + phasis = speech) impairment of speech, characterized by a lack of coordination and failure to arrange words in proper order.

ectoderm one of three germ cell layers in the developing gastrula.

Edinger-Westphal nucleus visceral motor nucleus in oculomotor complex; gives rise to preganglionic parasympathetic fibers of oculomotor nerves; plays a role in pupillary constriction and accommodation.

efferent conducting impulses away from.

emboliform nucleus (G., embolos = wedge) cerebellar nucleus located medial to dentate nucleus; receives Purkinje cell axons from paravermal or intermediate part of hemisphere; part of interposed nucleus.

encephalon (G., enkephalos) brain.

end artery artery carrying bulk of blood to given region.

endolymph fluid of the membranous labyrinth of the inner ear.

entorhinal area part of the parahippocampal gyrus adjacent to the hippocampus; provides sole input to the hippocampus.

ependyma (G., epi = upon + endyma = garment) epithelium lining the central canal of the spinal cord and the ventricles of the brain.

epidural space area external to dura; potential in cranial dura, actual in spinal dura.

epithalamus a small area of the diencephalon, dorsal to the posterior part of the thalamus, consisting of pineal gland, habenular trigones, and habenular commissure.

esotropia (G., eso = inward + trope = turn) inward deviation of the eye; frequently caused by abducens nerve lesion; syn. convergent or internal strabismus.

expressive aphasia see *nonfluent aphasia*.

extensor plantar response see *Babinski response*.

extrafusal muscle fibers large skeletal muscle fibers that produce muscular contraction and are innervated by alpha motor neurons; to be distinguished from intrafusal muscle fibers within muscle spindles, which are innervated by gamma motor neurons.

falx (L.) shaped like a sickle.

falx cerebelli dural fold lying between the cerebellar hemispheres.

falx cerebri dural fold lying between the cerebral hemispheres.

fasciculus (L., fascis = bundle) a bundle of nerve fibers within the CNS.

fasciculus retroflexus see *habenulointerpeduncular tract*.

fast pain sharp, pricking pain that is well localized; tested by pinprick.

fastigial nucleus most medial of the cerebellar nuclei; receives Purkinje cell axons from vermal region.

filtration angle see *iridocorneal angle*.

fimbria (L., fringe) longitudinal band of fibers coming from the alveus of hippocampus and continuing as the fornix.

final common path term used for the alpha motor neurons through which are funneled all impulses from multiple sources to the skeletal muscles; only connections between CNS and extrafusal muscle fibers.

fissure a deep furrow, cleft, or slit.

fissure of Sylvius deep groove on lateral surface of cerebral hemisphere; separates temporal lobe below from frontal and parietal lobes above; syn. lateral fissure.

fixation point point on which vision is focused.

flaccid paralysis muscle paralysis with hypotonicity; the cardinal sign of a lower motor neuron lesion.

flexion withdrawal reflex automatic motor response to withdraw from an ipsilateral painful stimulus.

flocculonodular lobe syndrome disorder characterized by instability of the trunk (truncal ataxia) usually caused by tumors near the midline of the vestibulocerebellum; syn. vestibulocerebellar midline syndrome.

floor plate ventral part of the developing neural tube. Although not involved with neurogenesis, it exerts a significant influence on the migration and differentiation of neurons in the basal plate and axonal guidance.

fluent aphasia type of language disorder in which words are formed rapidly but they do not make sense because of the loss of ability to comprehend spoken or written words; associated with lesion of Wernicke area; syn. sensory or receptive aphasia.

folium (L., a leaf) one of the folds of the cerebellar surface.

foramen of Luschka see *lateral aperture of the fourth ventricle*.

foramen of Magendie see *median aperture of the fourth ventricle*.

foramen of Monro opening between third ventricle and lateral ventricle; syn. interventricular foramen.

forceps (L. formus = warm + capere–to take) a pincerlike instrument.

forceps major fibers of the splenium of the corpus callosum that extend posteriorly into the occipital lobe.

forceps minor fibers of the genu of the corpus callosum that extend anteriorly into the frontal lobe.

forebrain most rostral subdivision of the brain consisting of the telencephalon and diencephalon; syn. prosencephalon.

fornix (L., arch) bundle of fibers continuous with fimbria of hippocampus that is the main output of the hippocampus; runs in the free margin of the septum pellucidum and divides at the anterior commissure into a small precommissural bundle (from the hippocampus proper) and a larger postcommissural bundle (from the subiculum), which end in the septal region and mamillary body, respectively.

fovea (L., pit) a cup-shaped depression or pit.

fovea centralis depression in the center of the macula lutea of the retina caused by displacement of the inner layers; contains only cones and is the area of most acute vision.

foveola minute pit in the center of the fovea centralis.

frontal eye field area of the cerebral cortex located mainly in the posterior part of the middle frontal gyrus and concerned with voluntary eye movements.

funiculus (L., little cord) one of three subdivisions of the spinal white matter.

GABA γ-aminobutyric acid, an inhibitory neurotransmitter.

gag reflex contraction of pharyngeal muscles on stimulation of the lateral part of the oral pharynx; dependent on intact afferent fibers in glossopharyngeal nerve and efferent fibers in vagus nerve.

gait ataxia ataxia affecting the muscles of the lower limbs.

gamma-loop three-neuron reflex arc, consisting of a gamma motor neuron and its fusimotor axon, which causes intrafusal muscle fibers to contract; a Ia afferent fiber and its dorsal root ganglion cell; and an alpha motor neuron and its motor endplates, which cause extrafusal muscle fibers to contract. Allows for initiation or influence of movements and tone by alpha motor neurons.

gamma motor neuron neurons located in same places as alpha motor neurons but which innervate intrafusal muscle fibers; maintain muscle spindle sensitivity; syn. γ-motor neuron.

ganglion (G., a swelling or knot) a collection of nerve cell bodies in the peripheral nervous system.

gemmule (L., gemma = a bud) cytoplasmic bud on surface of a dendrite for synaptic contact; syn. dendritic spine.

genu (L.) knee, any structure shaped like a bent knee.

genu of internal capsule that part of the internal capsule between the posterior part of the head of the caudate nucleus and anterior part of the thalamus medially and the lentiform nucleus laterally.

Gerstmann syndrome disorder characterized by finger agnosia, acalculia, right-left confusion, and agraphia; caused by lesion in dominant hemisphere near junction of inferior parietal lobule and occipital lobe.

glaucoma disorder of the eye characterized by increased intraocular pressure resulting from interference with absorption or excessive formation of aqueous humor.

glia (G., glue) interstitial, supportive cells within the central nervous system; syn. neuroglia.

glioblasts glial progenitor cells in the CNS.

global aphasia most severe aphasia combining deficits seen in Broca, Wernicke, and conduction aphasias.

globose nucleus cerebellar nucleus located lateral to fastigial nucleus; receives Purkinje cell axons from paravermal or intermediate part of hemisphere; part of interposed nucleus.

globus pallidus (L., globus = globe + pallidus = pale) inner part of the lentiform nucleus found between the putamen and the internal capsule; one of the basal ganglia; syn. pallidum.

glomus (L., a ball) the choroid plexus in the atrium (trigone) of the lateral ventricle; probably the most prolific producer of CSF; syn. choroid enlargement.

glutamate excitatory neurotransmitter.

Golgi neuron (of cerebellum) nerve cell of granular layer of cerebellar cortex whose dendrites in the molecular layer are excited by the granule cell axons and whose axon inhibits granule cells.

Golgi tendon organ proprioceptive ending found in tendons; its appropriate stimulus is an increase in tendon tension.

granule cell (1) nerve cell of the inner or granular layer of the cerebellar cortex; axon enters molecular layer and forms the parallel plexus; only excitatory neuron in the cerebellar cortex. (2) intracortical neurons found predominantly in layers II and IV of the neocortex.

graphesthesia ability to recognize and identify figures drawn on the skin.

Guillain-Barré syndrome acquired neuropathy caused by an immune-mediated demyelination of peripheral nerve axons that is treated by plasmapheresis or immunoglobulin therapy.

gustatory (L., gusto = to taste) relating to the sense of taste.

gustatory nucleus rostral part of the solitary nucleus receptive for taste fibers.

gyrus (L., gyros = circle) prominent, rounded elevations on surface of cerebral hemispheres separated by sulci; pl. gyri.

habenula cell mass found at dorsal and posterior edge of the third ventricle near the pineal gland; part of the epithalamus.

habenulointerpeduncular tract compact bundle of fibers arising in the habenula and passing ventrally to the interpeduncular nucleus of the midbrain and the adjacent reticular formation; syn. fasciculus retroflexus.

heat gain center neurons in posterior hypothalamus that initiate cutaneous vasoconstriction, piloerection, and shivering.

heat loss center neurons in preoptic and anterior hypothalamic nuclei that initiate sweating and cutaneous vasodilation.

helicotrema (G., helix = coil + trema = hole) area at the apex of the cochlea where the scala vestibuli and scala tympani communicate with one another.

hemi (G.) half.

hemianopsia blindness in half of the visual field in one or both eyes.

hemiparesis weakness or incomplete paralysis of one side.

hemiplegia paralysis of one side of the body.

heteronymous (G., having a different name) different visual fields of both eyes.

hindbrain pons, cerebellum, and medulla; syn. rhombencephalon.

hippocampus (G., sea horse) curved band of archipallium located in temporal lobe between choroidal fissure and parahippocampal gyrus; consists of dentate gyrus, hippocampus proper, and subiculum; concerned with learning and memory and processing of new information; syn. hippocampal formation.

homonymous (G., of the same name) same visual field of both eyes.

horizontal cell local circuit neuron in the internal nuclear layer of the retina that influences synaptic transmission between the photoreceptor cells and the bipolar neurons.

horizontal gaze center see *lateral gaze center*.

Horner syndrome disorder characterized by ptosis, miosis, and anhidrosis; caused by central or peripheral interruption of sympathetic impulses to face and eye.

Huntington disease hereditary disorder characterized by progressive increase in choreoid movements and dementia; inherited by a dominant gene that causes degeneration of striatal and cortical acetylcholine and GABA neurons.

hydrocephalus (G., hydro = water + kephale = head) excessive accumulation of CSF caused by obstruction of flow, interference with drainage, or increased formation.

hyper (G., hyper = above) prefix signifying above, beyond, or excessive.

hyperacusis (G., hyper + akousis = hearing) abnormal loudness of hearing.

hypercarbia increased carbon dioxide at the tissue level.

hyperkinetic disorders increased or excessive speed in the initiation or performance of a movement.

hyperthermia fever or increased body temperature.

hypertonia, hypertonicity (G., hyper + tonos = tension) excessive tone in skeletal muscles; results in increased resistance to passive stretch.

hypo (G., hypo = under) prefix signifying beneath, under, or deficient.

hypocarbia decreased carbon dioxide at the tissue level.

hypokinetic disorders (G., hypo = under + kinesis = movement) decrease or slowing in the initiation or performance of a movement.

hypophysial portal system vascular connection between the median eminence and adjacent infundibular stalk and the anterior lobe of the pituitary by means of which the hypothalamic releasing factors are transported.

hypothalamic regulatory hormones substances formed in hypothalamic neurons that are transported to the pituitary gland to regulate the release of its hormones.

hypothalamic syndrome disorder manifested by diabetes insipidus, endocrine disorders, impairment of temperature regulation, abnormalities in sleep patterns, and behavior changes; results from a lesion of the hypothalamus.

hypothalamohypophysial tract unmyelinated fibers from the supraoptic and paraventricular nuclei of the hypothalamus, which reach the posterior pituitary.

hypothalamus part of the diencephalon forming the ventral walls of the third ventricle; chief effector of the limbic system and the highest control center for the autonomic nervous system.

hypotonia, hypotonicity (G., hypo + tonos = tension) diminution or loss of muscular tonicity; results in decreased resistance to passive stretch.

hypoxia lack of adequate oxygen at the tissue level.

inferior cerebellar peduncle fiber bundle connecting the cerebellum and medulla.

inferior fronto-occipital fasciculus association bundle interconnecting frontal, temporal, and occipital lobes.

infranuclear lesion lower motor neuron lesion involving axon in peripheral nerve.

infundibulum (L., a funnel) median eminence and infundibular stem of neurohypophysis; syn. neural stalk.

insula (L., island) lobe of the cerebrum located deep to the lateral fissure; syn. island of Reil.

intention tremor to and fro shaking that occurs when a voluntary movement is made; associated with posterior cerebellar lobe dysfunction.

intercalated (L., intercalare = to insert) in between; syn. internuncial.

internal arcuate fiber secondary tactile, vibration, and proprioception sense axons from the dorsal column nuclei that arch around the central gray in the caudal half of the medulla.

internal capsule white matter between the caudate nucleus and diencephalon medially and the lentiform nucleus laterally; continuous rostrally with corona radiata, caudally with cerebral crus.

internuclear ophthalmoplegia (G., ophthalmos = eye + plege = stroke) disorder of eye movements caused by damage to the medial longitudinal fasciculus between the abducens and oculomotor nuclei; manifested during horizontal conjugate movements by lack of adduction in eye on same side as lesion.

interpeduncular fossa deep depression on the ventral surface of the midbrain between the cerebral peduncles.

interthalamic adhesion nuclear connection between the two thalami across the third ventricle; syn. massa intermedia.

intrafusal muscle fiber muscle fiber part of a muscle spindle, innervated by gamma motor neurons.

inverse myotatic reflex contraction of a muscle causes an increase in tension, which fires a Golgi tendon organ that carries this information by Ib fibers to excite the antagonists and inhibit the synergists.

iodopsin visual pigment of the cones.

ipsilateral (L., ipse = same + latus = side) on the same side; e.g., disorder occurring on the same side as the lesion.

iridocorneal angle angle of the anterior chamber of the eye through which aqueous humor drains into the scleral trabeculae; syn. filtration angle.

iris (G., rainbow) the circular pigmented membrane behind the cornea, perforated in the center by the pupil; it is the anterior division of the uvea and is attached marginally to the ciliary body; pl. irides.

Ishihara test determines whether there is an impairment of color vision by asking the patient to identify numbers formed by dots of a single color embedded with a background of different colored dots.

isthmus rhombencephali part of the pons rostral to the cerebellum that merges with the midbrain.

juxta (L.) near to.

juxtarestiform body fiber bundle in medial part of inferior cerebellar peduncle carrying primarily vestibular fibers.

kernicterus nuclear jaundice in which yellow pigment is formed in certain basal ganglia and limbic nuclei.

kinesthesia (G., kinesis = movement + aisthesis = sensation) awareness of position and movement of body parts.

kinocilium (G., kineo = to move + cilium) longest cilium found on hair cell in ampullary crest; bending of stereocilia toward or away from kinocilium results in excitation or inhibition (respectively) of vestibular nerve fibers.

Klüver-Bucy syndrome disorder characterized by a profound loss of fear, docility, oral tendencies, and hypersexuality; results from bilateral ablation of the amygdalae.

Korsakoff syndrome disorder involving memory loss, confusion, and often confabulation; lesions frequently found in the walls of the third ventricle involving the mamillary bodies, medial dorsal thalamic nuclei, or anterior thalamic nuclei.

labyrinth the fluid-filled intercommunicating spaces of the internal ear.

labyrinthectomy ablation of the vestibular membranous labyrinth to ameliorate the clinical signs of Ménière disease.

lamina (L., a plate) a thin layer.

lateral aperture lateral opening connecting fourth ventricle with subarachnoid space; syn. foramen of Luschka.

lateral fissure most prominent cleft on lateral surface of cerebral hemisphere; begins anteriorly and proceeds posteriorly separating the frontal and parietal lobes from the temporal lobe; syn. sylvian fissure.

lateral gaze center neurons in the paramedian pontine reticular nucleus that elicit horizontal eye movements to the ipsilateral side; formerly called parabducens nucleus; syn. horizontal gaze center.

lateral lemniscus tract in the lateral part of the pontine and midbrain tegmentum from the pontomedullary junction to the inferior colliculus; composed of the central acoustic fibers, although sometimes the spinothalamic tract is included.

lateral medullary syndrome disorder characterized by loss of pain and temperature sensations over ipsilateral half of face and contralateral half of body; nausea; vertigo; ipsilateral ataxia; ipsilateral paralysis of soft palate, pharynx, and vocal cord; and Horner syndrome. Caused by vascular lesion involving the vertebral or the posterior inferior cerebellar artery; syn. Wallenberg syndrome.

lead-pipe rigidity bidirectional hypertonicity resulting from increased tone in all of the muscles acting on a joint; associated with basal ganglia disorders.

lemniscus (G., lemniskos = ribbon or fillet) a secondary sensory tract ascending through the brainstem to the thalamus.

lenticular fasciculus bundle of fibers emerging from the medial pallidum and piercing through the posterior limb of the internal capsule to enter the subthalamus through which it travels medially to reach the prerubral field where it enters the thalamic fasciculus; syn. Forel's field H2.

leptomeninges (G., leptos = slender or delicate + meninx = membrane) arachnoid and pia mater, the two thin membranes covering the brain and spinal cord.

lesion-induced plasticity modification of surviving axonal connections in response to CNS injury.

light reflex constriction of pupil on increased light reaching the retina.

limbic lobe (L., limbus = border) structures on medial surface of cerebral hemisphere bordering the corpus callosum and rostral brainstem; includes chiefly the cingulate and parahippocampal gyri.

limbic system (L., limbus = border) cortical and subcortical structures that influence behavior and autonomic responses chiefly through the hypothalamus;

includes the limbic lobe, amygdala, hippocampus, septal region, and hypothalamus; some also include the anterior thalamic nucleus, medial part of the midbrain tegmentum, orbitofrontal cortex, and anterior cingulate gyrus.

Lissauer's tract a tract at the dorsolateral surface of the spinal cord that contains short (two segments or less) pain and temperature fibers from the dorsal roots and axons from the substantia gelatinosa neurons; syn. dorsolateral fasciculus.

lissencephalous smooth appearance of the cerebral cortex where gyri failed to develop.

locus ceruleus (L., locus = place + caeruleus = dark blue) pigmented nucleus in the rostral and lateral part of the floor of the fourth ventricle formed by catecholamine-containing neurons.

loop of Meyer those fibers of the optic radiation, which, after leaving the lateral part of the lateral geniculate nucleus and passing into the temporal lobe, arch over the anterior part of the inferior horn of the lateral ventricle before turning back toward the occipital lobe.

lower motor neuron brainstem or spinal cord alpha motor neuron; axon carries impulses to extrafusal muscle fibers; syn. final common pathway.

lower motor neuron syndrome disorder characterized by flaccid paralysis, decreased or absent reflexes, and severe atrophy; caused by loss of the final common path, i.e., the loss of the alpha motor neurons or their axons innervating a muscle.

lumbar puncture procedure by which the dural sac is entered by inserting a needle usually between LV3 and LV4 or LV4 and LV5 in adults and always below LV4 in infants.

macula lutea (L., macula = spot + luteus = saffron-yellow) yellowish area of retina lateral and slightly below the optic disc at a point corresponding to posterior pole of retina.

macula of saccule sensory neuroepithelium in anteromedial part of wall of saccule.

macula of utricle sensory neuroepithelium in anterolateral part of wall of utricle.

mamillary body (L., mamilla = little breast) eminence on ventral surface of hypothalamus containing mamillary nuclei.

mantle layer between the inner ventricular germinal epithelium and the outer marginal layer of the developing neural tube; contains postmitotic neurons; syn. intermediate layer.

marginal layer outermost part of the developing neural tube containing primarily the processes of underlying cells.

meatus (L.) a passage or opening.

mechanoreceptor receptor that is excited by its distortion as a result of touch, pressure, muscle or tendon stretch, and so forth.

medial eminence elevation at each side of the midline on the floor of the fourth ventricle.

medial forebrain bundle diffuse system of fibers located in the lateral hypothalamus; interconnects with septal region rostrally and midbrain reticular formation caudally.

medial lemniscus tract located medially in the medulla, ventrally in the pontine tegmentum, and dorsolaterally in the midbrain tegmentum; carries touch, pressure, and proprioception impulses from the contralateral gracile and cuneate nuclei to the ventral posterolateral nucleus of the thalamus.

medial longitudinal fasciculus bundle of fibers extending from the midbrain to the spinal cord; located close to the midline in the dorsal part of the tegmentum adjacent to the nuclei of the external ocular muscles; pontine and midbrain part composed largely of fibers ascending to motor neurons of the external ocular nuclei; medullary part composed of fibers descending to spinal motor neurons innervating the paravertebral musculature.

median aperture midline opening between posterior part of fourth ventricle and subarachnoid space; syn. foramen of Magendie.

median eminence circumventricular organ that is frequently considered to be the raised portion of the tuber cinereum; together with the infundibular stem and process (neural lobe) forms the neurohypophysis.

medulla oblongata (L., medulla = marrow + oblongus = oblong) that part of the brainstem that is continuous with the spinal cord; syn. myelencephalon.

medulloblastoma glioma consisting of neoplastic cells that arise from the neuroepithelial roof of the fourth ventricle.

Meissner corpuscle encapsulated tactile receptor in dermal papilla.

melanin dark brown or black pigment found in cytoplasm of neurons in some nuclei (substantia nigra, locus ceruleus, and so forth).

membranous labyrinth system of endolymph-containing ducts and chambers of the inner ear; includes utricle, saccule, semicircular ducts, cochlear duct, and their connections.

Ménière disease progressive disorder of the vestibulocochlear apparatus characterized by fluctuating sensorineural hearing loss, tinnitus, vertigo, and severe nausea. Symptoms are episodic and are generally progressively more severe in nature.

meninges (G., meninx = membrane) dural, arachnoid, and pial membranes enveloping the central nervous system.

meningioma (G., meninges + oma = tumor) benign tumor of arachnoid origin; tends to occur along superior sagittal sinus, sphenoid ridges, and near optic chiasm.

meningocele subcutaneous protrusion of meningeal sac filled with cerebrospinal fluid.

meningomyelocele subcutaneous protrusion of a meningeal sac that contains neural tissue in addition to cerebrospinal fluid.

Merkel disc tactile nerve ending in the epidermis.

mesencephalon midbrain portion of the developing brainstem.

metencephalon pontine and cerebellar portions of the brain; syn. after brain.

microgyria abnormally small cortical gyri.

microsmatic (G., mikros + osmasthia = to smell) having a feeble sense of smell.

midbrain middle segment of brain; syn. mesencephalon.

middle cerebellar peduncle fiber bundle connecting the cerebellum and the pons; syn. brachium pontis.

middle cerebral candelabra shape of trunks and branches of middle cerebral artery in lateral fissure as seen radiographically.

Mini Mental Status Exam brief standardized patient questionnaire used to assess cognition including arithmetic, memory, and orientation.

miosis (G., meiosis = a lessening) constriction of the pupil.

modiolus (L., hub of a wheel) bony central axis of the cochlea.

monoplegia (G., mono + plege = stroke) paralysis or paresis in one limb.

mossy fibers afferent axons arising from cerebellar input nuclei other than the inferior olive; branch repeatedly in white matter and granule layer and are excitatory to granule cells and cerebellar nuclei.

motor aphasia see *nonfluent aphasia.*

motor endplate acetylcholine synapse of alpha motor neuron on extrafusal muscle fiber; syn. myoneural junction.

motor unit alpha motor neuron, its axon, and the extrafusal muscle fibers it innervates.

Müller cell glial-like cells chiefly in the bipolar cell layer of the retina whose processes form the external and internal limiting membranes.

multiple sclerosis temporally progressive autoimmune inflammatory disorder affecting CNS myelin. Demyelinating plaques in the white matter appear in radiographic images of the brain.

muscle spindle mechanoreceptor in skeletal muscle.

muscular dystrophy myopathy affecting skeletal muscles more proximal than distal resulting in weakness. Muscular dystrophies may be acquired or inherited.

mutism inability to speak.

myasthenia gravis (G., mys = muscle + asthenia = weakness) autoimmune disease characterized by muscular weakness, beginning usually in the orofacial region, caused by increased turnover of acetylcholine receptors at the neuromuscular junction.

mydriasis extreme dilation of the pupil.

myelencephalon (G., myelos = marrow +enkephalos) medulla oblongata; syn., spinal brain.

myelin regularly alternating lipoprotein lamellae that ensheathe the axons of some nerve fibers.

myotatic reflex (G., myo = to shut + tasis = stretching) contraction of a muscle induced by stretching; syn. stretch, deep, or tendon reflex.

myotome skeletal muscles supplied by a single spinal cord segment.

near response convergence of the eyes when vision is directed from a far to a near target.

near triad convergence of the eyes, pupillary constriction, and thickening of the lens for accommodation.

negative signs functional deficits resulting from a lesion.

neglect syndrome perceptual disorder related to lack of recognition of the opposite side of the body and its surroundings.

neocerebellum (G., neos = new) newest portion of the cerebellum having strong connections with the cerebrum; syn. posterior lobe of cerebellum, cerebrocerebellum.

neospinothalamic system newer spinothalamic system, which carries fast pain to the ventral posterolateral thalamic nucleus; its peripheral fibers are of the A delta type and it arises chiefly from marginal neurons in the dorsal horn of the spinal gray.

nerve deafness perception deafness caused by damage to sensory cells of the inner ear or to the cochlear nerve; degree of hearing loss depends on amount of damage.

neural crest longitudinal band of cells of ectodermal origin found at each side of the junction of the neural plate with the body ectoderm from which develops sensory ganglion cells, autonomic ganglion cells; the leptomeningeal coverings of the brain and other structures.

neural folds thickenings of the neural plate that come together to form the neural tube.

neural plate specialized midline part of the ectoderm that gives rise to both the CNS and PNS.

neural tube most fundamental structure for the development of the CNS; formed by joining of the neural folds.

neurinoma benign tumor arising from Schwann cells.

neuroblasts progenitor cells for neurons.

neuroepithelium epithelial cells that serve as the special receptors in the auditory, vestibular, olfactory, and gustatory systems; syn. neurepithelium.

neurofibrillary tangles abnormal accumulations of insoluble intracellular filaments that become pathogenic to neuronal function leading to their death. Extracellular tangles accumulate in Alzheimer disease.

neurogenic bladder abnormal functioning of the urinary bladder as a result of a CNS or PNS lesion.

neuroglia (G., glia = glue) nonneuronal support cells of the CNS; 10 times more numerous than neurons; four types: astrocytes, oligodendrocytes, microglia, and ependymal cells; syn. glia.

neurolemma cytoplasmic sheath of Schwann cells surrounding a peripheral nerve fiber.

neurolemmal tube functional conduit composed of Schwann cells and surrounding basal lamina for intact and regenerating axons.

neuroma tumor formed by regenerating axons in the PNS that when activated can lead to inappropriate pain sensations.

neuropathies disorders involving peripheral nerves.

neuropil (G., pilos = felt) part of gray matter consisting of preterminal axons, dendrites, and glia in which nerve cell bodies are embedded.

neurotransmitter (L., neuro + transmitto = to send across) any specific chemical agent released by a presynaptic cell on excitation, which crosses the synaptic cleft to stimulate or inhibit the postsynaptic cell.

Nissl body plates of rough endoplasmic reticulum and free ribosomes found in cytoplasm of nerve cell perikaryon and large dendrites.

nociceptor (L., noceo = to injure, hurt + capio = to take) receptor that is stimulated by actual tissue injury or anticipated injury; a receptor for pain.

node of Ranvier discontinuity in the myelin sheath of a nerve fiber where one Schwann cell in peripheral nerves or one oligodendrocyte in central tracts meets the next.

nodulus (L., little knot) most posterior or caudal part of vermis of cerebellum.

Nogo receptor recognizes three proteins present in CNS myelin that are inhibitory to the growth of regenerating axons.

nonfluent aphasia language disorder characterized by difficulty in forming words; associated with lesion of Broca speech area; syn. motor or expressive aphasia.

nonreflex neurogenic bladder incontinence and severe retention; a "lower motor neuron" type resulting from lesions of sacral spinal cord or cauda equina.

notochord embryonic mesodermal cord that induces the neural plate; persists in adult as nucleus pulposus in central part of intervertebral disc.

NREM sleep stage in which the absence of rapid eye movements occurs; generated by groups of neurons in hypothalamus and medulla.

nuclear lesion lower motor neuron lesion involving cell body.

nystagmus (G., nystagmus = a nodding) involuntary rapid movements of the eyeballs consisting of fast and slow phases; named according to direction of fast phase.

obex (L., barrier) point at midline of dorsal surface of medulla marking caudal tip of the fourth ventricle.

obstructive hydrocephalus blockage of CSF flow within the ventricular system; syn. noncommunicating hydrocephalus.

occipital eye field primary visual and visual association areas of the cerebral cortex, which are concerned with vergence eye movements.

oculocephalic reflex turning of the eyes in the direction opposite to that of rotation of the head; signifies intact vestibulo-ocular reflex in comatose patient; syn. doll's eye movement.

off-center neurons retinal and lateral geniculate neurons activated by light applied to the surrounding area and inhibited by a dot of light striking them.

oligodendrocytes (G., oligos = few + dendron = tree + glia = glue) neuroglial cells with small electron-dense oval nuclei and scanty cytoplasm; form myelin sheath of CNS.

on-center neurons retinal and lateral geniculate neurons activated by a spot of light and inhibited by light applied to the surrounding area.

operculum (L., cover or lid) those parts of the cerebrum that cover the insula and form the margins of the lateral fissure.

ophthalmoplegia (G., ophthalmos = eye + plege = stroke) paralysis of the eye muscles.

optic disc or papilla area where the optic nerve fibers leave the retina.

optokinetic nystagmus nystagmus induced by looking at a moving object; syn. railroad nystagmus.

ora serrata (L., ora = edge + serratus = notched) serrated anterior edge of the optical portion of the retina, posterior to the ciliary body; marks the separation between neural and nonneural portions of the retina.

organ of Corti sensory end organ for hearing found in cochlear duct of internal ear; syn. spiral organ.

osseous labyrinth see *bony labyrinth*.

otoconia (G., otos = ear + konis = dust) crystalline particles of calcium carbonate and a protein adhering to the gelatinous otolithic membrane of the maculae of the utricle and saccule; syn. statoconia or otoliths.

otolith (G., otos + lithos = stone) one of the particles constituting the otoconia; syn. statoconium, otoconium, statolith.

otolithic membrane gelatinous substance overlying the maculae of utricle and saccule into which their cilia are embedded; contains calcium carbonate crystals, the otoliths.

oval window opening between tympanic cavity and scala vestibuli of cochlea; syn. fenestra vestibuli.

oxytocin hormone secreted by magnocellular neurons in the supraoptic and paraventricular nuclei of the hypothalamus that stimulates contraction of the smooth muscle fibers (cells) in the pregnant uterus and contractile cells around the ducts of mammary glands.

pachygyria abnormally large cortical gyri.

Pacinian corpuscle pressure-sensitive nerve ending of the subcutaneous tissue having a laminated capsule; associated with vibration sense.

paleo (G., palaios) old.

paleocerebellum anterior lobe of cerebellum having strong connections with the spinal cord; syn. spinocerebellum.

paleospinothalamic system older spinothalamic system, which carries slow pain to a broader area including the reticular formation and intralaminar and medial thalamic nuclei, therefore less localized than the neospinothalamic system; peripheral fibers are of the C type; arise from neurons chiefly in laminae IV, V, and VI of the dorsal horn.

pallidum globus pallidus.

palsy weakness or paralysis of muscles.

Papez circuit neural circuit concerned with consolidation of memory and learning and thought to be reverberating; includes hippocampus, fornix, mamillary bodies, mamillothalamic tract, anterior thalamic nucleus, cingulate gyrus, cingulum, and entorhinal area of parahippocampal gyrus.

papilledema see *disc edema*.

parallel plexus axons of cerebellar granule cells that travel through the molecular layer of the cerebellar cortex parallel to the longitudinal axis of the folium; excitatory to Purkinje, stellate, basket, and Golgi neurons.

paralysis agitans see *Parkinson disease*.

paraplegia (G., para = beside + plege = stroke) paralysis of the lower limbs.

parasympathetic division of the autonomic system concerned with maintenance of the organism; preganglionic component arises in cranial and sacral portions of the central nervous system.

paravermis the portion of the cerebellum lateral to the vermis and medial to the lateral hemisphere; its output is primarily to the interposed nucleus, which affects chiefly the red nucleus.

paresis (G., a letting go, slackening, relaxation) partial paralysis or weakness.

parietal eye field part of the superior parietal lobule that affects saccadic movements.

Parkinson disease neurologic syndrome characterized by tremors at rest, rigidity, bradykinesia, and postural instability ascribed to lesions of the substantia nigra; syn. paralysis agitans.

peduncle (L., pediculus = little foot) a footlike structure.

peri (G.) around.

photopic vision vision when eye is light adapted.

phototransduction conversion of a photic stimulus to a biochemical cascade that leads to an electrical propagation of an action potential signaling the stimulus.

pia mater innermost layer of the meninges.

pineal gland epithalamic circumventricular organ associated with melatonin secretion and sleep.

plasticity modifiability of brain structure and function to pathologic and normal stimuli.

pneumotaxic center neurons in dorsolateral tegmentum of rostral pons that inhibit inspiratory phase of respiration.

poikilothermy (G., poikilos = varied + therme = heat) a condition in which the body temperature varies with the environment; can result from a lesion in the posterior hypothalamus.

poliomyelitis viral infection that targets lower motor neurons resulting in paralysis; syn. polio.

polymyositis inflammatory disease of muscle fibers.

pons (L., a bridge) that part of the brainstem located between the medulla oblongata and the midbrain.

positive signs spontaneous, uncontrollable activity resulting from a lesion.

posterior lobe syndrome disorder characterized by ataxia, hypotonia, intention tremor, dysmetria, dysdiadochokinesia and, if bilateral, explosive speech; results from a lesion in the posterior lobe of the cerebellum, dentate nucleus, or dentatothalamic tract; syn. neocerebellar syndrome.

premotor cortex area chiefly on surface of precentral gyrus where postural adjustments to support skilled movements are planned in response to external stimuli.

projection fibers axons that connect the cerebral cortex with subcortical neurons.

proprioception (L., proprius = one's own + capio = to take) information concerning joint position and movement.

propriospinal neurons spinal cord cells whose axons make up the fasciculi proprii adjacent to the gray matter.

prosencephalon most rostral primary brain vesicle that gives rise to the diencephalon and telencephalon; syn. forebrain.

prosopagnosia difficulty in recognizing familiar faces.

ptosis (G., fall) drooping of the upper eyelid.

pulvinar (L., pulvinus = pillow) posterior portion of the thalamus that overlies the midbrain.

Purkinje neuron large efferent neuron of the cerebellar cortex whose massive dendritic tree spreads chiefly transverse to the long axis of the folium in the molecular layer, and whose axon inhibits neurons chiefly in the cerebellar nuclei.

putamen (L., to shell or husk) the larger, lateral part of the lentiform nucleus.

pyramidal cell large triangular neuron of cerebral cortex having apical dendrite extending toward pial surface as well as horizontally directed basal dendrites; axon emerges from base of cell and passes to the white matter as an association, commissural, or projection fiber.

quadriplegia (quadri + G. plege, stroke) tetraplegia; paralysis of all four limbs.

radial glia glia that guide migrating neurons to their destinations.

ramus (L., a branch) primary division of a nerve.

raphe (G., a seam) midline of pons and medulla.

raphe nuclei serotonergic nuclei clustered in the midline of the brainstem.

Rathke's pouch upward directed out-pocketing of the stomodeum of the oral cavity that joins with the downward extension of the third ventricle, the infundibulum, to develop into the pituitary gland.

reactive synaptogenesis formation of new synapses in response to injury of the CNS.

receptive aphasia see *fluent aphasia*.

reciprocal inhibition occurs during activation of a reflex circuit such as the patellar tendon reflex, in which the agonist muscle is excited monosynaptically and the antagonist muscle is inhibited disynaptically.

referred pain pain that is perceived as coming from a site other than its origin.

reflex an involuntary response to a stimulus.

reflex neurogenic bladder "upper motor neuron" type resulting from CNS lesions rostral to sacral spinal cord.

Reissner membrane see *vestibular membrane*.

REM sleep stage in which rapid conjugate eye movements occur. Generated by centers in dorsolateral pontine reticular formation.

Renshaw cell inhibitory spinal interneuron activated by collateral axon that reciprocally inhibits the parent neuron.

respiratory center neurons located bilaterally in the ventrolateral medulla at the caudal part of the fourth ventricle; descending projections activate inspiratory lower motor neurons to diaphragm and intercostal muscles. Bilateral damage results in respiratory arrest.

restiform body (L., restis = rope + forma = shape) fiber bundle connecting cerebellum and medulla; massive lateral part of inferior cerebellar peduncle.

reticular formation (L., reticulum = a net) groups of nerve cells and nerve fibers intermingling in the midbrain and pontine tegmentum and the medulla.

retina (L., dim of rete = a net) inner layer of the eyeball that contains the receptors for vision and gives rise to the optic nerve.

retinitis pigmentosa accumulation of photoreceptor cell debris between these cells and the pigment epithelial cell layer.

retrograde axonal transport movement of products of cellular metabolism from the distal nerve ending to the cell body.

rhodopsin visual pigment of the rods.

rhombencephalon (G., rhombos = rhomboid + enkephalos = brain) kite-shaped metencephalon and myelencephalon composed of pons, cerebellum, and medulla oblongata; syn. hindbrain.

rhombic lip that portion of the developing metencephalon giving rise to the cerebellum.

rigidity (L., rigidus = rigid, inflexible) stiffness or inflexibility manifested by pervasive resistance to passive movement.

Rinne tuning fork test vibrating tuning fork heard longer and louder when in contact with the skull (usually the mastoid process) than when held near the pinna—indication of some disorder of the sound-conducting apparatus.

rod photoreceptor of retina concerned with light sensitivity.

Romberg sign if a patient standing is more unsteady with the eyes closed, dorsal column ataxia rather than cerebellar ataxia is indicated.

roof plate dorsal part of the developing neural tube. Although not involved with neurogenesis, it exerts a significant influence on the migration and differentiation of neurons in the alar plates.

rostral (L., rostrum = beak) a position more toward a superior or higher center; cephalad.

round window opening between tympanic cavity and scala tympani of cochlea.

Ruffini ending a subcutaneous mechanoreceptor that provides information about stretching of the skin and shapes of objects.

saccade small, quick eye movements on changing point of fixation.

saccule (L., sacculus = a little bag) part of membranous labyrinth located in vestibule of bony labyrinth; located in front of utricle.

sacral sparing normal motor and sensory functions in sacral region after spinal cord injury more rostrally; associated with central cord syndrome, which spares external part of white matter that contains fibers carrying sacral impulses.

saltatory conduction (L., salto = leap) current flow limited to the nodes of Ranvier in myelinated axons, thereby greatly increasing the speed of action potential propagation; occurs as the result of ionic exchanges.

scala tympani (L., scala = stairway + G., tympanon = a drum) perilymphatic space of cochlea lying posterior to the spiral lamina and basilar membrane.

scala vestibuli (L., scala = vestibulum = vestibule) perilymphatic space of cochlear lying anterior to the spinal lamina and vestibular membrane.

Schwann cell cell of ectodermal origin that forms the neurolemma of a peripheral nerve fiber and contains the myelin if the axon is myelinated.

sclera (G., skleros = hard) the fibrous outer layer of the eyeball which is continuous with the cornea anteriorly; forms the white of the eye.

scotopic vision (G., skotos = darkness + opsis = vision) vision when the eye is dark adapted.

semicircular canals perilymphatic canals of the bony labyrinth that contain the semicircular ducts and their ampullae.

senile dementia impairment of higher cortical function and memory in senescence.

sensory aphasia see *fluent aphasia*.

septal area part of limbic lobe anterior to lamina terminalis and consisting of the paraterminal gyrus and subcallosal area.

septal region limbic system region anterior and lateral to lamina terminalis; includes the septal area and the septal nuclei; associated with reward or pleasurable feelings.

septum pellucidum (L., septum = a wall + pellucidus = transparent) thin sheet of tissue extending between corpus callosum and fornix; forms most of medial wall of anterior horns of lateral ventricles.

sheath of Schwann see *neurolemma*.

sinus venosus sclerae canal which drains aqueous humor; found encircling cornea at corneoscleral junction; syn. canal of Schlemm.

slow pain dull, burning pain that is diffuse rather than localized, resulting from tissue injury.

somatic (G., somatikos = bodily) pertaining to the body wall rather than the viscera.

somatosensory system pertaining to the general somatic senses: somatic pain and temperature, touch, vibration, and proprioception sensibility.

somatotopic related to particular regions of the body; describes localization of different body parts in functional pathways.

somesthetic (B., soma + aisthesis = sensation) denoting general senses of pain, temperature, touch, pressure, proprioception and vibration.

spasticity condition of increased muscle tone and exaggerated tendon reflexes.

spina bifida a congenital anomaly characterized by defective closure of the vertebral arches through which the spinal cord and meninges may protrude.

spinal shock spinal cord areflexia caused by sudden interruption of cortical input.

spinocerebellum anterior lobe of the cerebellum with strong connections with the spinal cord; syn. paleocerebellum.

spiral organ sensory end organ for hearing found in cochlear duct of internal ear; syn. organ of Corti.

splenium (G., splenion = bandage) posterior portion of corpus callosum.

split brain brain in which the corpus callosum and sometimes the anterior and hippocampal commissures have been severed in the median plane.

stereocilia groups of extremely long, slender, nonmotile microvilli projecting from neuroepithelial cells.

stereognosis (G., stereos = solid + gnosis = knowledge) ability to recognize an object by touch alone.

strabismus deviation of an eye as a result of impaired function of an extraocular muscle or nerve.

stria (L. furrow or groove) a longitudinal strand, stripe, or band of nerve fibers in the central nervous system.

striatum the caudate nucleus and putamen, the chief input nuclei of the basal ganglia; syn. neostriatum.

subarachnoid space beneath the arachnoid, refers to space filled with CSF.

subcommissural organ circumventricular organ beneath the posterior commissure.

subdural space beneath the dura, between the dura and the arachnoid; refers to a potential space containing a serous fluid.

subfornical organ circumventricular organ between the columns of the fornix.

substantia gelatinosa lamina II of the spinal gray consisting of interneurons that play a role in pain modulation.

substantia innominata gray matter of the anterior perforated substance; contains basal nucleus of Meynert.

substantia nigra nuclear mass located in the midbrain; one of the basal ganglia; consists of (1) a posterior compact part with dopaminergic melanin-containing neurons whose malfunction is associated with Parkinson disease, and (2) an anterior reticular part that is continuous with the medial pallidum.

subthalamic nucleus nuclear mass located in subthalamus; one of the basal ganglia; malfunction associated with ballismus.

subthalamus part of the diencephalon found between the thalamus dorsally, the cerebral peduncle ventrally, and the hypothalamus medially; composed of subthalamic nucleus, zona incerta, and prerubral field; syn. ventral thalamus.

sulcus (L., groove) a furrow or groove on the surface of the brain.

sulcus limitans longitudinal groove on the lateral wall of the developing neural tube separating the basal and alar plates.

superior cerebellar peduncle fiber bundle connecting the cerebellum and the midbrain; syn. brachium conjunctivum.

superior colliculus round, paired rostral or superior eminence on the dorsal surface of the midbrain; its major afferent connections are with the retina, visual association areas, frontal eye field, and brainstem ascending sensory paths; its efferent connections are with the brainstem and spinal cord (tectobulbar and tectospinal tracts), and visual association areas. It functions as a visuomotor integration center.

superior longitudinal fasciculus large association bundle connecting cortex on the lateral surfaces of the frontal, parietal, and occipital lobes; sometimes described as dorsal part of arcuate fasciculus.

superior medullary velum thin lamina of white matter between the superior cerebellar peduncles; forms the roof of the pontine part of the fourth ventricle in the midline, beneath the lingula of the cerebellum; syn. anterior medullary velum.

supplementary motor cortex area in superior frontal gyrus where self-initiated movements are planned and forwarded to the primary motor cortex.

supranuclear lesion upper motor neuron lesion.

suspensory ligament of the lens fibers running from the ciliary body to the capsule of the lens; holds lens in place and functions in accommodation; syn. ciliary zonule.

sylvian fissure see *lateral fissure*.

sympathetic (G., syn = with + pathos = suffering) that division of the autonomic system having the origin of its preganglionic component in the thoracic and lumbar cord segments and playing a role in the preparation of the organism for emergency situations.

synapse (G., syn = together + haptein = to touch) site of functional contact between neurons where impulses pass from one neuron to another.

synaptogenesis formation of new synapses.

syndrome (G., concurrence of symptoms) the aggregate of signs and symptoms associated with any morbid state.

syringomyelia (G., syrinx = tube + myelos = marrow) spinal cord abnormality in which cavitation occurs.

tabes dorsalis (L., tabes = a wasting away) deterioration of dorsal spinal roots and dorsal columns of the spinal cord resulting chiefly from syphilis or pernicious anemia and manifested by pain and paresthesia, impairment of postural and vibration sensibility, ataxia, and decreased stretch reflexes; syn. locomotor ataxia.

tachycardia heart hurry; rapid beating of the heart, usually applied to rates more than 100 beats per minute.

tapetum (L., tapete = carpet) fibers of the corpus callosum that pass laterally to form the roof of the posterior horn of the lateral ventricle and also sweep inferiorly to form the lateral walls of the posterior and inferior horns.

tectum (L., tectus = roof) a structure that covers as in the roof of the midbrain, consisting of the colliculi.

tegmentum (L. tegmen = a covering) the dorsal part of the cerebral peduncle and the pons.

telencephalon secondary brain vesicle formed from the prosencephalon that gives rise to the cerebral hemispheres; syn. end brain.

temporal eye field an area in the posterior part of the lateral surface of the temporal lobe that is associated with smooth pursuit and optokinetic eye movements.

thalamic fasciculus bundle composed of fibers from the cerebellar nuclei (chiefly the dentate) and the basal ganglia (chiefly the pallidum) that converge in the prerubral field and pass to the ventral lateral and adjacent part of the ventral anterior thalamic nuclei; syn. Forel's field H1.

thalamus (G., thalamos = a room) division of the diencephalon lying medial to the tail and body of the caudate nucleus and internal capsule and forming the dorsal part of the lateral walls of the third ventricle; syn. dorsal thalamus.

tic douloureux (F., painful spasm) trigeminal neuralgia.

tinnitus (L., a jingling) a ringing in the ears.

tonotopic localization of certain sound types within the auditory pathways.

tonsil (L., tonsilla = a stake) rounded lobule on inferior surface of each cerebellar hemisphere.

transcortical motor aphasia a disorder characterized by impaired fluency but normal repetition, naming, and reading; caused by a lesion in the left supplementary area or prefrontal area.

transcutaneous electric nerve stimulation (TENS) selective electrical stimulation of large cutaneous afferent fibers to inhibit slow pain conduction in spinothalamic neurons; used for treatment of chronic pain.

transient ischemic episodes or attacks brief periods of focal cerebral dysfunction lasting less than 24 hours; caused by carotid or vertebrobasilar ischemia; syn. TIA.

trapezoid body (L., trapezodes = table-shaped) nerve fibers chiefly from the ventral acoustic stria that course across the midline in the ventral part of the tegmentum in the caudal half of the pons.

tremor (L., tremere = to shake) involuntary trembling or shaking.

trichromatic vision normal color vision in which the three primary colors are perceived.

trigeminal (L., trigeminus = threefold) three born at a time.

trigeminal neuralgia pain of a severe, throbbing, or stabbing character in the course or distribution of the trigeminal nerve.

trigone (L., trigonum) a triangle.

trophic (B., trophe = nourishment) relating to nutrition. Substances that maintain the metabolism of a cell or its processes promoting neuronal survival.

trophic factors substances that guide the migration of developing neurons and axons and promote the regeneration of injured axons.

truncal ataxia ataxia affecting the muscles of the trunk; most often caused by a lesion of the vestibulocerebellar midline.

tuber cinereum (L., tuber = swelling + cinis = ashen or gray-colored) area on ventral surface of the hypothalamus between the mamillary bodies and optic chiasm.

tubercle (L., tuber) a swelling of a surface.

two-point sense the ability to distinguish two separate points applied to the skin simultaneously.

umami taste quality described by some as associated with monosodium glutamate or by others as meaty.

uncinate fasciculus (L., uncinatus = hook shaped) association bundle connecting the frontal and temporal lobes.

uncinate fits epileptiform stimulation of the primary olfactory cortex that causes olfactory sensations usually disagreeable in nature.

uncus (L., hook) thickening on the medial side of the parahippocampal gyrus overlying the amygdala and resting near the free edge of the tentorium cerebelli.

uninhibited reflex bladder incontinence but no retention; occurs after bilateral frontal lobe lesions.

upper motor nerve syndrome disorder characterized by spastic paralysis, exaggerated myotatic reflexes, and an extensor plantar (Babinski) response; caused by lesion of corticospinal system although some include other corticofugal paths also.

utricle (L., little womb) part of the membranous labyrinth located in the vestibule of the bony labyrinth.

uvea (L., uva = grape) middle or vascular layer of the eyeball; consists of choroid, ciliary body, and iris.

vallecula (L., vallis = valley) deep depression on the inferior surface of the cerebellum between the two hemispheres.

vascular dementia second leading cause of dementia that occurs as the result of numerous sublethal strokes in the cerebral cortex.

vasopressin see *antidiuretic hormone* (ADH).

velum (L., a veil or covering) a thin layer of tissue resembling a veil or curtain.

ventricular layer innermost layer of the developing neural tube where mitogenesis occurs, giving rise to all cells in the CNS except microglia.

vergence when both eyes simultaneously rotate medially or laterally as in convergence when an object approaches and divergence when an object moves away.

vermis (L., worm) the midline portion of the cerebellum; its connections are primarily with the fastigial nucleus, which affects the vestibular nuclei for equilibrium and eye movements.

vertical gaze center accessory oculomotor neurons at the rostral end of the medial longitudinal fasciculus in the midbrain that control vertical eye movements; upward movements represented more dorsally, downward more ventrally.

vertigo (L., dizziness) a sensation of irregular or whirling motion, either of oneself (subjective vertigo) or of external objects (objective vertigo).

vestibular membrane membrane within the cochlea that separates the scala vestibuli and the cochlear duct; syn. Reissner membrane.

vestibule (L., vestibulum = entrance court) middle part of the bony labyrinth that contains the saccule and utricle and communicates with the semicircular canals posteriorly and the cochlea anteriorly.

vestibulo-ocular reflex three-neuron reflex resulting in turning of eyes in a direction opposite to that of head rotation: (1) vestibular ganglion, (2) vestibular nuclei, (3) III, IV, and VI nuclei.

vibration sense awareness of deep touch and pressure tested with a high-frequency (256 vibrations/s) vibrating tuning fork.

Virchow-Robin space spaces that surround blood vessels where they enter the CNS.

vitreous body (L., vitreus = glass-like) gelatinous substance filling posterior compartment of the eye, posterior to the lens.

Wallenberg syndrome see *lateral medullary syndrome*.

Wallerian degeneration axonal degeneration occurring distal to axonal injury or after destruction of its cell body; syn. anterograde or secondary degeneration.

watershed areas areas supplied by most distal parts of cerebral cortical and spinal arteries that may anastomose and provide collateral circulation but are susceptible to ischemic injuries; syn. border zones.

Weber syndrome disorder characterized by contralateral spastic hemiplegia with ipsilateral ophthalmoplegia (with the eye turned down and out, ptosis, and mydriasis); results from a lesion of the cerebral crus and oculomotor nerve of one side in the midbrain; syn. ventral midbrain syndrome, superior alternating hemiplegia, or alternating oculomotor hemiplegia.

Weber tuning fork test application of a vibrating tuning fork to the midline of the forehead to ascertain in which ear the sound is heard better, the better heard ear being abnormal in conduction deafness or normal in sensorineural deafness.

Wernicke area posterior part of the superior temporal gyrus of the dominant hemisphere, which functions as a receptive speech center; fluent (sensory or receptive) aphasia attributed to its injury.

Wernicke zone triangular zone in retrolenticular part of the internal capsule lateral to the lateral geniculate nucleus containing the optic radiations.

zona incerta small, relatively clear nucleus located in the dorsal and lateral part of the subthalamus and continuous with the reticular thalamic nucleus.

Suggested Readings

Apuzzo MLJ. Surgery of the Third Ventricle, 2nd ed. Baltimore: Williams & Wilkins, 1998.

Bear MF, Connors BW, Paradiso MA. Neuroscience Exploring the Brain, 3rd ed. Baltimore: Lippincott Williams & Wilkins, 2006.

Blumenfeld H. Neuroanatomy Through Clinical Cases. Sunderland, MA: Sinauer Associates Inc, 2002.

Brazis PW, Masdeu JC, Biller J. Localization in Clinical Neurology, 5th ed. Philadelphia: Lippincott Williams & Wilkins, 2006.

Brodal A. Neurological Anatomy in Relation to Clinical Medicine, 3rd ed. New York: Oxford University Press, 1981.

Brodal P. The Central Nervous System: Structure and Function. New York: Oxford University Press, 2003.

Burt AM. Textbook of Neuroanatomy. Philadelphia: WB Saunders, 1993.

Crosby EC, Humphrey T, Lauer EW. Correlative Anatomy of the Nervous System. New York: Macmillan, 1962.

Haines DE. Fundamental Neuroscience for Basic and Clinical Applications, 3rd ed. Philadelphia: Churchill Livingstone Elsevier, 2005.

Heimer L. The Human Brain and Spinal Cord. Functional Neuroanatomy and Dissection Guide. New York: Springer-Verlag, 1994.

Kandel ER, Schwartz JH, Jessell TM. Principles of Neural Science, 4th ed. New York: McGraw-Hill Medical, 2000.

Kiernan JA. Barr's The Human Nervous System: An Anatomical Viewpoint, 8th ed. Baltimore: Lippincott Williams & Wilkins, 2004.

Kingsley, RE. Concise Text of Neuroscience, Baltimore: Williams & Wilkins, 1996.

Martin JH. Neuroanatomy Text and Atlas. New York: Elsevier, 2003.

Nauta WJH, Feirtag M. Fundamental Neuroanatomy. New York: WH Freeman, 1986.

Noback CR, Strominger NL, Demarest RJ. The Human Nervous System: Introduction and Review, 4th ed. Philadelphia: Lea & Febiger, 1991.

Nolte J. The Human Brain: An Introduction to its Functional Anatomy, 4th ed. St. Louis: Mosby-Year Book, 2002.

Parent A. Carpenter's Human Neuroanatomy, 9th ed. Baltimore: Williams & Wilkins, 1996.

Westmoreland BF, Benarroch EE, Daube JR, Reagan TJ, Sandok BA. Medical Neurosciences, 3rd ed. Boston: Little Brown & Co Inc, 1994.

Willis WD Jr, Grossman RG. Medical Neurobiology. Neuroanatomical and Neurophysiological Principles Basic to Clinical Neuroscience. 3rd ed. St. Louis: Mosby-Year Book, 1981.

Yasargil MG. Microneurosurgery, Vol. 1 Anatomy. Stuttgart: Georg Thieme, 1984.

Atlas of Myelin-Stained Sections

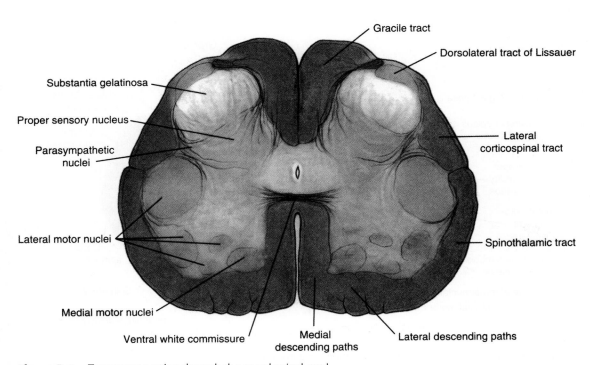

Gracile tract

Dorsolateral tract of Lissauer

Substantia gelatinosa

Proper sensory nucleus

Parasympathetic nuclei

Lateral corticospinal tract

Lateral motor nuclei

Spinothalamic tract

Medial motor nuclei

Ventral white commissure

Medial descending paths

Lateral descending paths

Figure D-1 Transverse section through the sacral spinal cord.

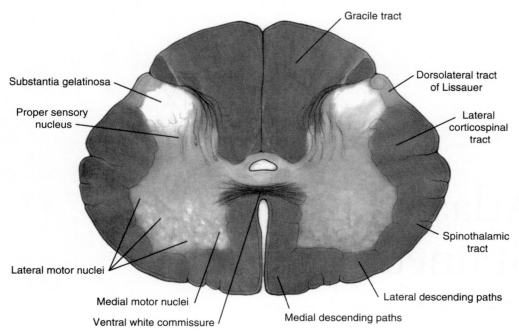

Gracile tract

Substantia gelatinosa

Proper sensory nucleus

Dorsolateral tract of Lissauer

Lateral corticospinal tract

Spinothalamic tract

Lateral motor nuclei

Medial motor nuclei

Ventral white commissure

Medial descending paths

Lateral descending paths

Figure D-2 Transverse section through lumbar spinal cord.

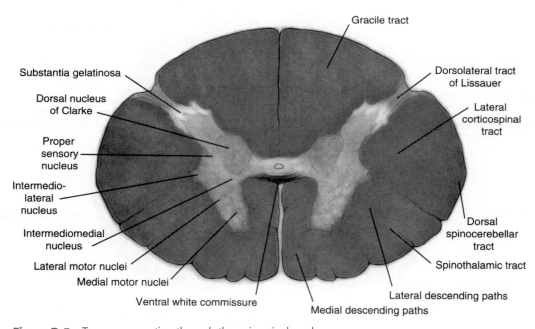

Gracile tract

Substantia gelatinosa

Dorsal nucleus of Clarke

Proper sensory nucleus

Intermedio-lateral nucleus

Intermediomedial nucleus

Lateral motor nuclei

Medial motor nuclei

Ventral white commissure

Dorsolateral tract of Lissauer

Lateral corticospinal tract

Dorsal spinocerebellar tract

Spinothalamic tract

Lateral descending paths

Medial descending paths

Figure D-3 Transverse section through thoracic spinal cord.

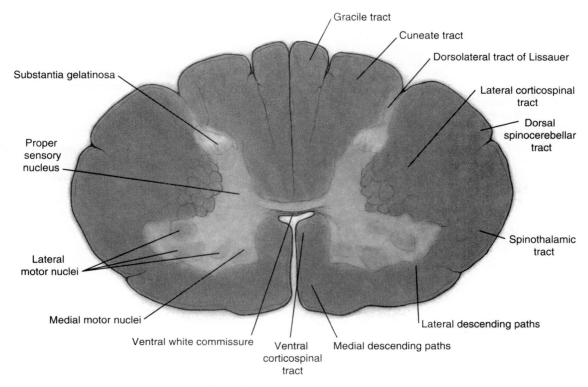

Figure D-4   Transverse section through cervical enlargement.

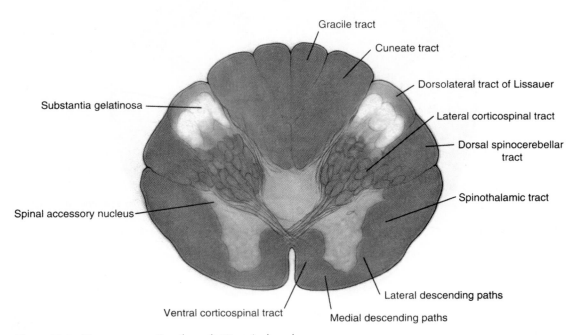

Figure D-5   Transverse section through C1, spinal cord.

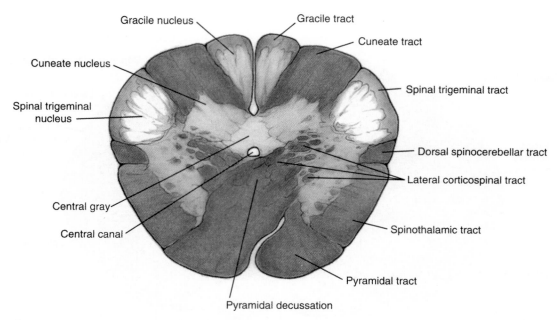

Figure D-6   Transverse section through medulla at pyramid decussation.

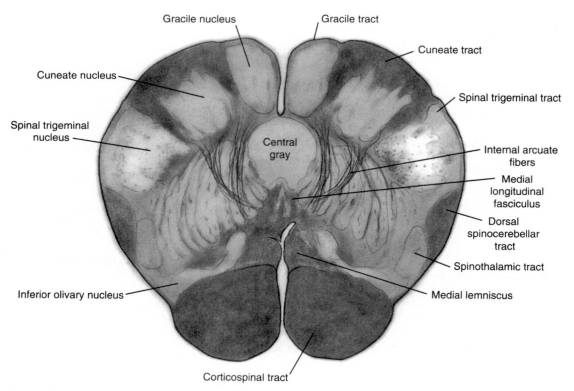

Figure D-7   Transverse section through medulla at dorsal column nuclei.

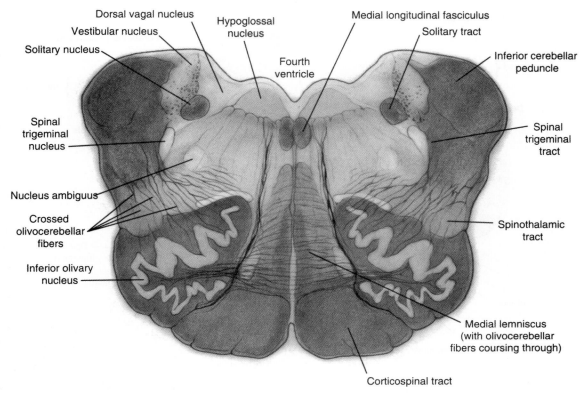

Figure D-8   Transverse section through medulla at hypoglossal and vagal nuclei.

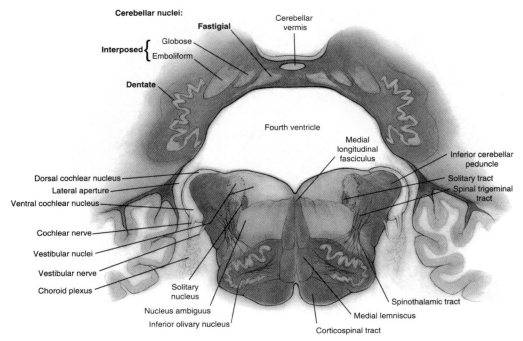

Figure D-9   Transverse section through medulla at lateral aperture.

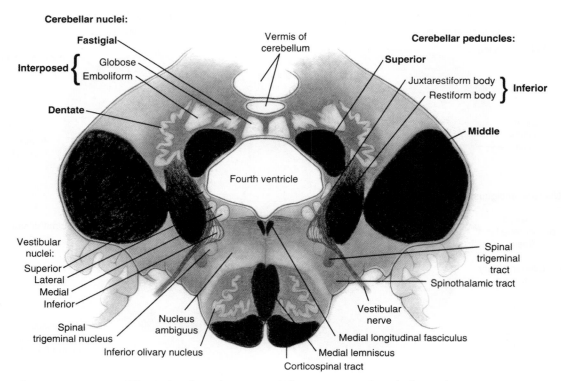

Figure D-10   Transverse section through pontomedullary junction and cerebellar nuclei.

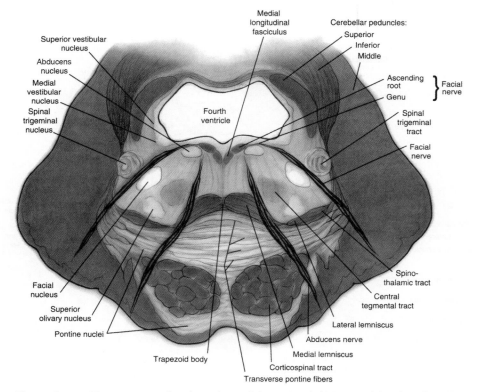

Figure D-11   Transverse section through caudal pons at abducens and facial nuclei.

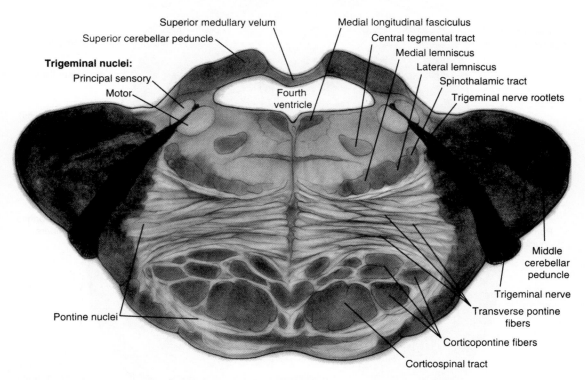

Figure D-12 Transverse section through midpons at motor and principal sensory trigeminal nuclei.

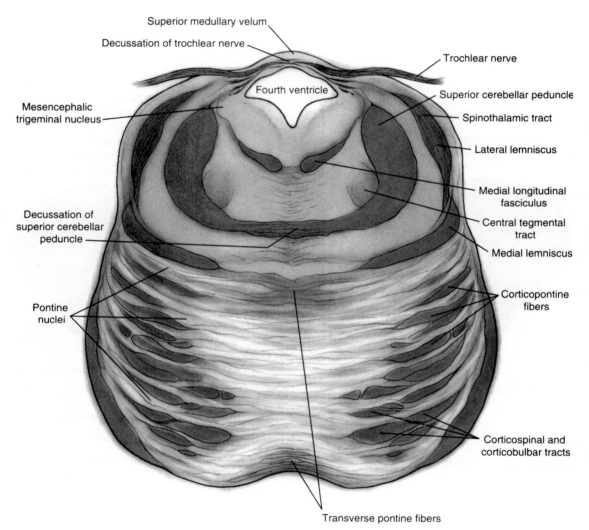

Figure D-13   Transverse section through rostral pons at decussation of trochlear nerves.

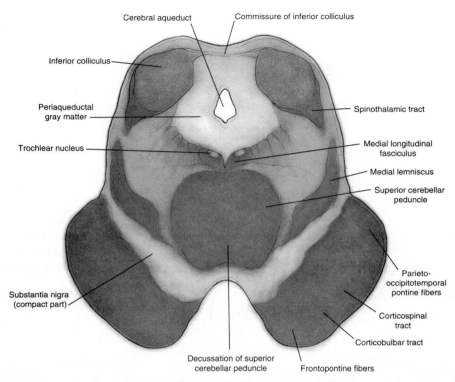

Figure D-14   Transverse section through midbrain at inferior colliculus.

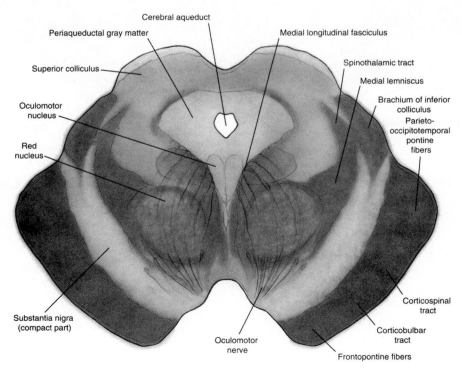

Figure D-15   Transverse section through midbrain at superior colliculus.

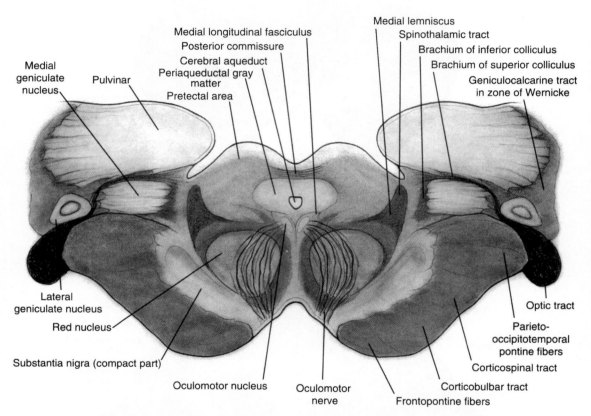

Figure D-16   Transverse section through midbrain at pretectal region and overlapping posterior thalamus.

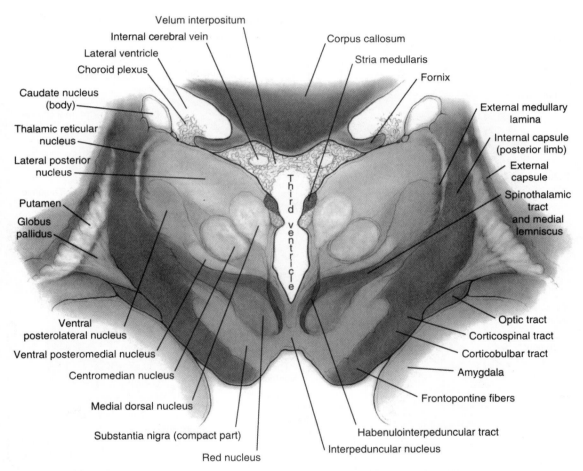

Figure D-17 Coronal section through posterior thalamus and overlapping midbrain and lentiform nuclei.

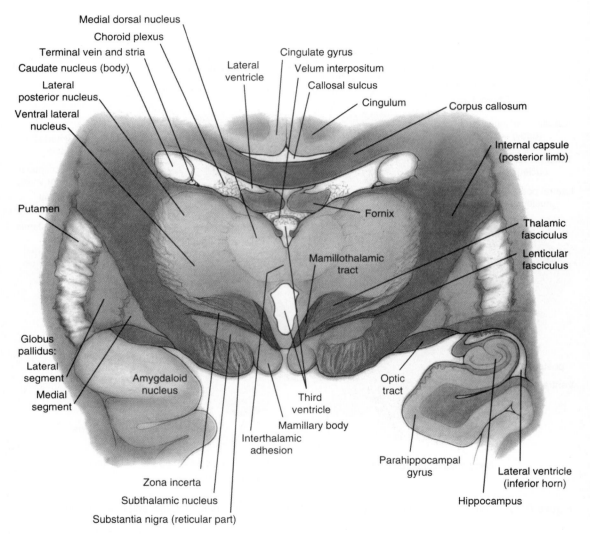

Figure D-18 Coronal section through deep forebrain at mamillary bodies level.

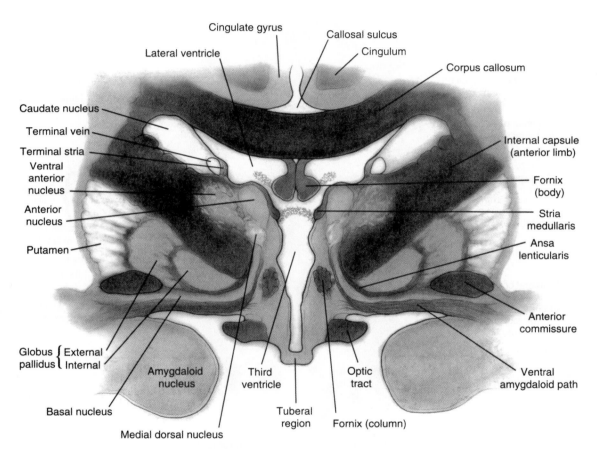

Figure D-19   Coronal section through deep forebrain at tuberal level of hypothalamus.

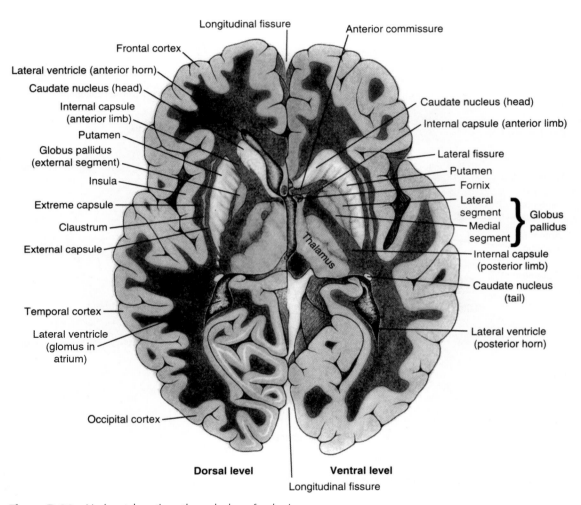

Figure D-20   Horizontal sections through deep forebrain.

INDEX

Page numbers in *italics* denote figures; those followed by a t denote tables.